Foundations of Respiratory Medicine

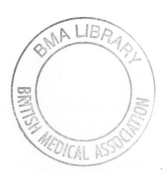

Foundations of Respiratory Medicine

Simon Hart • Mike Greenstone
Editors

Foundations of
Respiratory Medicine

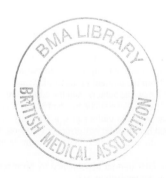

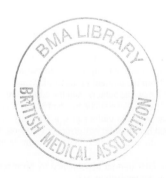

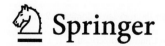 Springer

Editors
Simon Hart
Respiratory Research Group
Hull York Medical School
Castle Hill Hospital
Cottingham
East Yorkshire
United Kingdom

Mike Greenstone
Department of Respiratory Medicine
Hull and East Yorkshire Hospitals
NHS Trust, Castle Hill Hospital
Cottingham
East Yorkshire
United Kingdom

ISBN 978-3-319-94125-7   ISBN 978-3-319-94127-1   (eBook)
https://doi.org/10.1007/978-3-319-94127-1

Library of Congress Control Number: 2018949944

This Springer imprint is published by Springer Nature, under the registered company Springer International Publishing AG
The registered company address is: Gewerbestrasse 11, 6330 Cham, Switzerland

Foreword

Despite the proliferation of detailed online information and easy access to exhaustive review articles, trainee physicians often seek a concise and relevant text to support their everyday practice as well as preparation for knowledge-based examinations. In this book the authors, practising physicians and experts in their chosen topic areas, combine familiarity of recent advances with clinical guidelines and the realities of clinical uncertainty.

Comprehensive coverage of respiratory medicine knowledge is delivered in accessible topic chapters that include basic science, applied pathophysiology and imaging. The authors provide concise and clear explanation of clinical disease and its management, identifying the core knowledge that is required for both effective respiratory care and postgraduate examinations.

The blend of evidence-based medicine and real-world clinical experience provides the reader with an excellent foundation for specialist respiratory practice.

Newcastle upon Tyne, UK   Ian Forrest

Contents

Contributors

K. Suresh Babu, MD, DM, FRCP Respiratory Medicine, Queen Alexandra Hospital, Portsmouth, Hampshire, UK

Rachael Barton, DM, MRCP, FRCR Queen's Centre for Oncology and Haematology, Hull and East Yorkshire Hospitals NHS Trust, Castle Hill Hospital, Cottingham, UK

Anne Campbell, BMedSci, MBChB, MD, FRCPath Cellular Pathology, Hull and East Yorkshire Hospitals NHS Trust, Hull Royal Infirmary, Hull, UK

Robina K. Coker, BSc, MBBS, PhD, FRCP Respiratory Medicine, Hammersmith Hospital, Imperial College Healthcare NHS Trust, London, UK

Robin Condliffe, MD Pulmonary Vascular Disease Unit, Royal Hallamshire Hospital, Sheffield Teaching Hospitals NHS Trust, Sheffield, South Yorkshire, UK

Brendan G. Cooper, MSc, PhD Lung Function and Sleep Department, Queen Elizabeth Hospital, Birmingham, UK

Michael Cowen, FRCS Cardiothoracic Surgery Department, Hull and East Yorkshire Hospitals NHS Trust, Castle Hill Hospital, Cottingham, UK

Mark Elliott, MA, MB, BChir, MD Leeds Centre for Respiratory Medicine, St James's University Hospital, Leeds, West Yorkshire, UK

Shoaib Faruqi, MD Department of Respiratory Medicine, Hull and East Yorkshire Hospitals NHS Trust, Castle Hill Hospital, Cottingham, UK

Helen Fowles, MB BCh MRCP Respiratory Research Group, Hull York Medical School, Castle Hill Hospital, Cottingham, UK

Dipansu Ghosh, MBBS, MD, FRCP Leeds Centre for Respiratory Medicine, St James's University Hospital, Leeds, West Yorkshire, UK

Melanie Greaves, MBBS, MRCP, FRCR Radiology Department, Manchester University NHS Foundation Trust, Wythenshawe Hospital, Manchester, UK

Michael A. Greenstone, MB, ChB, MD, FRCP Department of Respiratory Medicine, Hull and East Yorkshire Hospitals NHS Trust, Castle Hill Hospital, Cottingham, East Yorkshire, UK

Seamus Grundy, MBChB, PhD Thoracic Medicine, University Hospital Aintree, Liverpool, UK

Simon P. Hart, PhD, FRCPE Respiratory Research Group, Hull York Medical School, Castle Hill Hospital, Cottingham, East Yorkshire, UK

Thomas P. Hellyer, MBBS, PhD Institute of Cellular Medicine, Newcastle University, Newcastle Upon Tyne, UK

Peter M. Hickey, MBChB, BSc(Hons) Pulmonary Vascular Research Group, Department of Infection, Immunity and Cardiovascular Disease (IICD), University of Sheffield, Sheffield, South Yorkshire, UK

Adam Hill, MBChB, MD, FRCPEd Royal Infirmary and University of Edinburgh, Edinburgh, UK

Jack A. Kastelik, BSc, MBChB, MD Department of Respiratory Medicine, Hull and East Yorkshire Hospitals NHS Trust, Castle Hill Hospital, Cottingham, UK

David G. Kiely, BSc Hons, MD, FRCP, FESC, FCCP Pulmonary Vascular Disease Unit, Royal Hallamshire Hospital, Sheffield Teaching Hospitals NHS Trust, Sheffield, South Yorkshire, UK

Allan Lawrie, BSc, PhD Pulmonary Vascular Research Group, Department of Infection, Immunity and Cardiovascular Disease, University of Sheffield, Sheffield, South Yorkshire, UK

Rod Lawson, BA, MA, MBBS, PhD, FRCP Sheffield Teaching Hospitals NHS Foundation Trust, Sheffield, UK

Michael Lind, MD FRCP Queen's Centre for Oncology and Haematology, Hull York Medical School, Castle Hill Hospital, Cottingham, UK

James L. Lordan, MB BChBAO, PhD, BSc Hons, DCH Cardiothoracic Block/Institute of Transplantation, Freeman Hospital, Newcastle upon Tyne, UK

Alyn H. Morice, MD, FRCP Respiratory Research Group, Hull York Medical School/University of Hull, Castle Hill Hospital, Cottingham, UK

Jaymin B. Morjaria, MBBS, FRCP, MD Royal Brompton and Harefield NHS Foundation Trust, Harefield, Middlesex, UK

Sega Pathmanathan, BM, MRCP Department of Respiratory Medicine, Hull and East Yorkshire Hospitals NHS Trust, Castle Hill Hospital, Cottingham, East Yorkshire, UK

Daniel Peckham, MBBS, DM, FRCP Leeds Centre for Respiratory Medicine, St James's University Hospital, Leeds, West Yorkshire, UK

Anthony J. Rostron, MB, BChir, PhD, MRCS, FRCA Institute of Cellular Medicine, Newcastle University, Newcastle Upon Tyne, UK

Anda Samson, MD Department of Infection, Hull and East Yorkshire Hospitals, Castle Hill Hospital, Cottingham, East Yorkshire, UK

Dejene Shiferaw, MD, MRCP(UK), MRCP(Resp) Department of Respiratory Medicine, Hull and East Yorkshire Hospitals NHS Trust, Castle Hill Hospital, Cottingham, UK

A. John Simpson Institute of Cellular Medicine, Newcastle University, Newcastle upon Tyne, UK

Pasupathy Sivasothy, PhD, MBBS, FRCP Department of Medicine, Cambridge University Hospitals Foundation Trust, Cambridge, UK

Hiten Thaker, MSc, MB, FRCP, FRCPI, DTM&H Department of Infection, Hull and East Yorkshire Hospitals NHS Trust, Castle Hill Hospital, Cottingham, East Yorkshire, UK

Muhunthan Thillai, BA, PhD, MBBS, MRCP Cambridge Interstitial Lung Disease Unit, Papworth Hospital, Cambridgeshire, UK

William Tunnicliffe, FRCP Respiratory and Critical Care Medicine, Queen Elizabeth Hospital, Birmingham, UK

Paul Whitaker, MBChB, DM, MRCP Leeds Centre for Respiratory Medicine, St James's University Hospital, Leeds, West Yorkshire, UK

Abbreviations

AAV	Anti-neutrophil cytoplasmic antibody (ANCA)-associated vasculitides
ABG	Arterial blood gas
ABPA	Allergic bronchopulmonary aspergillosis
ACCESS	A Case Control Etiological Sarcoidosis Study
ACCP	American College of Chest Physicians
ACE	Angiotensin converting enzyme
ACOS	Asthma-COPD overlap syndrome
ACR	American College of Rheumatology
ACTH	Adreno corticotrophin hormone
AEC	Alveolar epithelial cells
AE-IPF	Acute exacerbations of IPF
AEP	Acute eosinophilic pneumonia
AERD	Aspirin-exacerbated respiratory disease
AIP	Acute interstitial pneumonia
ALI	Acute lung injury
ALK	Anaplastic lymphoma kinase
AM(s)	Alveolar macrophage(s)
ANCA	Anti-neutrophil cytoplasmic antibody
Anti-GBM	Anti-glomerular basement membrane [disease]
AP	Antero-posterior [chest radiographs]
ARDS	Acute respiratory distress syndrome
ASL	Airway surface liquid
ASV	Adaptive servo-ventilation
ATG	Anti-thymocyte globulin
ATP	Adenosine triphosphate
BAL	Bronchoalveolar lavage
BAPE	Benign asbestos pleural effusion
BCC	*Burkholderia cepacia* complex
BHL	Bilateral hilar lymphadenopathy
BLT	Bilateral lung transplantation
BLVR	Bronchoscopic lung volume reduction
BMD	Bone mineral density
BOS	Bronchiolitis obliterans syndrome
BP	Blood pressure
BPI	Bacterial permeability inhibitor
BSI	Bronchiectasis Severity Index

BSR	British Rheumatology Society
BTS	British Thoracic Society
BVAS	Birmingham vasculitis assessment score
CABG	Coronary artery bypass graft
CAP	Community-acquired pneumonia
CAT	COPD assessment test
CDT(s)	Catheter-directed therapy(ies)
CDT	Catheter-directed thrombolysis
CEP	Chronic eosinophilic pneumonia
Cf	Cardiac frequency
CF	Cystic fibrosis
CFPA	Chronic fibrosing pulmonary aspergillosis
CFRD	Cystic fibrosis-related diabetes
CFTR	Cystic fibrosis transmembrane conductance regulator
CHART	Continuous hyperfractionated accelerated radiotherapy
CHD	Congenital heart disease
CHS	Cough hypersensitivity syndrome
CLAD	Chronic lung allograft dysfunction
CMR	Cardiovascular magnetic resonance
CMV	Cytomegalovirus
CNIs	Calcineurin inhibitors
CO	Carbon monoxide
CO2	Carbon dioxide
COP	Cryptogenic organising pneumonia
COPD	Chronic obstructive pulmonary disease
CPAP	Continuous positive airway pressure
CPET	Cardio-pulmonary exercise test(ing)
CPO	Cardiogenic pulmonary oedema
CRP	C-reactive protein
CSA	Central sleep apnoea
CSF	Cerebrospinal fluid
CT	Computed tomography
CTD	Connective tissue disease
CtDNA	Circulating tumour DNA
CTEPH	Chronic thromboembolic pulmonary hypertension
CTPA	Computed tomography pulmonary angiography
CUS	Compression venous ultrasonography
CWP	Coal workers' pneumoconiosis
CXR	Chest radiograph/chest X-ray
DAD	Diffuse alveolar damage
DCD	Donated after cardiac death
DEXA	Dual energy X-ray absorptiometry
DIOS	Distal intestinal obstruction syndrome
DIP	Desquamative interstitial pneumonia
DOAC(s)	Direct oral anticoagulant(s)
DOT	Directly observed therapy
DPB	Diffuse pan-bronchiolitis
DPI(s)	Dry-powder inhaler(s)

DVT	Deep venous thrombosis
EAA	Extrinsic allergic alveolitis
EBB	Endobronchial biopsies
EBUS	Endobronchial ultrasound
EBUS-TBNA	Endobronchial ultrasound-guided transbronchial needle aspiration
ECMO	Extra-corporeal membrane oxygenation
EDS	Excessive daytime somnolence
EEG	Electroencephalography
EGFR	Epidermal growth factor receptor
EGPA	Eosinophilic granulomatosis with polyangiitis
EIA	Exercise-induced asthma
ELISA	Enzyme-linked immunosorbent assay
ENT	Ear, nose and throat
ERV	Expiratory reserve volume
ESC	European Society of Cardiology
ESS	Epworth sleepiness score
EULAR	European League Against Rheumatism
EUS	Endoscopic ultrasound
EUVAS	European Vasculitis Study Group
EVLP	*Ex vivo* lung perfusion
FDG	Fluoro-2-deoxy-*d*-glucose
FeNO	Fractional expired nitric oxide
FISH	Fluorescent *in situ* hybridisation
FNA	Fine needle aspiration
FRAX	Fracture risk assessment tool
FRC	Functional residual capacity
FVC	Forced vital capacity
GM	Galactomannan
GMSCF	Granulocyte-monocyte colony-stimulating factor
GOLD	Global initiative for chronic obstructive lung disease
GORD	Gastro-oesophageal reflux disease
GPA	Granulomatosis with polyangiitis
HAP	Hospital-acquired pneumonia
Hb	Haemoglobin
HCAP	Healthcare-associated pneumonia
HDAC2	Histone deacetylase-2
HFNO	High flow nasal oxygen
HIT	Heparin-induced thrombocytopenia
HIV	Human immunodeficiency virus
HLT	Heart-lung transplantation
HP	Hypersensitivity pneumonitis
HRCT	High resolution computed tomography
HSCT	Haematopoietic stem cell transplant
IA	Invasive aspergillosis
IASLC	International Association for the Study of Lung Cancer
IC	Inspiratory capacity
ICOPER	International Cooperative Pulmonary Embolism Registry

ICS	Inhaled corticosteroids
ICU	Intensive care unit
IgG4-RD	IgG4-related sclerosing disease
IGRA	Interferon-γ release assay
IHC	Immunohistochemistry
ILD(s)	Interstitial lung disease(s)
IMRT	Intensity-modulated radiotherapy
INR	International normalised ratio
IPAF	Interstitial pneumonia with autoimmune features
iPAH	Idiopathic pulmonary hypertension
IPC	Indwelling pleural catheter
IPF	Idiopathic pulmonary fibrosis
IPH	Idiopathic pulmonary haemosiderosis
IRIS	Immune reconstitution syndrome
IRT	Immunoreactive trypsinogen
ISAAC	International Study of Asthma and Allergies in Childhood
ISHLT	International Society for Heart and Lung Transplantation
IVC	Inferior vena cava
JVP	Jugular venous pressure
KCO	Transfer coefficient
LABA	Long acting beta$_2$ agonists
LAD	Lung assist device
LAM	Lymphangioleiomyomatosis
LAS	Lung allocation scores
LCH	Langerhans cell histiocytosis
LDCT	Low dose CT
LDH	Lactate dehydrogenase
LF-LAM	Lateral flow lipoarabinomannan assay
LHD	Left heart disease
LLN	Lower limit of normal
LMWH	Low molecular weight heparin
LVEF	Left ventricular ejection fraction
LVRS	Lung volume reduction surgery
MAC	Mycobacterium avium complex
MAD(s)	Mandibular advancement device(s)
MAPPET	Management Strategy and Prognosis of Pulmonary Embolism Registry
MARS	Mesothelioma and radical surgery (trial)
MCBT	Multiple combination bactericidal testing
MDCT	Multidetector CT
MDR	Multi-drug resistant
MDR-TB	Multi-drug resistant TB
MEFV	Maximal expiratory flow volume
MEP	Maximal expiratory pressure
MERS-CoV	Middle East respiratory syndrome coronavirus
MIFV	Maximal inspiratory flow volume
MIP	Maximal inspiratory pressure
MMA	Maxillo-mandibular advancement

MMF	Mycophenolate mofetil
MND	Motor neurone disease
MPA	Microscopic polyangiitis
mPAP	Mean pulmonary arterial pressure
MPM	Malignant pleural mesothelioma
MRI	Magnetic resonance imaging
MRSA	Methicillin-resistant *Staphylococcus aureus*
MSLT	Multiple sleep latency test
MTB	*Mycobacterium tuberculosis*
mTOR	Mammalian target of rapamycin
MTX	Methotrexate
NETT	National Emphysema Treatment Trial
NFAT	Nuclear factor of activated T-cells
NIV	Non-invasive ventilation
NNT	Number needed to treat
NPD	Nasal potential difference
NPV	Negative predictive value
NREM	Non-rapid eye movement
NSCLC	Non-small cell lung cancer
NSIP	Non-specific interstitial pneumonia
NTM	Non-tuberculosis mycobacteria
NTM-PD	Non-tuberculosis mycobacteria pulmonary disease
OARs	Organs at risk
ODI	Oxygen desaturation index
OHS	Obesity hypoventilation syndrome
OP	Organising pneumonia
OPTN	Organ procurement and transplantation network
OS	Overall survival
OSA	Obstructive sleep apnoea
OSAS	Obstructive sleep apnoea syndrome
OTC	Over-the-counter
PA	Postero-anterior [chest radiographs]
PAH	Pulmonary arterial hypertension
PAP	Pulmonary alveolar proteinosis
PAR	Protease-activated receptor
PAS	Para-amino salicylic acid
PAS	Periodic acid Schiff [staining material]
PCI	Prophylactic cranial irradiation
PCR	Polymerase chain reaction
Pcrit	Intraluminal airway pressure
PDE4	Phosphodiesterase type 4
Pdi	Transdiaphragmatic pressures
PE	Pulmonary embolism
PEEP	Positive end-expiratory pressure
PEF	Peak expiratory flow
PEITHO	Pulmonary Embolism Thrombolysis [trial]
PERT	Pancreatic enzyme replacement therapy
PESI	PE Severity Index

PET-CT	Positron-emission tomography combined with CT
PFS	Progression-free survival
PGD	Primary graft dysfunction
PLM(s)	Periodic limb movement(s)
pMDI(s)	Pressurised metered-dose inhaler(s)
PMF	Progressive massive fibrosis
PORT	Post-operative RT
PPO	Predicted post-operative
PPV	Positive predictive value
PRES	Posterior reversible leuco-encephalopathy syndrome
PSP	Primary spontaneous pneumothorax
PTLD	Post-transplant lymphoproliferative disorder
PVCM	Paradoxical vocal cord motion
PVL	Panton-Valentine leukocidin
R_0	No residual disease
RAS	Restrictive allograft syndrome
RB-ILD	Respiratory bronchiolitis-ILD
RCOG	Royal College of Obstetricians and Gynaecologists
RCT	Randomised controlled trial
REM	Rapid eye movement
REMBD	REM sleep behaviour disorder
RER	Respiratory exchange ratio
RERA(s)	Respiratory effort-related arousal(s)
RFT(s)	Respiratory function test(s)
RIF	Right iliac fossa
RSD	Relative standard deviation
RT	Radiotherapy
RTKI	Receptor tyrosine kinase inhibitor
RT-PCR	Reverse transcriptase polymerase chain reaction
RV	Residual volume
RV	Right ventricular
SABA	Short-acting beta$_2$ agonists (salbutamol and terbutaline)
SABR	Stereotactic ablative body radiotherapy
SCC	Small cell carcinoma
SCLC	Small cell lung cancer
SIADH	Syndrome of inappropriate antidiuretic hormone secretion
SLE	Systemic lupus erythematosus
SLT	Single lung transplant
SMRP	Soluble mesothelin-related peptides
SNIP	Sniff nasal inspiratory pressure
SPECT	Single photon emission tomography
SR	Standardised residual
SVC	Superior vena cava
SWS	Slow wave sleep
TB	Tuberculosis
TBB or TBLB	Transbronchial (lung) biopsy
TLC	Total lung capacity
TLCO	Transfer factor

TLI	Total lymphoid irradiation
TOF	Tracheo-oesophageal fistula
t-PA	Tissue plasminogen activator
TPMT	Thiopurine methyltransferase
TR	Tricuspid regurgitant
TST	Tuberculin skin test
UACS	Upper airways cough syndrome
UAR	Upper airway resistance
UARS	Upper airway resistance syndrome
UFH	Unfractionated heparin
UIP	Usual interstitial pneumonia
URTI	Upper respiratory tract infections
USAT	Ultrasound-assisted thrombolysis
UVPPP	Uvulopalatopharyngoplasty
VA	Alveolar volume
VAP	Ventilator-associated pneumonia
VAT/S	Video-assisted thoracoscopy/thoracic surgery
VC	Vital capacity
VCD	Vocal cord dysfunction
Ve	Respiratory ventilation
VEGF	Vascular endothelial growth factor
VKA	Vitamin K antagonist
VO_2	Oxygen uptake
VOD	Veno-occlusive disease
VTE	Venous thromboembolism
WBC	White blood cell(s)
WHO	World Health Organization
XDR-TB	Extensively-drug-resistant TB

Applied Respiratory Anatomy

Melanie Greaves

Imaging Modalities

Chest Radiographs

The plain chest radiograph (CXR) is the most commonly performed imaging procedure. The standard, routine postero-anterior (PA) CXR examination consists of an erect radiograph taken with the patient upright and in full inspiration with the front of their chest positioned against the imaging plate. The beam passes through the patient from back to front, hence the name postero-anterior.

The left lateral chest radiograph used to be performed as a routine with a PA film but is now infrequently obtained and somewhat undervalued in the age of computed tomography. It can, however, be crucial in identifying abnormalities in the posterior costophrenic angles, within the mediastinum, and in areas closely related to the spine and sternum. Relatively blind areas on frontal views make up 40% of the lung area and 25% of the lung volume. It is important that if a lateral CXR is obtained it is reported with the PA CXR taken at the same sitting.

Chest radiographs are frequently required to be taken at the patient bedside or in the emergency department and consequently, antero-posterior

(AP) chest radiographs comprise almost 50% of chest radiographic examinations. Patients lie or sit with their back against the imaging plate and the X-ray beam passes through them from anterior to posterior.

AP radiographs are of inferior quality to PA CXRs for a variety of reasons. Patients are typically too ill to sit upright and are therefore positioned semi-recumbent or supine. They may find it difficult to hold their breath, and the divergent geometry of the X-ray beam results in magnification of structures at the front of the chest. Mobile equipment uses lower energy X-rays, and the exposure factors are longer, increasing the probability of image degradation by motion artefact. The above factors lead to magnification of the cardiomediastinal structures and poor visualisation of both mediastinal structures and pulmonary parenchyma. Diagnostic difficulty is increased for the reporting radiologist, particularly with respect to identifying pleural effusions and pneumothoraces, and excluding lesions behind the heart and beneath the diaphragm.

The Silhouette Sign

In conventional radiography it is possible to differentiate four basic physiological densities from one another: air, fat, soft tissue, and calcium. Non-physiological denser mediums such as iodine, barium, or metal add a fifth.

When looking at plain films it should be remembered that adjacent anatomical structures

M. Greaves
Radiology Department, Manchester University NHS
Foundation Trust, Wythenshawe Hospital,
Manchester, UK

© Springer International Publishing AG, part of Springer Nature 2018
S. Hart, M. Greenstone (eds.), *Foundations of Respiratory Medicine*,
https://doi.org/10.1007/978-3-319-94127-1_1

of different densities have a well-defined demarcating interface between them. For example, on a chest radiograph, the lateral border of the left ventricle can be clearly distinguished from the adjacent air-filled lung parenchyma. Conversely, anatomical structures that are contiguous and the same density (for example the soft tissue density chambers of the heart) will appear as one mass, with no line of demarcation between them. This is referred to as the silhouette sign and can be useful in locating abnormalities within the thorax.

Computed Tomography

Current computed tomography (CT) scanners have multiple rows of detector elements allowing for the simultaneous acquisition of data as the patient moves through the rotating gantry. The speed of scanning has markedly increased as a consequence of faster rotation times and the multiple detector arrays. The entire chest can now be imaged in a single breath hold, decreasing motion artefacts and allowing for optimization of contrast enhancement.

Multidetector CT scanners (MDCT) generate large volume data sets which enable sophisticated multiplanar and three-dimensional reconstructions. Multiplanar reconstructions (for example in coronal and sagittal planes) may enable better appreciation of anatomical structures than a series of individual cross-sectional transaxial images.

Volume rendering uses all of the data from the CT acquisition in the final image. This is a truly three-dimensional reconstruction that conveys depth perception. The images produced are particularly useful in clarifying vascular morphology and complex three-dimensional anatomic relationships. Their use can enable communication between radiologist and clinician by displaying scan information in a more familiar form to the non-imager.

Thoracic CT scans are routinely performed with the patient in the supine position during suspended full inspiration. Additional scans may be acquired in forced expiration, to demonstrate air trapping or central airway collapse, or with the patient prone, to differentiate true parenchymal disease from normal gravitational atelectasis in posterior basal lung.

CT evaluation can be performed with or without intravenous contrast administration. Iodinated contrast is essential for the diagnosis of pulmonary emboli and aortic dissection and can allow for easier discrimination of lymph nodes from vessels.

The normal thorax contains structures with a wide range of densities from bone to air, and in contrast to plain radiographs, a CT image can display a wider range of these in black, white, and shades of grey. Unfortunately the human eye can discriminate relatively few shades of grey and to evaluate all the available information, CT images are typically viewed on at least two, and usually three, different "window" settings optimised for soft tissue, lung, and bone.

High-Resolution CT

High-resolution CT is widely used for the evaluation of a variety of diffuse parenchymal and airway diseases, as it enables more detailed visualisation of the pulmonary parenchyma. It is performed using a conventional CT scanner with imaging parameters chosen to maximise spatial resolution. These include using a thin slice width (0.625–1.25 mm) reconstructed with a sharp, high-resolution image reconstruction algorithm. HRCT allows for depiction of lung morphology at a level comparable to gross macroscopic anatomy.

Conventionally, HRCT is performed by acquiring the thin slices at 1–2 cm gaps, as this is an examination typically used to diagnose diffuse lung disease. With the introduction of MDCT scanners, there has been a tendency to move towards volumetric acquisition through the entire thorax. This latter allows for detection of all abnormalities present, including small lung nodules, but at the price of higher patient radiation. Although there is improved diagnostic accuracy of volume HRCT for the diagnosis and exclusion of bronchiectasis when compared with conventional HRCT it is uncertain if this technique is better for evaluating diffuse interstitial lung disease.

Ultrasound

Thoracic ultrasound involves no ionising radiation, is relatively cheap, and readily available at the bedside.

It is more sensitive than a plain radiograph at detecting pleural fluid and is typically better than CT in differentiating pleural fluid from pleural thickening and in evaluating the complexity of pleural effusions. Ultrasound can also be used to diagnose pneumothoraces.

It is an invaluable tool for the detection and localization of pleural fluid. Ultrasound guidance during thoracentesis and chest drain placement can minimise complications, and it is increasingly used for peripheral lung, pleural, and supraclavicular nodal biopsies. Diaphragmatic paralysis can be diagnosed effectively with ultrasound as an alternative to X-ray fluoroscopy.

Imaging Anatomy and Interpretation

It is necessary to have a systematic approach to reading both chest radiographs and CT. The precise methodology can be very individual, but should include evaluation of the lungs, pleura, airways, hila, heart and great vessels, mediastinum, diaphragm, and chest wall, the anatomy of which are detailed below.

The Lungs, Lobes, and Fissures

Each lung is conical in shape, having a blunt apex which reaches above the sternal end of the first rib, a concave base overlying the diaphragm, a costovertebral surface moulded to the chest wall, and a mediastinal surface which is concave to accommodate the mediastinum.

The right lung is slightly larger than the left and is divided by the minor and major fissures into three lobes: upper, middle, and lower. The left lung only has a major fissure, and hence only two lobes: upper and lower. The lobes are further divided into segments, each of which is supplied by a segmental bronchus and a tertiary branch of the pulmonary artery. They are named according to the segmental bronchus that supplies them and are wedge-shaped with their apices at the hilum and bases at the lung surface.

The major or oblique fissures begin at the level of the fifth thoracic vertebra and extend downwards, obliquely and forward, roughly paralleling the sixth rib and ending at the diaphragm a few centimetres from the anterior pleural gutter. The right is more obliquely orientated, the left more vertical. The right contacts the minor fissure. This separates the anterior segment of the right upper lobe from the middle lobe and runs, roughly horizontally, from the edge of the lung towards the hilum at the level of the fourth anterior rib.

There are several accessory fissures. These are of little more than academic interest but it is worthwhile being able to recognise them as normal variants. The most easily identifiable is the azygos fissure, which occurs in approximately 0.5% of individuals. In early fetal life the embryonic precursor of the azygos vein migrates over the apex of the right lung to its usual position in the right side of the mediastinum. Occasionally, instead of migrating over the lung apex, it invaginates the apical right upper lobe, taking visceral and parietal pleura with it. The fissure is then seen as a curvilinear structure extending obliquely across the superomedial right upper lobe, terminating in a tear-drop shaped opacity caused by the vein itself.

Although the fissures may extend to the hilum resulting in complete lobar separation, they are commonly incomplete. This can be important, as regions of parenchymal continuity from lobe to lobe can provide a ready pathway for collateral air drift or disease spread. Fissural incompleteness can also reduce the effectiveness of bronchial valve placement for volume reduction procedures.

Fissures are easily seen on plain radiographs and CT and can be useful in identifying and localising volume loss. If the volume of a lobe is decreased, the adjacent fissure will be displaced towards the collapsed region. Fissures become reoriented and may appear as lines or interfaces, depending upon whether or not the partially collapsed lobe is air or fluid containing. The right upper lobe is bounded inferiorly by the minor fissure and posteriorly by the major fissure. As the right upper lobe loses volume, the minor fissure moves superiorly and medially on the frontal chest radiograph. Typically the lateral portion of the fissure is higher than the medial.

The Pleura

The normal visceral and parietal pleura are not visible on a CXR apart from the double layer of visceral pleura forming the interlobar fissures.

On CT, the pleural layers are visualised as part of the intercostal stripe, a 1–2 mm line of soft tissue attenuation seen at the point of contact between the lung and the chest wall. This is composed of the visceral pleura, the parietal pleura, normal pleural fluid, the endothoracic fascia and the innermost intercostal muscles; most of the visible stripe is due to the intercostal muscles. In the paravertebral regions, the innermost intercostal muscle is lacking and the thin line seen on CT represents pleura and endothoracic fascia. Extrapleural fat pads can be seen internal to ribs on both chest radiographs and CT, and can easily be confused with pleural thickening (as can the transverse thoracic and subcostal muscles on CT).

The costophrenic angles should be clearly defined and be sharp. It should be remembered that the posterior costophrenic angles are more inferior than the lateral. As such, small amounts of fluid will accumulate posteriorly and not blunt the lateral costophrenic recesses on a frontal radiograph. A lateral radiograph is therefore more sensitive for diagnosing tiny effusions blunting the posterior costophrenic angles.

On ultrasound the parietal and visceral pleura normally appear as a single bright line no wider than 2 mm, and normal air-filled lung can be seen sliding with respiration.

The lymphatic drainage of the pleura is important in the assessment of the spread of pleural malignancy. The visceral pleura drains to the same nodal groups as the lung parenchyma; bronchopulmonary, hilar, mediastinal, supraclavicular, and scalene. The parietal pleura however, has a different drainage into internal thoracic, subpleural, costophrenic, and cardiophrenic nodes.

The Airways

Only the trachea, main, and lobar bronchi can be identified with certainty on the plain radiograph, and are visible as black tubular structures containing air.

The trachea begins at the C6 level and is a midline structure that has a slight deviation to the right after entering the thorax. Its walls are parallel except for a smooth indentation on its left side produced by the aorta. If the trachea is significantly deviated it is important to establish if this is positional or a consequence of true pathology such as right upper lobe fibrosis or a thyroid goitre.

The trachea divides into the two main bronchi at the carina. This lies at the level of the sternal angle (T5). In adults the right main bronchus has a steeper angle than the left, hence aspiration is more frequent on the right. The carinal angle is in the region of 60°; greater than 90° is pathological.

On the frontal chest radiograph the upper lobe bronchi usually leave the main bronchi in a horizontal plane, the right lying higher than the left.

On a lateral chest radiograph the trachea can be easily seen descending slightly posteriorly. The anterior wall is often indistinct but the posterior wall can be seen as it abuts the air-filled lung. The posterior wall, together with fat, forms the posterior tracheal stripe. This is seldom useful clinically, as the normal oesophagus may be interposed thickening it. Thickening on serial chest radiographs is, however, more concerning.

The tracheal air column on a lateral radiograph often terminates in two rounded lucencies. The upper one represents the orifice of the right upper lobe bronchus, and the lower one the left upper lobe bronchus. The left upper lobe bronchus is typically more easily seen, as it is outlined by the left main pulmonary artery arching over it. Since the right and left main bronchi almost superimpose, the carina is difficult to identify on the lateral view, but usually approximates to the level of the sternal angle.

CT is used to evaluate the major airways and the images are typically viewed on lung windows.

On CT the trachea (Fig. 1.1) can be visualised extending from the inferior aspect of the cricoid cartilage to the carina. It contains 16–22 horseshoe-shaped cartilaginous rings which are

Fig. 1.1 Axial CT (lung window) at the level of the mid trachea

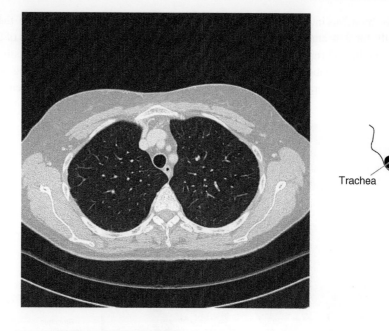

Trachea

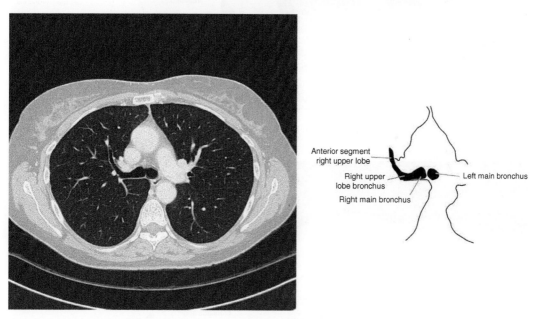

Anterior segment right upper lobe

Right upper lobe bronchus

Right main bronchus

Left main bronchus

Fig. 1.2 Axial CT (lung window) at the level of the right upper lobe bronchus

incomplete posteriorly, the posterior wall of the trachea being a thin fibromuscular membrane. It is most commonly seen as a round or oval structure on CT with a flattened posterior wall that becomes concave in expiration. Calcification of the cartilages becomes more common with age.

The right upper lobe bronchus arises from the lateral aspect of the main stem bronchus, approximately 2.5 cm from the carina (Fig. 1.2). It divides approximately 1 cm from its origin into three segmental branches: the anterior, posterior, and apical.

The bronchus intermedius (Fig. 1.3) continues distally for 3–4 cm and then bifurcates into the right middle and right lower lobe bronchi.

The middle lobe bronchus (Fig. 1.4) arises from the right lateral wall of the bronchus inter-medius almost opposite the origin of the superior segmental bronchus of the lower lobe. If you can find one you can easily identify the other. It is typically 1–2 cm long and bifurcates into its medial and lateral segmental branches.

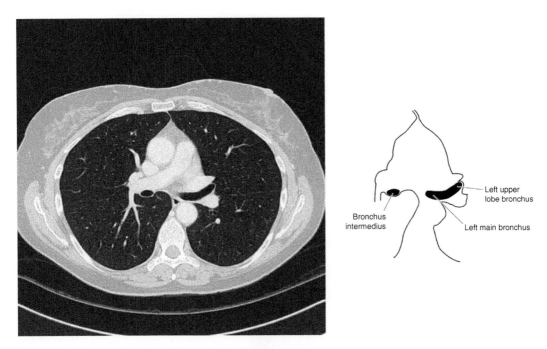

Fig. 1.3 Axial CT (lung window) at the level of the bronchus intermedius and left upper lobe bronchus

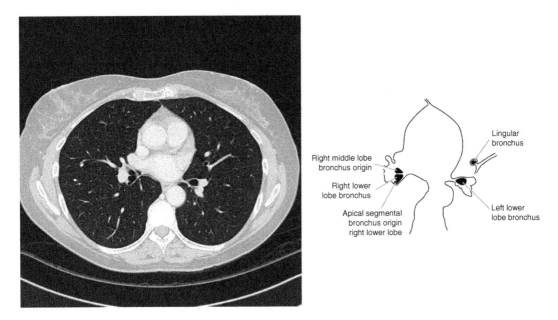

Fig. 1.4 Axial CT (lung window) at the level of the right middle lobe bronchus

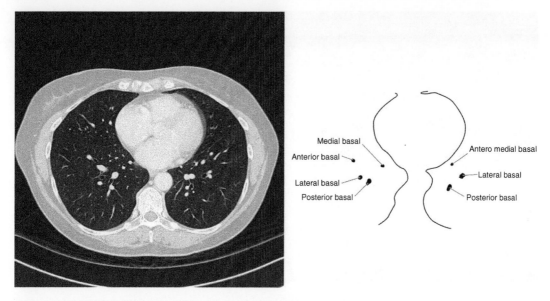

Fig. 1.5 Axial CT (lung window) at the level of the lower lobe basal segmental bronchi

The right lower lobe bronchus is the continuation of the bronchus intermedius beyond the right middle lobe bronchial take-off. The superior segmental bronchus arises from its posterior aspect (almost opposite the right middle lobe bronchus) and it then further divides into four basal segmental bronchi, the anterior, lateral, posterior and medial (Fig. 1.5).

The left upper lobe bronchus (shown in Fig. 1.3) usually trifurcates into the apico-posterior, anterior and lingular bronchi. The lingular bronchus (shown in Fig. 1.4) can usually be visualised at approximately the same level as the origin of the superior segmental bronchus of the lower lobe. Again, if you can find one you can usually identify the other.

The lingular bronchus extends for 2–3 cm before bifurcating into superior and inferior divisions. The left lower lobe branching pattern is similar to the right although there are typically only three segmental bronchi, anteromedial, posterior and lateral (shown in Fig. 1.5).

The bronchi divide in an asymmetric dichotomous manner. As they branch and get smaller their walls become thinner and less easy to identify, and in normal individuals it should not be possible to identify bronchi within 1 cm of the costal pleura on CT. Normal bronchioles cannot be visualised.

The Hila

The hila are complicated structures consisting mainly of the major bronchi and the pulmonary arteries and veins. They are not symmetrical but have the same components on each side. Normal hilar nodes cannot be visualised on plain radiographs but do become identifiable when enlarged. The hila should be checked for position, size, and density on every chest radiograph and closely evaluated on CT, as they are common sites for lymph node enlargement and tumours.

Each lung has a large pulmonary artery supplying blood to it, and typically two pulmonary veins. These comprise the majority of the hilar shadows on a chest radiograph but are clearly seen to best advantage on CT (Fig. 1.6).

The pulmonary arteries carry deoxygenated blood at low pressure. They supply 99% of the blood flow to the lungs and participate in gas exchange at the alveolar capillary membrane.

The main pulmonary artery originates in the mediastinum at the pulmonary valve and passes upwards, backwards, and to the left. On CT the diameter of the main pulmonary artery should be less than or equal to 29 mm, and is usually smaller than the ascending thoracic aorta at the

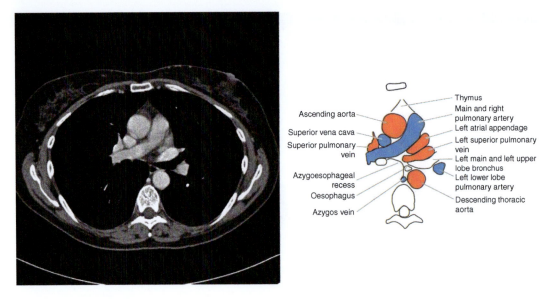

Fig. 1.6 Axial contrast-enhanced CT (soft tissue window) at the level of the right main pulmonary artery demonstrating hilar and mediastinal anatomy

same level. A larger calibre than this suggests pulmonary hypertension. The pulmonary trunk bifurcates within the pericardium, into a shorter left and longer right pulmonary artery.

The right pulmonary artery divides behind the superior vena cava into the artery to the right upper lobe (truncus anterior) and the right interlobar pulmonary artery. The interlobar pulmonary artery courses caudally in the major fissure anterolateral to the bronchus intermedius and right lower lobe bronchus giving segmental branches to the right middle and lower lobes.

On a frontal chest radiograph, the upper limit of the transverse diameter of the interlobar artery from its lateral aspect to the air column of the bronchus intermedius is 16 mm in men and 15 mm in women. Enlargement suggests increased pressure or flow.

The higher left main pulmonary artery passes over the left main bronchus and continues as the vertically orientated left interlobar pulmonary artery from which the segmental arteries to the upper and lower lobes arise. The left interlobar artery lies posterolateral to the lower lobe bronchus. On lateral radiographs the left pulmonary artery can usually be easily identified as it courses over the left main and upper lobe bronchi forming an arch smaller and parallel to the aortic arch.

The right pulmonary artery appears as a rounded density since it is viewed end on. The more posterior location of the left pulmonary artery with respect to the right explains why the bulk of the left pulmonary artery projects behind the upper lobe bronchial orifices and the right pulmonary artery projects in front of them.

The pulmonary veins carry recently oxygenated blood from the lungs to the left atrium.

The segmental pulmonary veins from the right upper lobe form the right superior pulmonary vein. The middle lobe vein usually joins the right upper lobe vein just prior to entry into the left atrium, although occasionally it may drain separately.

On the left, the upper lobe segmental veins join to form the left superior pulmonary vein incorporating the lingular vein also.

The horizontally orientated lower lobe segmental veins form the right and left inferior pulmonary veins which drain into the left atrium. The normal superior and inferior pulmonary venous confluences are sometimes large enough to simulate nodules on chest radiographs.

Whilst arteries and veins are relatively easily distinguished on CT, this can be very difficult on the chest radiograph. It is worth remembering, however, that the lower lobe veins are horizontally orientated, whereas the lower lobe arteries are more vertical.

The hilar point on chest radiographs is the angle formed by the superior pulmonary veins (draining the upper lungs) and the lower lobe pulmonary arteries. The more superior location of the left main pulmonary artery results in the left hilum lying higher than the right on a frontal chest X-ray. This relationship is seen in 97% of normal people; in the other 3% they are at the same level.

On CT the arteries can be seen to accompany the bronchi as they divide and progress distally. In addition to this there are additional pulmonary arteries which do not lie adjacent to a bronchus and these become more numerous peripherally.

The pulmonary veins are always separated from the bronchoarterial bundles. This relationship commences in the lung periphery where the bronchi and arteries are in the central portion of the secondary pulmonary lobule and the veins are located within the interlobular septa (see "Secondary Pulmonary Lobule").

The Heart and Great Vessels

The heart and pericardial sac are situated obliquely about two-thirds to the left and one-third to the right. On a frontal chest radiograph the position of the heart largely depends upon the patient's age and build. In younger, slim individuals the heart is more upright and central, whereas in older persons it tends to be more horizontally orientated and projects more to the left of midline. The cardiothoracic ratio is a commonly used measurement of overall heart size in relation to chest cavity. This is calculated as being the widest diameter of the heart to the widest internal diameter of the bony thorax on an erect PA chest radiograph. A cardiothoracic ratio larger than 50% has a sensitivity of approximately 80% for detecting left ventricular dilatation, but a specificity of only 50%. The heart size will appear larger on AP chest radiographs (as magnified by the divergent X-ray beam) and on chest radiographs taken at less than full inspiration.

The right heart border on a frontal chest radiograph is formed by the right atrium extending between the superior vena cava (SVC) and the inferior vena cava (IVC).

The left heart border is more complex, with three convexities above the left ventricle. These are formed by the aortic knuckle, the pulmonary trunk (above the left main bronchus), and the left atrial appendage (below the left main bronchus). This latter region should be straight or concave; any bulge in this region implies dilatation of the left atrial appendage. If the left atrium enlarges, it typically elevates the left main bronchus, widening the carinal angle.

The junction of the heart with the diaphragm produces cardiophrenic recesses on both sides. These contain fat and a few small nodes. Fat density is less than soft tissue, so the heart borders can usually be seen clearly though them.

The right ventricle forms the largest part of the anterior surface of the heart, and the left atrium is situated posteriorly, meaning that these chambers are not border forming on a frontal chest radiograph. They can, however, be seen on a left lateral view and on CT (Fig. 1.7). The right ventricle lies anteriorly and contacts the lower third of the sternum. If it contacts more than one-third of the sternum, right ventricular dilatation should be suspected. An enlarged left atrium can be seen to bulge posteriorly.

The pericardium (Fig. 1.8) is a double-walled fibro-serous membrane that encloses the heart and the roots of its great vessels. It helps optimise cardiac motion and chamber pressures and serves as a barrier to pathology. The tough fibrous outer layer is contiguous with the central tendon of the diaphragm, fused with the adventitia of the great vessels entering and leaving the heart and attached to the posterior surface of the sternum. The internal surface of the fibrous pericardium is lined with the parietal layer of serous pericardium, which is reflected onto the heart and great vessels as the visceral layer. The closer apposition of the visceral layer to the cardiac structures results in normal pericardial recesses which can be identified as containing small amounts of fluid. The pericardial cavity usually contains 15–50 ml of serous fluid.

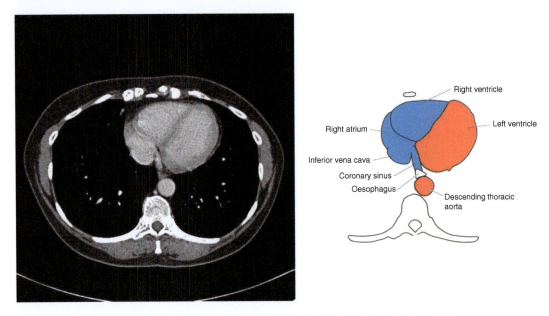

Fig. 1.7 Axial contrast-enhanced CT (soft tissue window) at the level of the right and left ventricles

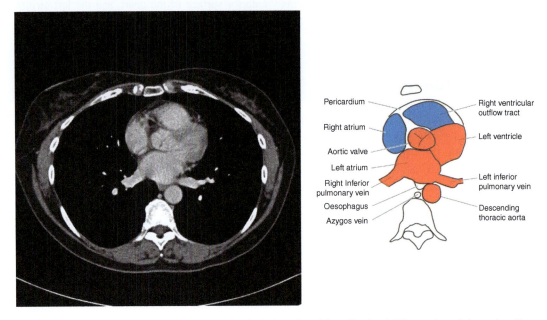

Fig. 1.8 Axial contrast-enhanced CT (soft tissue window) at the mid cardiac level. The portion of the pericardium anterior to the right ventricular outflow tract is seen as a fine line

The normal combined pericardial thickness is 2 mm or less; 4 mm is definitely abnormal, often suggesting a pericarditis. The normal pericardium cannot be appreciated on chest radiographs but can be easily identified on CT. Discrimination of pericardium from myocardium requires the presence of epicardial fat or pericardial fluid. It is usually easily visible over the right atrium and right ventricle, but often difficult to see adjacent to the lateral and posterior walls of the left ventricle.

Systemic Arterial Supply of the Thorax

The aorta provides the main systemic arterial supply of the thorax. This vessel is divided into the ascending aorta, arch, and descending aorta. It begins at the root of the aorta where the three aortic sinuses are located and courses upwards with a slight inclination forwards and to the right. The arch of the aorta (Fig. 1.9) lies in an almost sagittal plane in the upper mediastinum behind the lower part of the manubrium. It is visualised radiographically as the aortic knob or knuckle, and indents the left side of the trachea. A right-sided aortic arch is rare (less than 1%), may be associated with congenital heart disease, and typically indents the right side of the trachea.

Inferiorly, the arch is related to the pulmonary trunk (Fig. 1.10) and is connected to the left pulmonary artery by the ligamentum arteriosum (the fetal ductus arteriosum). The left recurrent laryngeal nerve is looped around this structure.

The three main branches of the arch are the right brachiocephalic trunk (also known as the innominate artery), the left common carotid artery, and the left subclavian artery (Fig. 1.11).

The brachiocephalic trunk divides behind the right sternoclavicular joint into the right subclavian and right common carotid arteries.

Variations in the branching patterns of the arch vessels are not uncommon. Frequently the right branchiocephalic trunk and the left common carotid artery have a common origin or trunk. It is not uncommon to see an aberrant right subclavian artery arising as the fourth branch of the aortic arch and passing behind the trachea from left to right to ascend to its normal position in the upper thorax.

The thoracic aorta descends in the posterior mediastinum to the left of the midline before moving centrally to lie behind the oesophagus. It traverses the diaphragm at the T12 vertebral level to become the abdominal aorta. The aorta gives off posterior intercostal arteries, subcostal, and phrenic arteries. It also supplies viscera via the bronchial, oesophageal, pericardial, and mediastinal arteries.

Bronchial Circulation

The bronchial arteries are responsible for supplying the majority of the oxygenated blood to

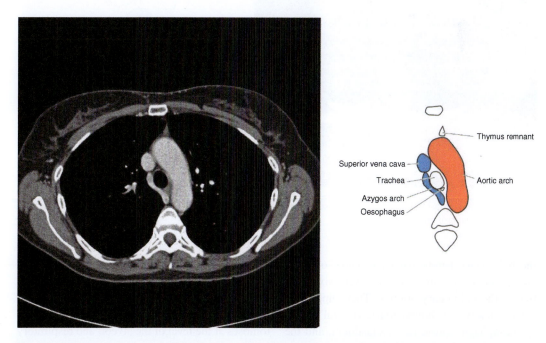

Fig. 1.9 Axial contrast enhanced CT (soft tissue window) through the upper thorax at the level of the aortic arch

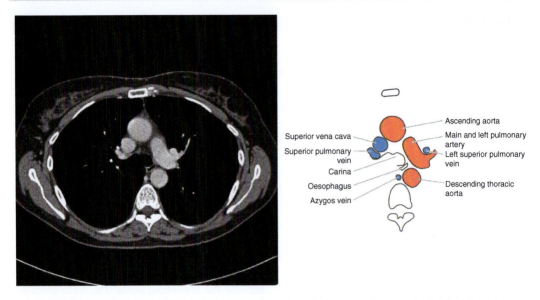

Fig. 1.10 Axial contrast-enhanced CT (soft tissue window) through the upper thorax at the level of the pulmonary trunk and left main pulmonary artery

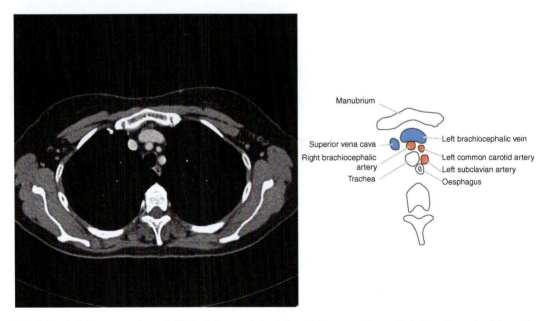

Fig. 1.11 Axial contrast-enhanced CT (soft tissue window) through the upper thorax just above the arch of the aorta demonstrating the proximal arch vessels

the pulmonary parenchyma and carry oxygenated blood to the lungs at a pressure six times that of the pulmonary arteries. They supply the central airways, the lymph nodes, visceral pleura, the oesophagus, posterior mediastinum, and the vagus nerves. They also supply the vasa vasorum of the aorta, pulmonary artery, and pulmonary veins. As a rule they do not participate in gas exchange. Bronchial arteries are connected to the pulmonary arteries through microvascular anastomoses at the level of the alveoli and respiratory bronchioles.

There is considerable variability in their number and precise site of origin; usually from the thoracic aorta between the T3 and T6 vertebral levels. In 70% of patients, two arise from the left and one from the right. On the right the bronchial artery usually arises from the right posterolateral aspect of the aorta in conjunction with an intercostal artery as an intercostobronchial trunk. On the left, superior and inferior bronchial arteries arise from the anteromedial arch and the thoracic aorta, respectively. The superior lies posterior to the left main bronchus, the inferior below it. The normal bronchial arteries can usually be identified on contrast-enhanced CT scans as they arise from the aorta.

Bronchial arteries may also arise from the internal mammary arteries, the thyrocervical trunk, the subclavian artery, and the coronary arteries. This has implications for the interventional radiologist when performing diagnostic and therapeutic procedures.

The intraparenchymal bronchial arteries branch with the airways, continuing as distally as the terminal bronchioles.

Normal bronchial arteries are small, measuring less than 2 mm at their origin, and are seen on CT as small undulating enhancing structures. The right bronchial arteries run to the right of the oesophagus and the left to the left. The bronchial and other collateral vessels (such as the intercostal and internal mammary arteries) hypertrophy in response to chronic inflammatory lung diseases such as bronchiectasis and aspergilloma, and the total systemic cardiac output through the bronchial arteries can increase dramatically. Bronchial arteries become very much more conspicuous on CT when hypertrophied and their visualisation should prompt the exclusion of longstanding ischaemic states, congenital cardiovascular anomalies, and chronic inflammatory conditions.

Systemic Veins of the Thorax

The superior vena cava (shown in Fig. 1.10) drains all the blood from the head and neck, the upper limbs, and the walls of the thorax and upper abdomen. It is formed by the union of the right and left brachiocephalic veins behind the sternal end of the first right costal cartilage. The right brachiocephalic vein descends vertically, whereas the left crosses in an oblique orientation anterior to the branches of the arch of the aorta. The SVC ends in the superior part of the right atrium at the level of the third right costal cartilage close to the sternum. It receives the azygos vein (shown in Fig. 1.9) which enters its posterior aspect at its mid-point, just before it enters the pericardium. The SVC lies on the right, anterolateral to the trachea and lateral to the ascending thoracic aorta. Occasionally, a left superior vena cava may persist and drain into the right atrium via the coronary sinus.

The intrathoracic inferior vena cava is short and can occasionally be seen on PA and lateral chest radiographs. It pierces the central tendon of the diaphragm at the approximate level of T8.

The azygos vein drains blood from both sides of the diaphragm to the heart. In the thorax it receives blood from the bronchial veins, the posterior intercostal veins, and the mediastinal structures.

Identification of the azygos vein on plain chest radiographs can be useful in confirming or helping to exclude pathology. Its course as it ascends in the mediastinum can be seen on the frontal chest radiograph as the azygo oesophageal line (see lines and stripes). The vein itself can be identified as a small oval density adjacent to the inferior right lateral wall of the trachea as it arches from front to back to join the SVC.

The Mediastinum and Its Contours

The mediastinum is the central component of the thoracic cavity containing all the thoracic viscera (except for the lungs), blood and lymphatic vessels, nodes, connective tissue and fat. It is covered on each side by the mediastinal pleura and is bounded by the two lungs, the sternum and the vertebral column. For diagnostic and descriptive purposes it is usually divided into several compartments, as many mediastinal lesions have characteristic locations, and it enables development of a compact differential diagnosis. There are, however, no physical boundaries between

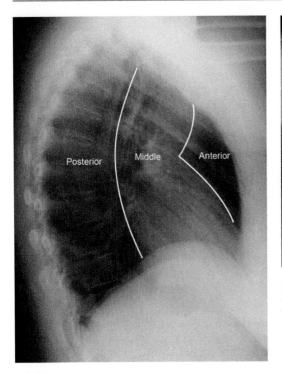

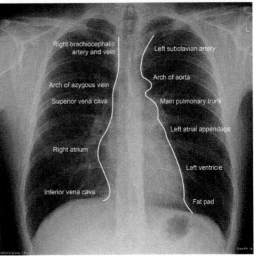

Fig. 1.13 Frontal chest radiograph with line tracing the various anatomic components forming the mediastinal borders

Fig. 1.12 Lateral chest radiograph demonstrating a basic anatomic method of dividing the mediastinum into compartments. This process is useful for the differential diagnosis of mediastinal pathology

compartments, and disease can spread freely between them.

There are many different ways of dividing up the mediastinum, but one of the most practical and simplest is the modified anatomical method, which identifies three compartments: anterior, middle, and posterior (Fig. 1.12). The anterior mediastinal compartment is bounded anteriorly by the sternum and posteriorly by the pericardium, aorta, and brachiocephalic vessels. It merges superiorly with the anterior aspect of the thoracic inlet and extends inferiorly to the diaphragm. It contains the thymus, branches of the internal mammary artery and vein, lymph nodes, and fat.

The middle mediastinum contains the pericardium and its contents, the ascending aorta and the arch, the superior and inferior vena cava, the brachiocephalic arteries and veins, the phrenic nerves and upper portions of the vagus nerves, the trachea, and main bronchi with their lymph nodes and the central pulmonary arteries and veins.

The posterior mediastinum includes the paraspinous area and is bounded anteriorly by the pericardium, laterally by mediastinal pleura, posteriorly by the bodies of the thoracic vertebra, and includes the paravertebral gutters. It contains the descending thoracic aorta, the oesophagus, the thoracic duct, the azygos and hemiazygos veins, autonomic nerves, fat, and lymph nodes.

On a frontal chest radiograph (Fig. 1.13) the right superior mediastinal border is formed by the right brachiocephalic vessels, and the SVC with the contour of the lower mediastinal border being formed by the heart. On the left, the convexity of the mediastinum is formed by the aortic arch, a small concavity called the aortopulmonary window and inferior to that the main pulmonary trunk. A small round bump on the lateral wall of the aortic knuckle is seen on approximately 1% of chest radiographs and represents the left superior intercostal vein. Its sudden appearance, particularly in patients who have had instrumentation of their veins, raises the possibility of SVC or left brachiocephalic venous obstruction. The outer border of the left mediastinum more inferiorly is formed by the left heart.

Mediastinal pathology is often difficult to appreciate directly on plain radiographs as most lesions will be of soft tissue density and therefore

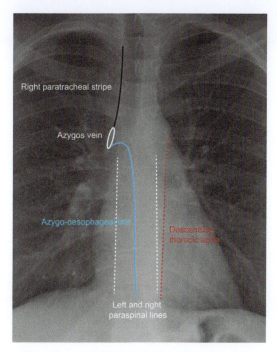

Right paratracheal stripe

Azygos vein

Azygo-oesophageal line

Descending thoracic aorta

Left and right paraspinal lines

Fig. 1.14 The normal mediastinal lines and stripes as seen on a frontal chest radiograph. Displacement or loss of these can indicate disease

inseparable from normal structures. They may, however, change the appearance of mediastinal contours, and it is for this reason that interpreting physicians should have an awareness of normal contours and interfaces. Displacement or loss of clarity of these interfaces can indicate disease. Mediastinal contours and lines that should be routinely checked are as follows.

The right paratracheal stripe (Fig. 1.14) is an easy to identify, linear opacity produced by the right upper lobe abutting the right lateral wall of the trachea. Air within the tracheal lumen and the right upper lobe contrast with the soft tissue density of the tracheal wall and the mediastinal soft tissue. It can be seen on the majority of normal chest radiographs and projects as a well-defined line extending from the level of the sternoclavicular joint to the azygos arch. The width of this line should not exceed 4 mm (the thickness of the visceral and mediastinal pleura, the tracheal wall, and the soft tissues in between). Widening most typically is secondary to right paratracheal lymphadenopathy although

tracheal wall disease and primary mediastinal masses are other causes.

The aortopulmonary window. This is the space between the aortic arch and the main pulmonary trunk and has a concave contour. It contains fat, the ligamentum arteriosum, the recurrent laryngeal nerve, and lymph nodes. A convexity in this region is usually abnormal and most commonly due to lymphadenopathy.

The paraaortic stripe. This is the interface of the descending thoracic aorta with the air in the left lower lobe. Distortion of this line may be caused by thoracic aneurysms and obliteration by parenchymal disease in the adjacent left lower lobe.

The azygo-oesophageal interface or recess is produced by a tongue of right lower lobe lying anterior to the vertebral bodies and adjacent to the azygos vein and oesophagus. It can frequently be identified as a long interface that extends from the diaphragm to the level of the azygos arch. Its right side is sharply delineated by air in the right lower lobe, the left side is of soft tissue density produced by the adjacent vein, oesophagus, aorta, and surrounding posterior mediastinal connective tissue. Viewed from the front its superior aspect forms a deep arc concave to the right. Any loss of concavity or increased density of this region below the azygos arch should be regarded with suspicion, as it most commonly results from lymphadenopathy in the subcarinal region.

Paravertebral stripes are a consequence of contact between lung and paravertebral soft tissues, and usually parallel the thoracic spine. The left is usually longer and more conspicuous than the right, being seen halfway between the lateral margin of the descending thoracic aorta and the spine. Displacement or focal contour abnormalities of these lines may result from vertebral pathology, such as osteophytes or fracture, paravertebral masses such as neurogenic tumours, or lymph node enlargement.

CT is almost invariably used to localise and characterise mediastinal abnormalities further, with diagnosis based on the location of the lesion, its shape, constituent tissues, and additional features such as its interaction with the surrounding structures.

Intrathoracic Lymph Nodes

Enlargement of intrathoracic lymph nodes is a manifestation of many diseases, and is frequently found in patients with bronchogenic carcinoma and other malignancies. Infections, particularly of mycobacterial and fungal origin, and non-infectious granulomatous diseases, such as sarcoidosis and pneumoconiosis, are other common causes.

Enlarged nodes can often be identified on plain chest radiographs, particularly when attention is focussed on the mediastinal interfaces as described above. Comparison with previous chest radiographs can be extremely useful in identifying subtle new disease.

CT is, however, the primary non-invasive technique for the diagnostic evaluation of thoracic lymph nodes, the location of which are described below.

Anterior Mediastinal Nodes

The internal mammary nodes lie with the internal mammary vessels close to the anterior chest wall. These nodes cannot be seen on a chest radiograph unless enlarged, and then only easily demonstrated on a lateral view. They receive lymph from the medial portion of the breast, the intercostal spaces, diaphragm, and the upper abdominal wall. Identification of these nodes is easy on CT, with the node being medial to the internal mammary vessel. Enlargement is often seen in lymphoma, pleural mesothelioma, and metastatic breast carcinoma.

Anterior diaphragmatic lymph nodes are located on the anterior aspect of the superior surface of the diaphragm and drain to the internal mammary nodes. They are more regularly seen at CT than on CXR. The paracardiac nodes are the more medial component of this group and again are most easily seen on CT. If visible they suggest abnormality.

Prevascular nodes are located anterior to the great vessels. The lowest of these nodes lies in the aortopulmonary window near the ligamentum arteriosum. Nodal enlargement may be identified by obscuration of the contour of the aortic knuckle on the frontal chest radiograph. As mentioned above, nodal enlargement in the AP window will produce a convex bulging of this region.

Middle Mediastinal Nodes

The right paratracheal nodal chain ascends along the anterolateral wall of the trachea, draining the right upper lobe and the middle and lower lobes indirectly via hilar and subcarinal nodes. The left lower lobe also drains to the right paratracheal nodes via the subcarinal nodes. The lowest node in this chain is the azygos node, lying near the azygos arch in the tracheobronchial angle. Nodal enlargement in this region is usually easily identified on a chest radiograph, with widening and lobulation of the right partracheal stripe and azygos vein area.

Left paratracheal nodes are smaller, generally fewer in number, and are rarely involved in isolation.

Subcarinal nodes lie below the carina and extend along the inferior margins of the main bronchi. They usually drain to the right paratracheal nodes. Enlarged subcarinal nodes are difficult to see on a chest radiograph as they lie in the centre of the chest, however, distortion of the azygo-oesophageal line is often a pointer to their presence.

Tracheobronchial nodes and bronchopulmonary nodes surround the mainstem bronchi and the pulmonary vessels medial to the mediastinal surface of the lung. They drain the lung and visceral pleura. Their enlargement produces a lobulated hilar contour and an increase in density, which is easier to appreciate if unilateral.

Posterior Mediastinal Lymph Nodes

These lie along the descending thoracic aorta and drain the posterior mediastinum (including diaphragm, oesophagus, and pericardium) to the thoracic duct. It is unusual to identify these nodes on a frontal chest radiograph even when markedly enlarged, but they may produce focal bulges in the paraspinous lines. This group of nodes is affected in lymphomas, and may be the site of metastases from lung and oesophageal carcinomas as well as tumours spreading from retrocrural and para-aortic abdominal nodes. Efferent lymphatics from this entire group drain to the thoracic duct, subcarinal, and intra-abdominal nodes.

The accurate identification of thoracic lymph node involvement is a crucial component of evaluation of a number of diseases, probably the most important of which is lung cancer staging. The most widely used criteria for predicting the presence or absence of disease in a lymph node is size. In general, the larger the node, the more likely it will be involved in the disease process. Unfortunately, no CT nodal size cut-off has proved entirely satisfactory.

The long transverse diameter on axial CT (long axis) is very dependent on the orientation of the typically sausage-shaped node to the scan plane. Nodal short axis (perpendicular to the measured long axis) has been shown on autopsy studies to be a more accurate predictor of nodal involvement. Most normal size nodes are less than 1 cm in short axis diameter.

Although the size of normal nodes may vary depending on their location, nodes in the para-tracheal, aortopulmonary window, hilar, subcari-nal, and paraoesophageal regions are considered abnormal if the nodal short axis is greater than 1 cm. Peridiaphragmatic and internal mammary nodes are considered abnormal if their short axis is greater than 0.5 cm. Nodes in the retrocrural and extrapleural regions are not normally visible on CT and should be considered abnormal when present. PET-CT and histological sampling are advised if the presence of disease in a node will affect therapy.

Lymph node maps have been used for at least 40 years and provide a method of precisely local-ising nodal involvement. They are required for accurately recording and communicating the presence of abnormal nodes. Lymph node loca-tions have been traditionally divided into 14 sta-tions based on surgical landmarks. Stations 1–9 correspond to mediastinal nodal groups. Stations 10–14 represent hilar and peribronchial nodal groups. Scalene and supraclavicular nodes are not represented, as they are extrapleural. The nodal map proposed by the International Association for the Study of Lung Cancer (IASLC) has been widely implemented since 2009.

The nodal stations are shown in Fig. 1.15:

1. Supraclavicular (low cervical, supraclavicu-lar and sternal notch nodes)
2. Upper paratracheal 2R and 2L; right and left
3. Prevascular 3A right and left. Retrotracheal 3P.
4. Lower paratracheal 4R and 4L right and left.
5. Subaortic
6. Paraaortic
7. Subcarinal

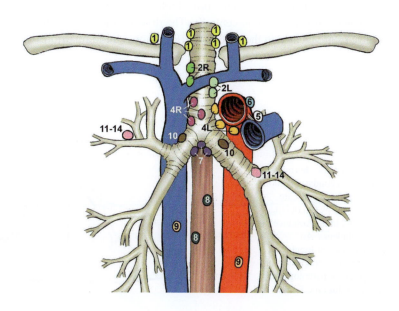

Fig. 1.15 IASLC mediastinal nodal map

8. Paraoesophageal (below carina)
9. Pulmonary ligament
10. Hilar
11. Interlobar
12. Lobar
13. Segmental
14. Subsegmental

Pulmonary Parenchyma

Beyond the segmental bronchi there are 20–25 generations of branches that end in terminal bronchioles. A terminal bronchiole gives rise to several generations of respiratory bronchioles, each providing 2–11 alveolar ducts and thence 5–6 alveolar sacs. The alveolus is the basic structural unit of gas exchange in the lung.

The secondary pulmonary lobule (Fig. 1.16) is the smallest unit of lung that can be seen on HRCT, and an understanding of its anatomy is a prerequisite for accurate HRCT diagnosis. This is because they have clearly defined anatomy, and many pathological abnormalities specifically affect components of the lobules and can be diagnosed on that basis.

Lobules contain 5–7 acini and are separated from the adjacent pulmonary lobule by an interlobular septum. They are typically irregularly polyhedral in shape and 1–2.5 cm in size. Each lobule is supplied by a lobular bronchiole and pulmonary artery which lie centrally. The draining veins are located in the septa. On HRCT nor-

mal interlobular septa are identified as straight lines 1–2.5 cm in length and slightly more than 0.1 mm in width (0.1 mm is typically the limit of HRCT resolution). The central largest lobular artery is normally visible as a dot-like or branching structure about 5 mm from the pleural surface. The largest lobular bronchiole can usually not be seen, as its walls are beyond the limit of resolution of the scan. The pulmonary parenchyma between the interlobular septa and the centrilobular core contains small vessels, airways, and alveoli which are below the resolution of CT. It is seen as a region of homogeneous attenuation slightly greater in attenuation than the air within the bronchi.

The lobules are usually easily defined in the supleural regions where the interlobular septa are well developed.

The components of the secondary pulmonary lobule become much more conspicuous when diseased, for example interlobular septa are easily identified when thickened by oedema fluid or tumour. Pathology related to small airways or arteries usually produces abnormality confined to the central portion of the lobule. Centrilobular emphysema, as expected by its name, is visualised as a small punched-out lucency in the central portion of the secondary pulmonary lobule surrounding the lobular artery. Infectious bronchiolitis will render the central lobular bronchioles visible by virtue of mucus plugging and peribronchiolar inflammation.

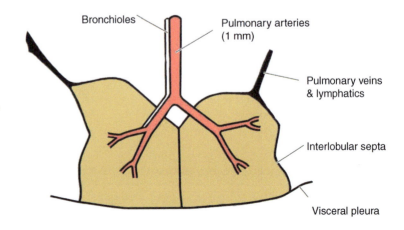

Fig. 1.16 Diagrammatic depiction of two normal adjacent secondary pulmonary lobules. The lobules are marginated by interlobular septa and in this instance the visceral pleura. An appreciation of lobular anatomy is prerequisite for diagnosis of pathology on high-resolution CT

Bronchioles

Pulmonary arteries (1 mm)

Pulmonary veins & lymphatics

Interlobular septa

Visceral pleura

The Diaphragm

The diaphragm is a musculotendinous sheet that separates the thoracic and abdominal cavities. It has both peripheral and central attachments. Its costal muscle fibres arise from the xiphoid process and the 7th–12th ribs. Posteriorly, tendinous fibres arise from the upper lumbar vertebrae forming crura. The right arises from L1–L3 and fibres from it surround the oesophageal hiatus, acting as a physiological sphincter limiting reflux of gastric contents. The left crus arises from L1 and L2.

Centrally the muscles of the diaphragm converge to form a central tendon which superiorly fuses with the fibrous pericardium. On a chest radiograph the upper surface of the dome-shaped diaphragm is visualised as it forms an interface with the air-filled lung. The soft tissues of the abdomen are indistinguishable from its inferior margin. The right hemidiaphragm is a few centimetres higher than the left in approximately 90% of adults. On a left lateral view of the chest the right hemidiaphragm is seen from front to back, whereas the anterior portion of the left is obscured by the overlying heart.

The diaphragm on CT is seen only where the upper surface interfaces with the lungs and the inferior surface abuts retroperitoneal or intraperitoneal fat. Its position can usually be inferred, as the lungs and pleura lie adjacent and peripheral to it and the abdominal viscera central to it. Multiplanar reconstructions can be very helpful in further evaluation of the diaphragm, particularly if a hernia or traumatic rupture is suspected.

The Chest Wall

Bones are the densest tissue seen on a normal plain radiograph. Those visualised on a chest radiograph include the ribs, clavicles, scapula, and vertebral bodies. A lateral radiograph is necessary to view the sternum and the vertebral bodies clearly.

Ribs are typically orientated obliquely, with their anterior portions angling downwards. The upper borders of the ribs are usually well defined, but the lower borders, particularly in the mid- and lower thoracic regions, are often difficult to see clearly. This is a consequence of the thinner bone of the subcostal groove in these regions accommodating the intercostal vessels and nerves.

Calcification of the costal cartilages is common, with the first costal cartilage calcifying shortly after the age of 20. The pattern of calcification differs between the two sexes. In men the upper and lower borders calcify first, whereas in women it is more central in location. Rib anomalies are not uncommon, and are usually not clinically relevant. It is worth checking for cervical ribs routinely as these occur in up to 1 in 150 individuals, arise from the seventh cervical vertebra, and may result in thoracic outlet syndrome.

The sternum is made up of the manubrium, the body, and the xiphoid process. The manubrium articulates with the clavicles. The sternum is most easily assessed on a lateral view or CT. The commonest congenital abnormality of the sternum is a pectus excavatum, when the sternum is depressed towards the thoracic vertebrae, narrowing the AP diameter of the chest. If severe, the heart is rotated and pushed to the left, and the right heart border appears indistinct on a PA chest radiograph. The anterior ribs appear more vertically orientated and the posterior ribs more horizontal than normal.

On a lateral view it is possible to see a retrosternal stripe of soft tissue interposed between the posterior border of the sternum and the lung. This is usually 1–3 mm thick with a characteristic lobulated contour with the lobulations at the levels of the ribs. A widening of this line or irregular lobulation may reflect internal mammary nodal involvement.

The bones of the thorax are seen in much greater detail with CT, as are the adjacent soft tissues of the chest wall. Multiplanar and volume-rendered 3D reformations can be invaluable for detecting subtle traumatic injuries and in planning chest wall reconstructive surgery.

Further Reading

El-Sherief AH, Lau CT, Wu CC, Drake RL, Abbott GF, Rice TW. International association for the study of lung cancer (IASLC) lymph node map: radiologic review with CT illustration. Radiographics. 2014;34(6):1680–91.

Gibbs JM, Chandrasekhar CA, Ferguson EC, Oldham SA. Lines and stripes: where did they go?—from conventional radiography to CT. Radiographics. 2007;27(1):33–48.

Hayashi K, Aziz A, Ashizawa K, Hayashi H, Nagaoki K, Otsuji H. Radiographic and CT appearances of the major fissures. Radiographics. 2001;21(4):861–74.

Müller NL. Imaging of the pleura. Radiology. 1993;186(2):297–309.

Nason LK, Walker CM, McNeeley MF, Burivong W, Fligner CL, Godwin JD. Imaging of the diaphragm: anatomy and function. Radiographics. 2012;32(2):E51–70.

Walker CM, Rosado-de-Christenson ML, Martinez-Jimenez S, Kunin JR, Wible BC. Bronchial arteries: anatomy, function, hypertrophy, and anomalies. Radiographics. 2015;35(1):32–49.

Webb WR. Thin-section CT of the secondary pulmonary lobule: anatomy and the image. The 2004 Fleischner Lecture 1. Radiology. 2006;239(2):322–38.

Whitten CR, Khan S, Munneke GJ, Grubnic S. A diagnostic approach to mediastinal abnormalities. Radiographics. 2007;27(3):657–71.

Applied Lung Physiology

Brendan G. Cooper and William Tunnicliffe

Introduction

The application and understanding of respiratory function tests (RFTs) form an integral component of the management of respiratory disorders. They are most frequently employed in the diagnosis and monitoring of patients with symptomatic disease, but may also be used to screen for early asymptomatic disease in high-risk groups, in prognostication, and in monitoring responses to treatment. The interpretation of pulmonary function tests requires knowledge of respiratory physiology. In this chapter we describe investigations routinely used and discuss their clinical implications.

General Considerations

Guidelines for performing pulmonary function tests have been published by the European Respiratory and American Thoracic Societies [1–6].

B. G. Cooper (✉)
Lung Function and Sleep Department,
Queen Elizabeth Hospital, Birmingham, UK
e-mail: brendan.cooper@uhb.nhs.uk

W. Tunnicliffe
Respiratory and Critical Care Medicine,
Queen Elizabeth Hospital, Birmingham, UK

Indications for performing RFTs include:

- Investigation of patients with clinical features suggesting pulmonary disease
- Monitoring patients with known pulmonary disease for progression and response to treatment
- Investigation of patients with disease that may have a respiratory complication
- Pre-operative evaluation
- Evaluating patients at risk of lung disease
- Surveillance following lung transplantation
- Research

Performing RFTs is generally safe, but contra-indications include:

- Myocardial infarction in the preceding month
- Unstable angina
- Recent ophthalmic surgery
- Thoracic or abdominal aortic aneurysm
- Current pneumothorax

The use of a risk management approach to decide whether lung function testing is appropriate is best for routine clinical practice [7]. Patients with active respiratory infections such as tuberculosis are not precluded from testing, though ideally RFTs should be deferred until the risk of cross contamination is reduced. If such patients must undergo testing, then extra precautions in addition to standard decontamination of equipment should be considered.

© Springer International Publishing AG, part of Springer Nature 2018
S. Hart, M. Greenstone (eds.), *Foundations of Respiratory Medicine*,
https://doi.org/10.1007/978-3-319-94127-1_2

For safety, RFTs are performed with the subject in the sitting position, and while nose clips are not routinely applied, they may be of benefit in some circumstances. Patients are advised not to smoke for a minimum of 1 h prior to testing, not to eat a large meal 2 h before testing, and not to wear tight-fitting clothing. Dentures are generally left in place unless they prevent the subject from forming an adequate seal around the mouthpiece. In routine practice, most manoeuvres are performed three times to ensure the test results are reproducible and accurate. Dynamic studies are performed first, followed by lung volumes, bronchodilator testing, and finally diffusion capacity.

What Constitutes a Normal or Abnormal Value?

Many factors influence lung function in healthy people. The most important are height, sex, and age, and account for around 70% of group variability. Ethnic differences also exist: subjects of Afro-Caribbean origin tend to have shorter trunk:leg ratios than Caucasians, and consequently tend to have smaller spirometric parameters relative to their overall height. In general, differences for other races do exist, but are smaller. Environmental influences that add to the variability include habitual activity; nutrition; body mass index; and exposure to altitude, climate, air pollution, and smoking, though to a considerably lesser degree.

Normal or reference ranges of values are generally derived from large population studies of healthy subjects. Ideally a normal reference population should include equal numbers of men and women in each age cohort, who are never smokers, free from respiratory disease, and who live locally. In assessing whether a test result is abnormal (assuming technically satisfactory data) the value measured is compared to the predicted normal value. The *percent predicted* value can falsely indicate the degree of abnormality and does not show the probability that a result is abnormal. In a heterogeneous but otherwise normal population, the values recorded for a particular parameter for height-, sex-, and age-matched individuals will be scattered either side of the mean value in a normal distribution. The scatter is measured as the standard deviation, SD, such that 90% of points will lie within ±1.645 SD of the mean and 95% within ±1.96 SD. Therefore 5% of the population, although normal, will have a value lower than −1.645 SD relative to the mean. This value is arbitrarily defined as *the lower limit of normal*. For certain parameters such as *residual volume*, +1.645 SD defines the *upper limit of normal*. The number of SDs above or below the predicted value is given by the standardised residual (SR) or Z-score:

$$\text{Standardized residual}\,(\text{SR})$$
$$= \text{observed} - \text{predicted value} / \text{SD}$$

An SR from −1.65 to −2.5 represents mild abnormality, between −2.5 and −3.5 moderate abnormality, and beyond −3.5 severe abnormality.

Traditionally, the observed value as *percent predicted* has been used as an intuitive index of deviation from normal (80% of predicted is often incorrectly used as an arbitrary cut off) but this has **no** scientific validity. The use of lower limit of normal (LLN) and SRs should always be used to interpret lung function data. Considerable caution should be exercised in using "percent predicted of normal" to determine if a test result is abnormal, especially when considering small, elderly subjects.

Purpose of Pulmonary Function Tests

RFTs provide measures of airflow, lung size, gas exchange, response to bronchodilators, respiratory muscle function, and breathing control. Basic tests available in the ambulatory setting include spirometry and pulse oximetry, and these can often be used to quickly narrow a differential diagnosis and suggest a subsequent strategy of additional testing. More complex testing includes measurements of lung, chest wall, and respiratory system compliance, measures of gas exchange and breathing control, and simple exercise testing through to complex cardiopulmonary exercise testing. The choice and sequence of testing are guided by information taken from the patient's history and physical examination.

As a diagnostic test RFTs help classify diffuse lung disease into one of three broad categories:

Obstructive lung disease	COPD
	Asthma
	Bronchiectasis
	Cystic Fibrosis
	Upper airway obstruction
Restrictive lung disease	Interstitial lung disease
	Chest wall disease
	Obesity
	Neuromuscular disease
Pulmonary vascular disease	Primary pulmonary hypertension
	Chronic thromboembolic disease

These categories are not mutually exclusive, for example COPD may have obstructive and vascular disease features, and sarcoidosis can have restrictive, obstructive, and vascular features.

It is important to understand how the volume of gas contained within the lung is divided into different parts (Fig. 2.1):

Tidal Volume (TV) The volume of air inspired or expired with each normal breath at rest.

Expiratory Reserve Volume (ERV) The maximum volume of air that can be expired after the expiration of the tidal volume.

Inspiratory Reserve Volume (IRV) The maximum volume of air that can be inspired after the inspiration of a tidal volume.

Residual Volume (RV) The volume of gas that remains in the lungs after maximal exhalation.

Functional Residual Capacity (FRC) The volume of air in the lungs following exhalation of the tidal volume (ERV + RV).

Vital Capacity (VC) or Forced Vital Capacity (FVC) The total volume of gas that can be forcefully exhaled following a maximal inspiratory effort (IRV + TV + ERV).

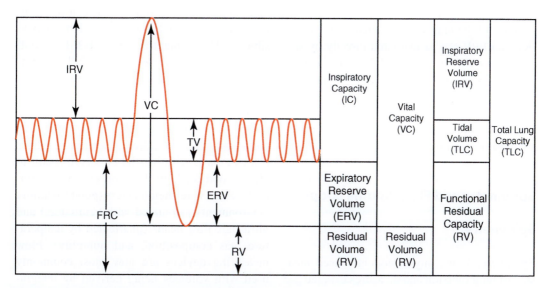

Fig. 2.1 Graphical depiction of lung volumes and capacities

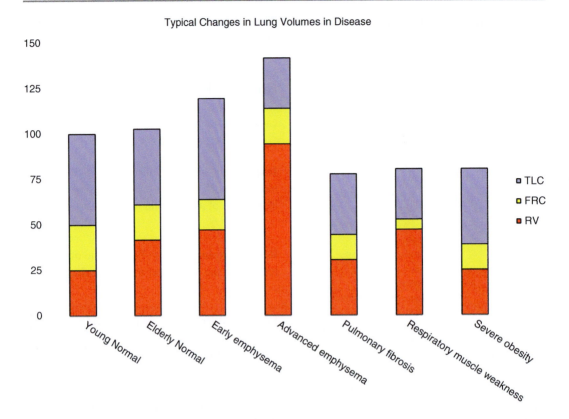

Fig. 2.2 Effects of age and disease on lung volumes

Total Lung Capacity (TLC) The volume of air in the lungs at maximal inspiration (IRV + TV + ERV + RV).

Some of the lung volumes such as TV, FVC, IRV, and ERV can be measured directly by spirometry. Others, including FRC and RV, cannot be so easily measured and must be obtained via other techniques such as body plethysmography, helium dilution, or nitrogen washout (see later). The effects of age and disease on lung volumes are illustrated in Fig. 2.2.

Spirometry and Flow Volume Loops

Spirometry

Spirometry is the most frequently used measure of lung function and measures exhaled gas volume as a function of time. It should be a relatively simple and quick procedure to perform, but in practice, without adequate training this is seldom the case; subjects are asked to take a maximal inspiration and then to forcefully exhale as quickly and for as long as possible. The mantra is F-F-F: Full inspiration-Forceful expiration-Full expiration. Forced expiratory manoeuvres may be measured with a range of devices, including volume spirometers (cumbersome and now rarely used), pneumotachographs (no moving parts and easy to calibrate), rotating vanes (moving parts with inertial effects, difficult to clean, good for high flows on exercise, portable), heated wire anemometers (good for humid environments associated with ventilators) and ultrasonic flow heads (unaffected by temperature, gas composition, and humidity). Flow measuring devices are now most commonly used with volumes being derived by integration of the flow signal.

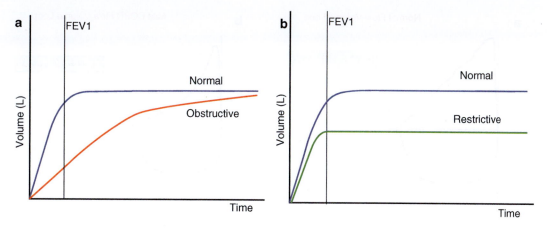

Fig. 2.3 Spirometry traces showing (**a**) obstructive and (**b**) restrictive defects

Measurements that are made include:

- Forced Expiratory Volume in 1 s (FEV$_1$)
- Forced Vital Capacity (FVC)
- The ratio of FEV$_1$/FVC
- VC (the "relaxed" non-forceful Vital Capacity)

These measurements allow the identification of obstructive and restrictive defects (Fig. 2.3a, b). In obstructive disease the FEV$_1$ is reduced as is the FEV$_1$:FVC ratio. In contrast, in restrictive disease the FEV$_1$ is reduced but the FEV$_1$:FVC ratio is normal or increased. Normal subjects (and those with restrictive disease) achieve a plateau on the spirogram, whereas in those with obstructive disease the volume plateau occurs late or not at all. In small airways obstruction the VC can often be much larger than the FVC because there is no dynamic airway collapse.

VC was the first lung function measurement to be used to assess the health of the lungs. It declines with age due to the loss of elastic lung recoil and airway closure in the dependent lung zones. Any pathology affecting the airways, alveoli, pleura, chest wall, or respiratory muscles will tend to lower VC (in both obstructive and restrictive lung disease). A high VC is usually a normal variant, but a high VC with a high TLC occurs in acromegaly. A normal VC does not exclude respiratory disease; it may occur in pulmonary vascular disease, quiescent asthma, early emphysema, bullous lung disease without gas trapping, and in early respiratory muscle disease.

FEV$_1$ is one of the most reproducible lung function measures and is more reliable than peak expiratory flow (PEF) in airflow obstruction. It is frequently used to monitor disease progression and is a strong predictor of mortality. Of note, when measuring FEV$_1$, maximal effort is associated with a significant fall in FEV$_1$ (up to 5%) in around 7% of subjects because of gas compression and a fall in thoracic gas volume caused by high alveolar and pleural pressures. PEF monitoring over weeks is a useful way to categorise asthma and monitor therapeutic control.

FEV$_1$/FVC or FEV$_1$/VC is the best diagnostic test for airflow obstruction, but does tend to decline with age. FEV$_1$ itself is the best parameter for following disease progression and bronchodilator response.

Flow Volume Loops

These are produced when the subject performs a maximal inspiratory manoeuvre (maximal inspiratory flow volume [MIFV] curve) followed by a maximal expiratory manoeuvre (maximal expiratory flow volume [MEFV] curve). The resultant graph displays flow on the vertical axis, against volume on the horizontal axis; expiratory flow is recorded above the horizontal axis and expiratory

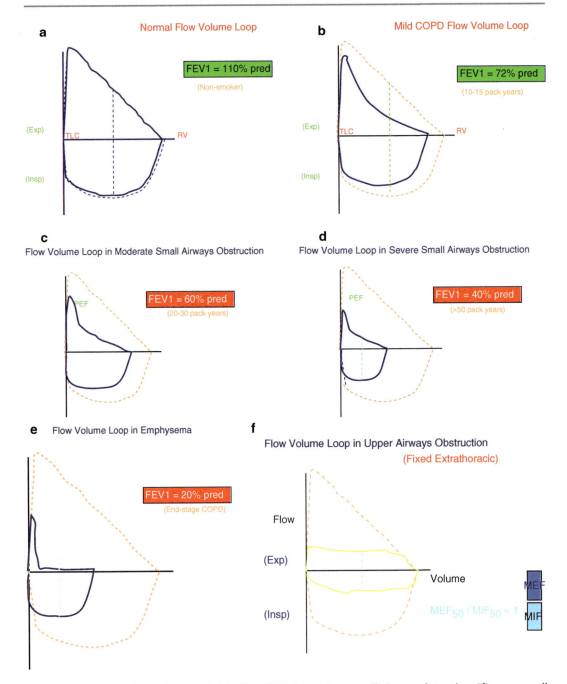

Fig. 2.4 Flow volume loops. (**a**) normal; (**b**) mild COPD; (**c**) moderate small airways obstruction; (**d**) severe small airways obstruction; (**e**) emphysema; (**f**) upper airway obstruction

flow below it (Fig. 2.4a–f). The maximal flow rate during expiration (peak expiratory flow [PEF]) can be measured, as can the maximal flows between 25% and 75% of the vital capacity (FEF 25–75%).

The MEFV curve complements spirometry and its diagnostic value lies predominantly in its shape. MEFV shapes for individuals are very repeatable, provided expiratory effort is consistent. Concavity in the descending component of the curve is a feature of airflow obstruction.

MEFV curves in normal subjects may show marked individual differences in the first 33% of expired volume, but thereafter there is generally a linear decrease in flow over the last 66% of the FVC. In contrast, airflow obstruction results in profound curvature in the latter portion of the curve.

To produce an MEFV curve, maximal expiratory effort must be applied. Paradoxically, a submaximal effort may lead to flows which are higher at a given expired volume and sometimes to a higher FEV_1. This is not true negative effort dependence, rather the effects of compression of thoracic gas, so that absolute lung volume (at a given expired volume) may be reduced by up to 10%.

Patients with peripheral obstructive lung disease typically have a concave appearance of the descending portion of the expiratory limb rather than a straight line, reflecting reduced expiratory flow in the peripheral airways. In patients with emphysema, the loss of elastic recoil and radial support results in pressure dependent collapse of the distal airways, producing more pronounced scalloping of the expiratory limb and, in the worst cases, the "church steeple" shape. Even if the morphology of the flow volume loop is normal, a reduction in PEF may be an indication of asthma.

Peak Expiratory Flow

PEF is the maximum flow recorded when expiration, delivered with maximal effort, is started from maximal inflation (total lung capacity, or TLC). The measurement of PEF became popular as an alternative to FEV_1 with the development of simple, portable, stand-alone peak flow meters allowing a measurement of airflow obstruction to be performed at the bedside, in the outpatient setting or in the patient's home. Peak flow meters are now used extensively in the self-monitoring of airflow obstruction in asthma.

In general, peak flow meters have relatively high equipment resistance; PEF readings are up to 10% less than when measured with a pneumotachograph screen. This reduction is not due to the resistance of the meter itself, but due to the higher alveolar pressure at which the PEF is achieved when the peak flow meter is used (PEF is very volume dependent).

PEF is reduced in airflow obstruction and in volume loss, due to pneumonectomy and pleural effusions. PEF is also reduced in respiratory muscle weakness, but is relatively well preserved in diffuse pulmonary fibrosis. It is non-specific and cannot distinguish obstruction from restriction.

Lung Volumes

The measurement of lung volumes is essential to confirm the following clinical phenomena:

1. Restrictive lung disease
2. Hyperinflation/gas trapping
3. Lung volume change after surgery/ intervention
4. Normal lung physiology

Lung volumes result from the mechanical balance of the lung recoil and chest wall expansion, and are dependent on the integrity of the chest wall (connective tissue, spine, ribcage, respiratory muscle function, and pleura) and the lung tissue itself (compliance, pulmonary blood content) as well as the size of the heart (the other object in the thorax that encroaches on availability of lung space!).

There are several methods of measuring lung size, but the most commonly found methods are (1) helium (He) dilution; (2) nitrogen (N_2) washout; and (3) body plethysmography (or "body box"). The first two methods can only measure the *ventilated* lung spaces, whereas the body box measures all the air in the thorax (and abdomen). This can be exploited in severe airflow obstruction or patients with non-ventilated large bullae, since the normal difference of 200 mL between methods is greater when comparing the ventilated/non-ventilated values. Subsequently, in patients with severe emphysema, the body box value is usually much higher than the He dilution/N_2 washout method. The body box can give enormously large values in severe emphysema.

Lung Volumes and Capacities

Measurement of lung volumes essentially requires the measurement of **functional residual capacity** (FRC), which is the volume of the lungs at the end of a normal expired breath when the balances of the lung and chest wall are opposite and equal (Fig. 2.1). **Inspiratory capacity** (IC) is the maximal amount of air that can be inspired following a normal tidal expiration. By the addition of the **inspiratory capacity,** the **total lung capacity** (TLC) can be calculated. If the (expired) vital capacity (VC) is measured by performing a full relaxed expiration, the **residual volume** (RV) can be calculated. These should all be measured in a linked series of manoeuvres for better accuracy:

$$FRC + IC = TLC; \quad TLC - VC = RV$$

Alternatively, from FRC, if a full expiratory reserve volume (ERV) manoeuvre is performed, this will produce the RV. By adding the VC to this, the TLC is calculated:

$$FRC - ERV = RV; \quad RV + VC = TLC$$

There is little to choose between the various methods, and usually the chosen method of measurement is given as a subscript of the volume nomenclature (e.g. TLC_{box}, TLC_{N2}, TLC_{He} for body box, nitrogen washout, and helium dilution methods, respectively.) A good lung function physiology service will quality control values for lung volume calculations, but when reporting the tests it is important to check for any obvious discrepancies. One useful "quality check" is to ensure that the alveolar volume (VA) from gas transfer testing and the TLC from lung volumes are within 10% of each other (i.e. almost equal). If there is a large discrepancy, there is an error in one or other test, or the patient has airway obstruction and gas-trapping.

Gas Transfer Test

Most routine lung function tests measure either the size of the lungs (lung volumes) or assess airway function (spirometry, airways resistance, oscillometry), but only a few physiological tests measure the ability of the lungs to exchange gases. The simplest test is probably the blood gas measurement, which measures the net oxygen/carbon dioxide level in the arteries (or capillaries). The cardio-respiratory exercise test can assess the oxygen uptake and carbon dioxide production, but this is a specialist test that many patients struggle to complete, and abnormalities may not become apparent until peak exercise is achieved. The most widespread standardised test for assessing gas exchange in the lungs is the single breath transfer test for carbon monoxide. The transfer factor (TLCO) is the total measure of the rate of uptake of carbon monoxide (CO) and is derived from the product of the measurements of alveolar volume (VA) and transfer coefficient (KCO):

$$TLCO = VA \times KCO$$

The test has its origins in the early 1900s when physiologists [8] were developing techniques to understand the physiology of the lung and used carbon monoxide as a marker gas because of its similar properties to oxygen, its combination with haemoglobin, and the fact that there is usually little back pressure of CO in blood. The technique was not fully standardised until the 1950s. Roughton and Forster [9] showed that the transfer of gas from the lung to haemoglobin (Hb) relies upon several components including (1) the diffusion across the alveolar capillary and other membranes; (2) the capillary blood volume available for transfer; and (3) the reaction rate on CO with Hb. This is captured by the equation:

$$1 / TL = 1 / Dm + 1 / \Theta Vc$$

TL = transfer factor, Dm = membrane diffusion, Θ = reaction rate of CO with Hb and Vc = pulmonary capillary blood volume.

Diffusion can be summarised by Fick's law:

$$V_{gas} = \frac{AD\left(P_1 - P_2\right)}{t}$$

This shows that the rate of gas diffusion (V gas) is proportional to the surface area (A), difference in gas tension across the alveolar capillary membrane D (P1–P2), all divided by the breath-hold time (t).

The test requires the subject to empty their lungs close to residual volume, then inhale the test gas (CO and a marker gas, e.g. helium) rapidly to TLC, followed by a breath-hold (8–10 s) before exhaling for the analysis of the expired CO left after some of the CO has been absorbed by the lung. The marker gas is used to adjust for the dilution factor of the residual volume.

Several pathophysiological processes can affect any of these components, which makes the interpretation of gas transfer more complex compared to spirometry. It was Ogilvie [10] who standardised the test by controlling the following components of the technique:

- Measurement of breath-hold time
- Portion of the expired air sample representing the alveolar level
- Intrathoracic pressure
- Effect of variation in lung volume
- Position of the body
- Variation of TLCO with alveolar O_2 tension
- Importance of venous COHb
- The interval at which TLCO can be repeated
- Effect of exercise
- Hyperventilation

The transfer factor (TLCO) describes the rate of transfer of a gas between alveoli and the erythrocytes in the alveolar capillaries, in the units of gas per unit time per unit pressure difference between the two sites. For clinical purposes it is necessary to know the pattern of TLC, VA, and KCO in different conditions (Table 2.1) and to be aware of some of the correction factors that can affect the test.

The TLCO and KCO can be affected by the following, for which there are appropriate corrections:

- Background carboxyhaemoglobin (COHb)
- Altitude
- P_AO_2 variation with altitude
- Variables including alcohol consumption, vigorous exercise, smoking, diurnal variation, bronchodilators

Most of these corrections will be performed by the qualified lung function staff and are usu-

Table 2.1 Patterns of TLCO and KCO in disease

Condition	TLCO	KCO
COPD	Decreased	Decreased
Emphysema	Decreased	Decreased
Asthma	Variable (decreased, increased, or no change)	Increased
IPF	Decreased	Decreased
Sarcoidosis	Decreased	Mildly decreased or No change
Extrapulmonary restriction	Decreased	May increase
Pulmonary vascular disease	Decreased	Decreased
Pulmonary oedema	Decreased	Decreased
Mitral valve disease	Decreased	Decreased
Congenital R to L shunts	Decreased	Decreased
Anaemia	Decreased	Decreased
Collagen diseases (RA, SLE)	Decreased	Decreased
Pneumonectomy	Decreased or No change	Increased
L to R shunts	Increased	Increased
Polycythaemia	Increased	Increased
Lung haemorrhage	Increased	Increased

ally indicated on any report forms. The most important clinical correction is probably the haemoglobin correction (for instance bone marrow transplantation patients, post heart/lung transplant). Recently new reference values (GLI 2016) have been derived for gas transfer, but are currently only applicable to Causcasians.

Assessing the Respiratory Muscles

By far the most common cause of extrapulmonary restriction is respiratory muscle weakness (e.g. myotonic dystrophy, motor neurone disease, Guillain-Barré syndrome, etc.). The mechanics of breathing requires both the integrity of the lung tissue and the chest wall functioning together. The chest wall comprises the skeletal components (spine and ribs), the muscular components (diaphragms, intercostals, and accessory muscles), and the elastic tissues of the skin and

Table 2.2 Summary of respiratory muscle function tests

Test	Normal values	Weakness	Notes
Sitting-supine VC	<20% decrease	>20% decrease (or > 15% with COPD)	Quick, cheap and simple screening test
MIP	More negative than -70 cm H_2O	Less negative than -40 cm H_2O	Offered by most UK labs, relatively cheap test, requires experienced staff
MEP	>$+70$ cm H_2O	<$+40$ cm H_2O	
Sniff nasal pressures SNIP	More negative than -70 cm H_2O	Less negative than -70 cm H_2O	Require repeated tests (up to 8–12 efforts), but easier for patients
Transdiaphragmatic pressures Pdi	More negative than -70 cm H_2O	Less negative than -40 cm H_2O	Consider phrenic nerve conduction studies EMG, muscle biopsy, neurological opinion

MEP maximum expiratory pressure, *MIP* maximum inspiratory pressure, *SNIP* sniff inspiratory pressure, *Pdi* pressure differential indicator

cartilage. During tidal breathing the diaphragm dominates the muscular activity, but at the extremes of ventilation (exercise, coughing) the diaphragm is complemented with the other respiratory muscle groups. Indeed, it is muscle function that determines total lung capacity (TLC) and determines the ability to ensure the forced manoeuvres to measure FEV_1 and FVC.

Simple screening in an outpatient setting to detect the presence of respiratory muscle weakness can be performed using sitting and supine vital capacity (VC) measures to see if a greater than 20% decrease (or >15% if COPD is present) between sitting and supine is observed [11].

Beyond this, a diagnosis of weakness is best confirmed using maximum respiratory pressures during inspiration (MIP) measured at FRC and expiration (MEP) measured at TLC (Table 2.2). A simple pressure meter requiring blowing or sucking against an occlusion (with a small leak) for at least 3 s can be repeated until the variability is less than 5 cm H_2O, or 5% of the highest two values. Whilst the test is usually performed using a flanged mouthpiece, the reference values for the test have wide ranges [12–14]. If MIP is < -70 cm H_2O (that is, more negative than -70 cm), and MEP greater than $+70$ cm, then weakness can be excluded. If MIP is less negative than -40 cm H_2O and MEP is less than $+40$ cm H_2O, then respiratory muscle weakness is probably present. Expiratory pressures between 40 and 70 cm H_2O should prompt con-

sideration of a further test. Remember that the larger the numerical value of the MIP or MEP, the stronger (more normal) the muscles are.

The gold standard test for respiratory muscle strength is transdiaphragmatic pressures (Pdi) using a gastric/oesophageal catheter, but nationally few centres provide this semi-invasive technique. MIP and MEP measures can be used to serially monitor respiratory muscle weakness, but in acute neurological illness, for example in Guillain-Barré, it is enough to look for a fall in VC to judge when intubation should occur.

The sniff nasal inspiratory pressure (SNIP) is a good test for monitoring decreasing muscle function over time [15, 16]. The pressure catheter is inserted in one nostril and the patient sniffs sharply so the peak inspiratory pressure can be recorded. Reference ranges are wide for this test, too, [17] but SNIP values are often higher than MIP because the sniff is a more natural and easy manoeuvre for patients to make. Values more negative than -70 cm H_2O can exclude weakness.

Finally, it should be noted that all of these methods of respiratory muscle assessment are volitional tests that require considerable patient effort and coaching to be repeatable and accurate, and poor effort can easily mimic weakness. There are electromagnetic stimulatory tests available, usually using Pdi, which remove the volitional effort, but they are used mainly as research tools and only a few clinical laboratories in the UK can offer this service. Experienced staff routinely performing these techniques get good results, but skills need to be maintained for reliable results.

> **Causes of Respiratory Muscle Weakness**
> - Motor neurone disease
> - Polyneuropathy
> - Phrenic injury (iatrogenic or neuralgic amyotrophy)
> - Spinal cord injury (trauma, vascular, demyelination)
> - Myasthenia gravis
> - Muscular dystrophies
> - Inflammatory myositis
> - Metabolic or endocrine muscle weakness
> - Nutritional muscular atrophy

Cardio-Pulmonary Exercise Testing (CPET)

CPET is an increasingly popular way to examine the integrative physiology of the lungs, heart, and circulation under stress, and to simulate the effects of surgery. Comparing the respiratory ventilation (Ve) and cardiac frequency (Cf) responses against the effort (workload) can show predictable patterns. Workload is best estimated by the measurement of oxygen uptake (VO_2). However, since metabolism plays a crucial role in exercise, it is necessary to understand the carbon dioxide (CO_2) production (VCO_2) and hence metabolic stresses on the exercise test. The ratio of VCO_2/VO_2 is the respiratory exchange ratio (RER) and reflects the fuel being metabolised, where 0.8 is close to mainly fat metabolism and 1.0 is pure carbohydrate.

The relative patterns of the test are complex and are summarised in Table 2.3. It takes a lot of experience to understand the principles and patterns of CPET results, but common reasons for requesting the tests include:

1. Known cardiac and respiratory disorder causing symptoms—apportioning relative contributions.
2. Unexplained breathlessness after normal "full tests" and other physiological tests.
3. Suspected hyperventilation or functional disorders causing dyspnoea.
4. Pre-operative assessment to determine probable outcome of surgery in a variety of surgical procedures (cardio thoracic, cardiovascular, gastrointestinal, some lung cancers, lobectomy, LVRS, etc.).

Table 2.3 Interpretation of CPET (reproduced with permission from Prof Mike Morgan)

	VO_2 PEAK	AT	VD/VT	SaO_2	O_2 pulse VO_2/Cf	VE/VO_2	HRR
Cardiac disease (may be limited by chest pain)	Low	Low	Normal	Normal	Low	High	Nil
Pulmonary vascular disease	Low	Low	High	Low	Low	High	Nil
Airway obstruction	Low	High or absent	High	Normal	Normal	High	High
Interstitial lung disease	Low	High or absent	High	Low	Normal	High (high Bf and low VT)	High
Chest wall restriction	Low	High or absent	Normal	Normal/low	Normal	Normal (high Bf and low VT)	High
Poor effort	Low	High or absent	Normal	Normal (or high)	Normal	Normal	High

VO_2 peak is the peak oxygen uptake, *AT* anaerobic threshold, *VD/VT* dead space to tidal volume ratio, SaO_2 oxygen saturation, *Oxygen pulse* oxygen uptake/cardiac frequency (VO_2/Cf), Ventilatory equivalent for oxygen (VE/VO_2), *HRR* heart rate reserve

There is a complex interaction of respiratory and cardiac processes that enable gas exchange from the mouth to the cell/mitochondrion for oxygen and vice versa for waste gas (CO_2). It is important to have a subjective measure of exhaustion/effort and document clearly the reason the test was stopped.

The key aspects of a CPET are:

1. Resting data
   (a) Were the resting data stable and within expected limits?
   (b) Was the RER stable and between 0.75 and 0.85?
2. Was it a maximal effort?
   (a) Plateau of VO_2 Peak
   (b) Patient exhaustion (Borg score)
   (c) Peak heart rate and ventilation close to predicted maximum
   (d) An sustained RER of greater than 1.3
3. Ventilation
   (a) What was the pattern of minute ventilation in terms of tidal volume and breathing frequency (Bf)?
   (b) Was the peak ventilation close to the MVV (maximum voluntary ventilation and usually $35.5 \times FEV_1$)?
   (c) What was the respiratory reserve (difference between MVV and the observed maximal ventilation VEmax)?
   (d) Was a ventilatory threshold (VT or AT) achieved (RER >1.3, inflection point on the VCO_2 vs VO_2 graph, Ve/VCO_2 rises after nadir)?
   (e) How breathless was the patient and were there any respiratory symptoms?
   (f) The Ve/VO_2 should be normal.
4. Cardiac response
   (a) Was the maximum heart rate (HR) achieved? (usually $210 - (0.33 \times age)$)
   (b) What was the heart rate reserve (predicted maximum HR-maximum observed HR)?
   (c) Was the oxygen pulse (VO_2/HR) which reflects stroke volume > 13 at VT or peak exercise? Did it plateau early?
   (d) What happened to blood pressure?
   (e) Where there any ECG changes of note?
5. Oxygen
   (a) Was the peak VO_2 near 90% predicted?
   (b) Was there an RER >1.3 at peak?
   (c) Was there any desaturation of oxygen by oximetry (SaO_2 or SpO_2) or by blood gas?
   (d) Was the $D(A-a)O_2$ difference within the normal range at rest and only slightly elevated at peak exercise?

The best CPET services are run by advanced physiologists who are experienced at performing the tests safely, getting reliable results, and being able to interpret the data. Physicians, surgeons, and anaesthetists should be trained in advanced exercise physiology to understand the limitations and interpretation of CPET. Using multidisciplinary team approaches improve learning, standards, and quality of CPET.

References

1. Miller MR, Crapo R, Hankinson J, Brusasco V, Burgos F, Casaburi R, et al. General considerations for lung function testing. Eur Respir J. 2005;26(1):153–61.
2. Pellegrino R, Viegi G, Brusasco V, Crapo RO, Burgos F, Casaburi R, et al. Interpretative strategies for lung function tests. Eur Respir J. 2005;26(5):948–68.
3. Macintyre N, Crapo RO, Viegi G, Johnson DC, van der Grinten CP, Brusasco V, et al. Standardisation of the single-breath determination of carbon monoxide uptake in the lung. Eur Respir J. 2005;26(4):720–35.
4. Wanger J, Clausen JL, Coates A, Pedersen OF, Brusasco V, Burgos F, et al. Standardisation of the measurement of lung volumes. Eur Respir J. 2005;26(3):511–22.
5. Miller MR, Hankinson J, Brusasco V, Burgos F, Casaburi R, Coates A, et al. Standardisation of spirometry. Eur Respir J. 2005;26(2):319–38.
6. American Thoracic Society. Lung function testing: selection of reference values and interpretative strategies. Am Rev Respir Dis. 1991;144(5):1202–18.
7. Cooper BG. Review: an update on contraindications for lung function testing. Thorax. 2011;66:714–23.
8. Krogh M. The diffusion of gases through the lungs of man. J Physiol. 1914;49:271–300.
9. Roughton FJW, Forster REJ. Relative importance of diffusion and chemical reaction rates in determining rate of exchange of gases in the human lung, with special reference to true diffusing capacity of pulmonary membrane and volume of blood in the lung capillaries. J Appl Physiol. 1957;11(2):290–302.

10. Blakemore WS, Forster RE, Morton JW, Ogilvie CM. A standardized breath holding technique for the clinical measurement of the diffusing capacity of the lung for carbon monoxide. J Clin Investig. 1957;36:1–17.

11. Polkey MI, Green M, Moxham J. Measurement of respiratory muscle strength. Thorax. 1995;50:1131–5.

12. Black L, Hyatt R. Maximal respiratory pressures: normal values and relationships to age and sex. Am Rev Respir Dis. 1969;99:698–702.

13. Wilson SH, Cooke NT, Edwards RH, Spiro SG. Predicted normal values for maximal respiratory pressures in caucasian adults and children. Thorax. 1984;39:535–8.

14. Bruschi C, Cerveri I, Zoia MC, Fanfulla F, Fiorentini M, Casali L, et al. Reference values of maximal respiratory mouth pressures: a population based study. Am Rev Respir Dis. 1992;146:790–3.

15. Miller JM, Moxham J, Green M. The maximal sniff in the assessment of diaphragm function in man. Clin Sci. 1985;69:91–6.

16. Hamnegard CH, Wragg S, Kyroussis D, Mills GH, Polkey MI, Moxham J, et al. Sniff nasal pressure measured with a portable meter. Am J Respir Crit Care Med. 1995;151:A415.

17. Uldry C, Fitting JW. Maximal values of sniff nasal inspiratory pressure in healthy subjects. Thorax. 1995;50:371–5.

Asthma

K. Suresh Babu and Jaymin B. Morjaria

Introduction

Asthma is a heterogeneous disease characterised by fluctuating symptoms of cough, wheeze, dyspnoea and/or chest tightness, as well as variable expiratory airflow limitation. Both the symptoms and airflow limitation typically change in intensity and over time. These variations may be triggered by factors such as atopy (allergen or irritant exposure), exercise, respiratory tract infections (commonly viral), or changes in the weather. Asthma symptoms and the associated airflow limitation may resolve spontaneously or in response to treatment, and may be absent for varying degrees of time (weeks to months) or present episodically (flare-ups or exacerbations), with wide-ranging severity (mild to life-threatening).

Chronic airway inflammation and airway hyper-reactivity to direct and indirect stimuli are the underlying pathophysiological hallmarks of asthma. Appropriate treatment can suppress these two processes, which may still be present despite the absence of symptoms and in the presence of normal lung function. Longterm failure to control asthma pathophysiology may result in airway remodelling and irreversible disease progression. This is termed "the asthma cycle" [1].

Asthma Phenotypes

Despite the marked heterogeneity of asthma due to the various underlying disease processes, recognisable clusters of clinical and/or pathophysiological parameters may be identified. These are called "asthma phenotypes." Commonly identified phenotypes include allergic asthma, non-allergic asthma, exercise-induced asthma, late onset asthma, asthma with fixed airflow limitation, asthma with obesity, and asthma-COPD overlap syndrome (ACOS).

Allergic asthma is the most common phenotype. It starts in childhood and is associated with a past and/or family history of allergic disease including eczema, allergic rhinitis, or food or drug allergy. These patients have underlying eosinophil-based airway inflammation and respond well to treatment with inhaled corticosteroids (ICS). Non-allergic asthma is not associated with atopy. It is characterised by the presence of neutrophilic, eosinophilic, or paucigranulocytic (few inflammatory cells) inflammation and is poorly responsive to ICS treatment. Exercise-induced asthma (EIA) typically occurs with worsening following exercise cessation. Late-onset asthma is typically found in women and presents with asthma symptoms for the first time in adult life. Often, patients

K. S. Babu
Respiratory Medicine, Queen Alexandra Hospital,
Portsmouth, Hampshire, UK

J. B. Morjaria (✉)
Royal Brompton and Harefield NHS Foundation Trust,
Harefield, Middlesex, UK

© Springer International Publishing AG, part of Springer Nature 2018
S. Hart, M. Greenstone (eds.), *Foundations of Respiratory Medicine*,
https://doi.org/10.1007/978-3-319-94127-1_3

respond poorly to ICS due to their tendency to be non-allergic. Asthma with fixed airflow limitation arises in patients with long-standing asthma with associated airway remodelling. Asthma with obesity occurs in patients with increased body mass index having asthma symptoms and little, if any, eosinophilic inflammation and a poor response to ICS. Recently a new phenotype (ACOS) has been described. Although there is limited mechanistic data on this phenotype, it is thought to occur in smokers and older adults who have clinical features of both asthma and COPD, the latter characterised by persistent airflow limitation.

Epidemiology

Asthma occurs in people of all ages. Across the world, it is estimated that 334 million people have asthma, with an increased burden of disability [2]. The age-old assumption of asthma being commoner in affluent countries no longer holds true—most of the world's asthmatics are found in low- and middle-income countries where its prevalence continues to increase. Factors responsible for the increasing asthma rates are not fully understood, but environmental and lifestyle changes have been implicated. The burden of asthma, as measured by disability and premature death, is greatest in children approaching adolescence (ages 10–14) and in the elderly (ages 75–79) with the lowest impact in 30- to 34-year-olds. The burden is similar in both sexes below 30–34 years, however, in older ages it is higher in males.

The International Study of Asthma and Allergies in Childhood (ISAAC) established that 14% of the world's children were likely to suffer asthmatic symptoms within the last year. Importantly, this study demonstrated that the prevalence of childhood asthma varied markedly between countries as well as between centres within countries studied. The highest prevalence of wheeze (>20%) was observed in Latin America and in English-speaking countries of Australasia, Europe, North America, and South Africa. The lowest prevalence (<5%) was noted in the Indian subcontinent, Asia-Pacific, Eastern Mediterranean, and northern and eastern Europe. In Africa the prevalence was 10–20%. The prevalence of severe asthma symptoms in the preceding 12 months was reported to be >7.5% in many centres. The World Health Organisation's World Health Survey (2002–2003) in 18- to 45-year-olds showed a 4.3% prevalence for a doctor's diagnosis of asthma, 4.5% taking asthma treatment, and 8.6% experiencing asthma symptoms in the preceding 12 months. The highest prevalence was observed in Australia, northern and western Europe, and Brazil.

In the UK, 5.4 million people (1.1 million children and 4.3 million adults) suffer from asthma, that is, 1 in 11 people and one in five households [3]. In 2013, the incidence rate for developing asthma was 237 people per 100,000, down from 518 per 100,000 in 2004. A quarter of a million people with severe asthma are unable to even climb a flight of stairs. Every 10 s an asthmatic suffers a potentially life-threatening asthma flare-up and every day there are three asthma-related deaths. Of the deaths, more than 80% are in those aged over 65, and approximately two-thirds are females [4]. Despite a greater than 50% decline in incidence, the prevalence of asthma overall has increased, and the NHS spends close to £1 billion in treating and caring for patients with asthma [3].

Pathophysiology

The hallmarks of asthma include airway inflammation, bronchoconstriction, bronchial hyper-responsiveness, and sometimes airway remodelling orchestrated by cellular and inflammatory mediators implicated in asthma [5].

Bronchoconstriction due to bronchial smooth muscle contraction is a prominent physiological event which usually results in symptoms in response to a variety of stimuli, including allergens and irritants. Allergen-induced bronchoconstriction is usually immunoglobulin (Ig) E-mediated, however, in aspirin- and other non-steroidal anti-inflammatory drugs (NSAIDs) induced events, it is non-IgE-mediated. Airway oedema is accompanied by progressive inflammation, mucus hypersecretion, and structural changes (including airway smooth muscle hypertrophy and hyperplasia) that enhance airway obstruction. These elements may contribute to airway hyper-responsiveness (AHR), which is an exaggerated bronchoconstrictor response to a variety of stimuli. This may be quantified using challenge testing. Inflammation, dysfunctional neuro-regulation, and structural changes are thought to influence AHR.

Airflow limitation in some asthmatics may only be partially reversible, due to permanent structural changes in their airways which are non-responsive to treatment. These changes include thickening of the basement membrane, sub-epithelial fibrosis, airway smooth muscle hypertrophy and hyperplasia, blood vessel proliferation and dilation, and mucous gland hyperplasia and hypersecretion. This constellation of changes is referred to as airway remodelling.

The pathophysiological mechanisms of airway inflammation are pivotal in asthma. Here we discuss the key inflammatory cells and mediators.

Lymphocytes

Around the turn of the millenium, subpopulations of lymphocytes, T-helper (Th1 and 2 cells) with their specific inflammatory mediator profiles as well as effects on airway function were described. Asthma emerged as an example of eosinophilic inflammation driven by Th2 cytokines including interleukin (IL)-4, IL-5 and IL-13, with resultant IgE overproduction and AHR. Additionally, regulatory T cells (Tregs), which normally inhibit Th2 cells as well as increase natural killer cells, may be attenuated. More recently, other pathogenic mechanisms have come to light (discussed under pathogenesis), including the identification of Th17 and Th0 cells.

Mast Cells

The activation of airway mast cells releases bronchoconstrictor mediators such as histamine, cysteinyl-leukotrienes, and prostaglandin D2. Allergen activation of mast cells occurs through high-affinity IgE receptors but may also be activated by osmotic stimuli (a probable mechanism in exercise-induced bronchospasm).

Eosinophils

Airway eosinophilia is present in most patients with asthma and often correlates with asthma severity. Eosinophils contain inflammatory enzymes, and generate leukotrienes and multiple pro-inflammatory cytokines. Corticosteroid therapy depletes airway eosinophilia and improves asthma symptoms.

Neutrophils

Neutrophilia is noted in the sputum of severe asthmatics during acute exacerbations, bacterial infections, and in chronic smokers. Their role in asthma is not clearly understood, but airway neutrophilia is associated with a poor response to corticosteroid therapy.

Dendritic Cells

DCs are antigen-presenting cells that interact with allergens in the airway. Subsequently, they migrate to regional lymph nodes where they present antigens to regulatory T cells and stimulate Th2 cell maturation from naive T cells.

Macrophages

Macrophages are the most abundant resident airway cells. They are activated by allergens through low-affinity IgE receptors to release pro-inflammatory mediators and cytokines, hence amplifying the inflammatory response.

Resident Airway Smooth Muscle Cells

ASMCs contribute to the inflammatory process in asthma, in addition to bronchoconstriction and AHR.

Epithelial Cells

Airway epithelial cells have been linked to the generation of inflammatory mediators and recruitment and activation of pro-inflammatory cells. During viral infections these cells may be injured or produce pro-inflammatory mediators, perpetuating airflow limitation and obstruction.

Inflammatory Mediators

Cytokines orchestrate and modify the inflammatory response in asthma. Th2-derived cytokines and their functions include: IL-5, eosinophil differentiation and survival; IL-4, Th2 cell differentiation; IL-13, IgE formation. Th1 cytokines include IL-1β and TNF-α that amplify the inflammatory process. Individual cytokine antagonists have been assessed as asthma treatments with mixed results. Anti-IL-5 and anti-IL-13 therapeutics have shown efficacy in distinct, well-characterised populations of patients. Chemokines such as eotaxin, TARC, and IL-8 are vital in the recruitment of inflammatory cells to the airways and maintaining the inflammatory process in asthma. Cysteinyl-leukotrienes are mainly generated from mast cells and are potent bronchoconstrictors. Inhibiting their production (using anti-leukotriene agents) is associated with improved asthma outcomes.

Nitric Oxide (NO) is a potent vasodilator that is mainly synthesised from the action of inducible NO synthetase (iNOS) in airway epithelial cells. Measurements of fractional exhaled NO (FeNO) can be used as a surrogate marker of inflammation in asthma, especially eosinophilic airways disease.

Immunoglobulin E-IgE is pivotal in the pathogenesis of allergic conditions and the development and persistence of inflammation. Mast cells express numerous IgE receptors, which when activated through cross-linking by antigen result in the release of a variety of pro-inflammatory mediators perpetuating airway inflammation and bronchoconstriction. Basophils, dendritic cells, and lymphocytes also contain high-affinity IgE receptors. Omalizumab, an anti-IgE therapy delivered subcutaneously, is the first licensed monoclonal antibody with good efficacy and tolerability for use in uncontrolled atopic asthma.

Asthma Pathogenesis

It is unclear as to why or how the inflammatory process in asthma is actually initiated. It is thought to depend on the interplay of host factors and environmental exposures.

Host Factors

Innate Immunity
Research suggests that there is an imbalance between Th1 and Th2 cytokine/inflammatory profiles, with a move to a more Th2-predominant response. The "Hygiene Hypothesis" may explain the increase in asthma prevalence in westernized countries. The hypothesis is based on a Th2-predominant state at birth following which exposure to environmental stimuli (including infections, exposure to other children and, less frequent, antibiotic use) activates the Th1 response, bringing an appropriate Th1/Th2 balance. In the absence of such life events the genetic profile of the child with a Th2-favoured imbalance will result in the production of IgE to key environmental antigens (e.g. house-dust mite, cockroach, Alternaria fungi).

Genetics
There is an inheritable component to asthma. However, the genetics concerned are complex. Polymorphisms affecting adrenergic and glucocorticoid receptors have been identified, though their relevance is under investigation.

Sex
In early life, asthma prevalence is higher in boys; at puberty and subsequently there is a female predominance.

Environmental Factors
Allergens The role of allergens in the development of asthma is unclear. Sensitization and exposure to dust mites and Alternaria fungi are important determinants in the development of

asthma in children. Additionally, exposure to allergens can result in airway inflammation and likelihood of an exacerbation.

Respiratory Infections Parainfluenza and respiratory syncytial virus (RSV) infections result in bronchiolitis which is similar to asthma in childhood; longitudinal studies have reported that around 40% of infants admitted to hospital with RSV infection continue to wheeze or develop asthma in later childhood.

Other Environmental Exposures

Smoking, air pollution, certain occupations, and diet have been associated with the likelihood of developing asthma. In adult asthmatics, tobacco use is associated with increased asthma severity and an attenuated responsiveness to inhaled corticosteroids.

Diagnosis of Asthma

When diagnosing asthma, taking a good clinical history is pivotal [2, 6]. The suspicion of asthma is based on the presence of characteristic respiratory symptoms, which exhibit variation. Symptoms include wheezing, shortness of breath, chest tightness, and cough. Typically, more than one symptom may be present, is worse at night or in the early mornings, varies over time and in intensity, and be triggered by various situations such as exercise, allergen exposure, change in temperature, viral infections, or irritants (exhaust fumes, smoking, or strong scents). Within the history, details of the initiation of respiratory symptoms in childhood, a history of allergic rhinitis or eczema, or a family history of asthma and allergy raises the probability that the respiratory symptoms are due to asthma. However, none of these features is unique to asthma, and may not be seen in all asthma phenotypes. Respiratory symptoms unlikely to be due to asthma include an isolated cough, chronic sputum production, dyspnoea with dizziness, light-headedness or paraesthesia, chest pain, and exercise-induced dyspnoea with noisy inspiration. Physical examination in patients with asthma is often normal. Expiratory wheezes on auscultation may be absent in severe

asthma exacerbations. Importantly, wheezing may also be heard in other conditions such as vocal cord dysfunction, COPD, respiratory infections, tracheomalacia, or inhaled foreign bodies. Crackles/crepitations and inspiratory wheeze are not characteristic features of asthma. Nasal examination may reveal signs of allergic rhinitis or nasal polyposis.

Both documented airflow limitation and variability in lung function are essential for the diagnosis of asthma (at least one episode of low FEV1 and an obstructive expiratory ratio (<0.75)) [1, 6]. The greater the variation and/or the more the occasions of excess variation in lung function, the more certain the clinician may be with the diagnosis. Variability in lung function may be assessed in a number of ways including:

1. Positive response to an inhaled bronchodilator (BD)—if possible withholding short-acting bronchodilators (SABA) for ≥4 h and long-acting bronchodilators (LABA) for ≥15 h—with an increase in FEV1 after 10–15 min of >12% and 200 mL from baseline following 200–400 mcg of inhaled salbutamol (more confidence if >15% and >400 mL respectively)

2. Increased variability (>10%) during twice-daily peak expiratory flow monitoring (PEF) over a 2-week period (daily diurnal PEF variability = the difference between PEF [day's highest—day's lowest]/mean of day's highest and lowest, and averaged over 1 week)

3. A marked increase in lung function after 4 weeks of anti-inflammatory treatment described as an increase in FEV1 by >12% and 200 mL (or PEF >20%) from baseline when free of respiratory infection

4. A positive exercise challenge described as a decrease in FEV1 >10% and 200 mL from baseline

5. A positive bronchial challenge test described as a fall in FEV1 from baseline of ≥20% with standard doses of methacholine or histamine, or ≥15% with standardised hyperventilation, hypertonic saline or mannitol challenge

6. Excessive variation in lung function between visits described as a variation in FEV1 >12% and >200 mL between visits, outside respiratory infections

Of note, FeNO is also a useful monitoring tool rather than a diagnostic one.

There may be a wide differential diagnosis in patients suspected with asthma [1]. This includes chronic upper-airway cough syndrome, inhaled foreign body or central airway obstruction, vocal cord dysfunction, hyperventilation and dysfunctional breathing, bronchiectasis, cystic fibrosis, congenital heart disease, alpha-1 antitrypsin deficiency, cardiac failure, obesity, medication-related cough, parenchymal lung disease, pulmonary embolism, etc.

Specific Populations/Situations

Occupational Asthma

Occupational or work-exacerbated asthma can easily be missed unless a detailed history is obtained. Symptoms may be induced by exposure to allergens or other sensitising irritants at work, or sometimes from a single massive exposure.

Although as many as one in ten asthmatics report that their condition is worsened by work (so called work-exacerbated asthma), in some the disease is *caused* by the workplace namely true occupational asthma (OA). The diagnosis is often delayed, but should be considered in all cases of adult-onset asthma, particularly if symptoms are better on days away from work or on holiday. The most frequently reported agents in the UK, and in descending order, are isocyanates, flour or grain dust, colophony and fluxes, latex, animals, aldehydes, and wood dust, as shown below [7].

Isocyanates
Flour and grain
Cleaning products
Enzymes, amylase
Solder/colophony
Wood dusts
Laboratory animals
Cutting oils and coolants
Hardening agents
Stainless steel welding
Latex

There are two types of OA which are distinguished by whether there is a latency period (months or years) between the exposure and the onset of symptoms:

1. OA caused after a latency period by most high molecular-weight (HMW) and certain low molecular-weight (LMW) agents (mediated by IgE), or certain specific occupational agents such as wood dust, where the allergic mechanisms have not been characterised. Occupational rhinitis is common with HMW agents and may declare itself in the year before OA presents.
2. OA without a latency period (non-allergic), which may occur after a single large exposure such as RADS (reactive airways dysfunction syndrome) or multiple exposures (so called irritant asthma)

To diagnose OA, serial peak flow measurements should be recorded at least four times a day for 4 weeks and should include three or more consecutive days at work and away from work. Computer-based software such as OASYS II (obtainable from www.occupationalasthma. com) has good sensitivity and excellent specificity, and calculates a work-effect index. Skin prick testing or specific IgE can confirm sensitisation (but not OA) to high molecular-weight agents such as enzymes, cereals, animals, or latex, or the occasional low molecular-weight agent such as platinum or acid anhydrides, but in most cases of LMW asthma the mechanism is unknown.

Inhalational challenges with HMW agents cause immediate and often dual responses, whereas LMW agents can cause isolated late or atypical responses, and it is recommended that specific inhalational challenge should only be attempted in specialist occupational lung disease units. Once a diagnosis of OA has been made, relocation should be immediate, but sometimes local working conditions and economic considerations make this difficult to implement. Even after exposure has ceased, persisting symptoms are common and a pattern of asthma triggered by non-specific stimuli may emerge.

Pregnancy

Diagnosis in pregnancy using bronchial provocation testing or stepping down controller medication is not recommended. Ideally, any confirmatory diagnosis should be conducted in the post-natal period.

Elderly and Obese

Asthma is infrequently diagnosed in the elderly due to poor perception of airflow limitation, age-related dyspnoea, lack of fitness, and reduced activity. Often the presence of other co-morbid conditions (especially cardiovascular disease) may complicate the diagnostic process.

Asthma is more common in obese patients, however, respiratory symptoms mimicking asthma are also found in obesity. Hence, appropriate objective investigations to confirm or refute asthma are essential.

Athletes

In athletes, bronchial provocation testing may be essential to confirm the diagnosis of asthma [1].

Patients Already on Treatment

Confirming a diagnosis of asthma in patients already on controller medications is important, and objective testing should be pursued [2, 6]. This may be conducted using bronchodilator reversibility, bronchial provocation testing (in patients with FEV1 >70% predicted), or reducing (stepping down or stopping) inhaled controller treatment with close supervision.

Asthma Monitoring

Asthma control has two main domains: symptom control and future risk of adverse outcomes [2, 6]. Lung function is an important aspect of future risk assessment, hence needs to be assessed at treatment onset and regularly thereafter. Poor symptom control is also strongly associated with an increased risk of asthma exacerbations.

Asthma symptom control tools have been developed. Simple screening tools include the Royal College of Physicians (RCP) Three Questions, asking about daytime symptoms, activity limitation, and difficulty sleeping in the previous month; and the 30-s Asthma Test, which also includes asthma-related time off work or school. Categorical symptom control tools include the consensus-based GINA symptom control tool, which is similar to the RCP tool but also includes reliever use, and may be used in association with the risk assessment tool to guide treatment decisions.

There are two main numerical "asthma control" tools with scores and cut-off points to delineate different levels of symptom control. They are the Asthma Control Questionnaire (ACQ), with scores ranging from 0 to 6 (high scores indicate poor control). A score in the range 0–0.75 is classified as well-controlled asthma, 0.75–1.5 as "grey zone," and >1.5 as poorly controlled asthma, with a minimum clinically important difference (MCID) of 0.5. The score is normally an average of five, six (includes reliever use) or seven (includes reliever use and pre-bronchodilator FEV1) items, with all versions having five symptom questions. The Asthma Control Test (ACT) scores range from 5 to 25 (high scores indicate good control). Score ranges of 5–15 are classified as poor control, 16–20 as not well-controlled and 20–25 as well-controlled asthma. The ACT includes a subjective assessment of control as well as symptom and reliever questions with a MCID of 3 points.

Asthma control is an important predictor of future exacerbations, but a more complete assessment requires identification of factors which are associated with adverse outcomes:

> **Independent Risk Factors for Asthma Exacerbations**
> - Ongoing exposure to allergens or irritants (e.g. smoking, occupational)[1]
> - Increased SABA use
> - Pregnancy
> - Uncontrolled asthma symptoms
> - Marked airflow limitation (esp <60%)[1]
> - Lack of or insufficient ICS (poor concordance, inhaler technique)[1]
> - Previous asthma-related intensive care (with or without intubation)
> - Severe asthma exacerbation in previous 12 months
> - Other co-morbid conditions (psychological, sino-nasal disease, allergies, obesity)
> - Sputum or blood eosinophilia[1]
> - Poor socio-economic status

---

[1]Risk factors associated with the development of fixed airflow limitation.

Peak expiratory flow (PEF) is a useful tool in monitoring response to treatment and for evaluating triggers, especially when an occupational aetiology is suspected. Routine long-term monitoring is now only recommended for patients with severe asthma or those with lack of perception of airflow limitation. In these situations diurnal measurements depicted on a standardized chart are useful. Response to ICS treatment with PEF will reach personal best values in around 2 weeks. Spirometry is the best tool in the diagnostic process of asthma (either using reversibility, bronchial provocations, etc.), which can be used at hospital clinic visits as well as annual follow-up visits in primary care.

In patients with difficult-to-treat and severe asthma, alternative monitoring and treatment-associated assessments may focus on markers of eosinophilic inflammation (FeNO and sputum eosinophils). It is important to remember that both FeNO and induced-sputum are principally monitoring tools for asthma. These monitoring tools may only be available in specialist centres and are useful in establishing whether the aetiology of a patient's symptoms may be asthma-related or not. For example, in cases of elevated sputum eosinophils (>2% of total cell count), additional corticosteroid therapy may be indicated.

Asthma Management

Primary Prevention

Asthma inception and persistence is thought to be driven by gene-environment interactions, most of which occur in early life and even in utero. Hence, there may be opportunity to intervene during pregnancy and in early life. Environmental risk factors for the development of asthma include:

Nutrition Breastfeeding and maternal intake of vitamins D and E are associated with reduced wheezing episodes in early life, yet interventions do not prevent the development of persistent asthma. Probiotic use has no role in preventing asthma.

Allergens and Pollutants/Irritants The development of asthma is more likely to occur due to sensitisation to inhaled indoor aero-allergens (for example house dust mite). Smoking during pregnancy has been associated with the development of asthma in young children.

Microbes and Medications According to the "hygiene hypothesis" (vide supra) human interaction with microbes may be vital in preventing asthma, and antibiotic use in pregnancy may be implicated in the development of asthma. Similarly, the use of paracetamol and NSAIDs has not only been implicated in promoting asthma exacerbations, but also in its development.

Psychosocial Factors Maternal distress in a child's early life has been associated with the risk of developing asthma, and likewise, a child's social environment may contribute to asthma severity.

Non-Pharmacological Strategies/Interventions

Smoking Cessation In asthmatic smokers attempts should be made at every visit to encourage smoking cessation. Family members who smoke should be discouraged from smoking in cars and in rooms alongside adults or children with asthma.

Occupational Exposure Avoidance In adult-onset asthma, an occupational cause should be considered, and every attempt should be made to identify and eliminate irritants/sensitizers, or consider referring to a specialist centre.

Allergen Avoidance Indoor allergen avoidance is not recommended in asthma, especially single-strategy allergen (e.g. house dust mite) avoidance in sensitised patients. For sensitized asthmatic pet owners, removing the pet from the house is often advised, although there is a lack of data to support this approach. In cat-owning households, removal of the cat leads to 50% reduced allergen levels after 6 months on average, but there is much variation, and it is unclear how allergen reduction relates to asthma symptoms. Furthermore, animal allergens can also be detected in schools and in non-pet-owning households. For outdoor allergens such as pollen and mould, sensitised patients may benefit from their avoidance (closing windows and doors, remaining indoors, and using air conditioning).

Air Pollution Patients with asthma should be discouraged from using heating and cooking sources that result in pollutants, or at least have appropriate ventilation facilities for fume extraction. During periods of high pollution and/or viral infections, asthmatics should be encouraged to avoid strenuous outdoor activity and preferably stay indoors.

Medication Avoidance Paracetamol, aspirin, and NSAIDs are not generally contraindicated unless there is a history of asthma deterioration with their use. Beta-blockers, be they oral or topical, should be avoided in asthma, and this applies to all compounds, even the more cardioselective β1 antagonists. If there is no alternative to their use, then vigilant monitoring is crucial.

Food Avoidance This is not recommended unless an allergy or food chemical sensitivity has been demonstrated by supervised oral challenges.

Physical Activity and Breathing Exercises Encouraging regular physical activity improves cardio-pulmonary fitness, but has little impact on lung function or asthma symptoms. Breathing exercises may be a useful adjunct to asthma pharmacotherapy, *particularly if an element of dysfunctional breathing is present.*

Diet and Weight Reduction Diets high in fruit and vegetables are generally beneficial. Weight reduction, if possible, in obese patients can be pivotal in asthmatics.

Psychosocial Factors Asthmatics at the severe end of the spectrum frequently have emotional/anxiety/depressive co-morbidities. Identifying goals and strategies to deal with these may help to attenuate asthma exacerbations/improve control, although no specific strategy has been shown to be superior over another.

Vaccinations Although there is little evidence for influenza vaccination, patients with moderate-to-severe asthma may be advised to have one annually. Routine pneumococcal vaccination is not recommended in asthmatics, though may be useful in children and the elderly.

Inhaler and Asthma Self-Management

Inhaler Choice, Training, and Management

The delivery of effective concentrations of inhaled asthma therapies, which work rapidly and with acceptable side effects, is important. Using an inhaler is a skill that needs not only to be learnt but also maintained. Poor inhaler technique results in poor asthma control and increased risk of exacerbations and adverse events. Both patients and healthcare professionals (HCP) often have a poor understanding of correct inhaler technique, and there is no "perfect" inhaler.

In choosing the most suitable inhaler for the patient, the HCP must consider any mechanical disabilities (e.g. arthritis), avoiding the confusing use of multiple inhaler types/devices, patient choice, cost, and the need for adjuncts such as spacer devices. Inhaler technique should be assessed at each opportunity, errors rectified by physical demonstration, and alternative devices considered.

There is increasing awareness that lack of concordance with asthma therapies may result in poor control and/or risk of exacerbation. This needs to be identified by empathic questioning, and checking prescription collections and inhaler dose counters. There may be a number of factors contributing to poor adherence, including challenges in using the inhaler device (e.g. arthritis), complex dosing regimes, different inhaler devices, forgetfulness, cost, poor insight and/or inappropriate expectations of therapy, denial or frustration about the diagnosis of asthma or its treatment, concerns about side effects (perceived or real), stigmatisation, cultural or religious issues, and patient dissatisfaction or disagreement with HCPs.

Self-management

Per se, guided self-management may range broadly from patient-directed to HCP-directed self-management. The former involves patients making amendments according to a prior written action plan in the absence of first contact with a HCP, while the latter would involve a written action plan but involve communication with the HCP in a planned or unplanned consultation. Personalised asthma action plans improve patient outcomes. An effective asthma self-management plan involves patient-monitoring of symptoms and/or peak flow, a written asthma action plan on how to recognise and respond to asthma worsening, and a HCP review of asthma control and treatment.

Pharmacotherapy of Stable Asthma

The drugs available for management of asthma can be divided into two broad categories—controller medications and reliever medications. Controller medications need to be taken regularly (irrespective of symptoms) and are primarily meant to prevent and control symptoms, reduce airway inflammation and/or decrease the risk of exacerbations. These include inhaled corticosteroids (ICS), leukotriene receptor antagonists (LTRAs), mast cell stabilisers, and long-acting bronchodilators (LABAs). Reliever medications, also known as rescue medications, are fast-acting bronchodilators that are taken as and when required to relieve acute symptoms.

The aim of asthma management is complete control of disease and is defined as:

- No daytime symptoms
- No nocturnal awakenings
- No need for rescue medications
- No asthma attacks
- No activity limitation
- Normal lung function
- Minimal side effects from medications

A stepwise approach is used for the management of asthma. Patients should be started on the most appropriate step according to their initial severity. The aim is to achieve early control and maintain it by either stepping up or stepping down treatment. The stepwise management of asthma is based on the BTS-SIGN guidelines 2016 [6].

Mild Intermittent Asthma

Inhaled SABAs should be prescribed *as relievers* to all patients with asthma. Using SABAs as required is at least as good as regular daily use. SABA-only treatment should be reserved for patients with infrequent, short-lived daytime symptoms, no nocturnal awakenings, and normal lung function. The GINA 2015 guidelines suggest early consideration of regular low-dose ICS in addition to SABAs in patients at risk of exacerbations.

Regular Preventer Therapy

ICS are the cornerstone in the management of asthma. They improve airway inflammation, lung function, and symptom scores, reduce exacerbations, and reduce need for reliever use. Regular ICS should be considered for patients who have had an asthma attack in the past 2 years, use SABA $\geq$3 times/week, have symptoms $\geq$3 times/week or wake one night/week. There is increasing evidence that at recommended doses ICS are safe and effective in children under 5 years. Most of the benefits of ICS are obtained at low doses equivalent of beclomethasone dipropionate (BDP) 400 mcg/day. Increasing the dose provides little further improvement in terms of asthma control, but increases the risk of side effects.

BDP and budesonide are approximately equipotent in clinical practice and a 1:1 ratio should be assumed when changing between BDP and budesonide. Fluticasone propionate and mometasone provide equal clinical efficacy to BDP at half the dosage (Table 3.1). ICS should be used twice daily except ciclesonide, mometasone, and fluticasone furoate, which are used once daily. Once good control is established, reducing

Table 3.1 Dosage per day (micrograms) for ICS in asthma

	Low dose	Medium dose	High dose
BDP-generic-MDI	400	800	1600
BDP-Clenil-MDI	400	800	1000
BDP-Qvar-MDI	200	400	
Ciclesonide-MDI	160	320	
Fluticasone propionate-MDI	200	500	1000
Budesonide easyhaler-DPI	400	800	1600
Budesonide turbohaler-DPI	400	800	
Fluticasone propionate accuhaler-DPI	200	400	1000
Mometasone twisthaler-DPI	400	800	

from twice daily to once daily ICS at the same total daily dose can be considered. Current or ex-smokers may require higher doses of ICS as smoking reduces the effect of ICS.

Initial Add-on Therapy

A proportion of patients on low dose-ICS alone may not be adequately controlled. This group of asthmatics need an add-on therapy. Before additional therapy is considered, it is prudent to ensure that the patient is adherent to treatment, uses the inhalers appropriately and that any obvious asthma triggers are eliminated.

LABAs are the initial add-on therapy to ICS in patients with poor asthma control. This should be considered prior to increasing the ICS dose. LABAs should only started in patients who are already on ICS treatment. In clinical studies there were no differences in efficacy when ICS and LABA were given in separate inhalers or in a combination inhaler, but use of ICS/LABA in a combination inhaler improves adherence and guarantees that LABAs are not taken without ICS. Therapy with LABAs may be associated with headaches or cramps, but more serious systemic side effects such as cardiovascular stimulation, tremor, and hypokalemia are uncommon.

Clinical studies have shown that the onset of action of formoterol is comparable to salbutamol, which provides an opportunity to use a single

ICS/LABA combination inhaler for maintenance and reliever therapy (MART).

Additional Add-on Therapy

If asthma control remains sub-optimal despite the addition of LABA, then the dose of ICS should be increased from low to medium. Other add-on therapies such as a LRTA or a long-acting muscarinic antagonist (LAMA) should be considered if asthma control is inadequate. Clinical studies have shown that LTRAs have a small and variable bronchodilator effect, improve lung function, reduce symptoms including cough, and reduce exacerbations. LTRAs can reduce the dose of ICS required by patients but are less effective than LABAs as initial add-on therapy. Tiotropium bromide, a LAMA, is licenced for use in adults with asthma. A review of randomised controlled trials (RCTs) in adults on LAMA in addition to ICS/LABA compared with ICS/LABA alone reported fewer asthma exacerbations, improved lung function, and some benefits relating to asthma control in those taking LAMA, but no improvement in quality of life. Mast cell stabilisers (cromoglycate and nedocromil) are sometimes used as add–on treatment, as prophylaxis against EIA, or occasionally in mild asthma when inhaled steroids are not tolerated.

The escalation of treatment for patients with asthma is based on a stepwise approach for increasing the therapy to obtain optimal asthma control (Fig. 3.1) based on the BTS-SIGN asthma guidelines. Once asthma control is achieved and when patients are stable on current therapies, stepping down treatment should be considered. Patients should be maintained on the lowest possible dose of ICS and reductions should be considered every 3 months to retain best possible control of their asthma.

Higher Level Therapies and/or Add-on Therapies

In a proportion of patients, despite correct inhaler technique and good adherence to therapy, their symptoms remain poorly controlled. If ICS are used at higher doses via pMDI it is recommended

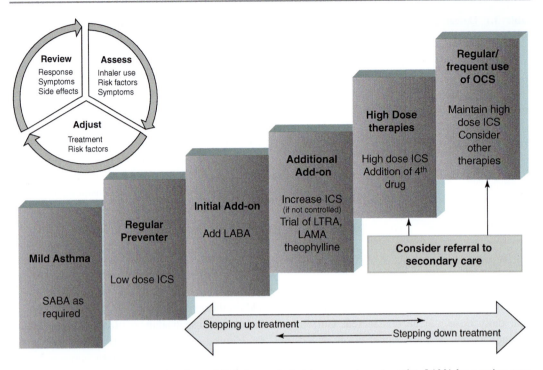

Fig. 3.1 Stepwise management of asthma. *SABA* short acting beta 2 agonist, *LABA* long acting beta 2 agonist, *ICS* inhaled corticosteroid, *OCS* oral corticosteroid, *LTRA* leukotriene receptor antagonist, *LAMA* long acting muscarinic antagonist

to use a spacer. If patients remain symptomatic on high-dose ICS and are taking LABA and/or LTRA, the treatment options would include addition of oral corticosteroids (OCS). The lowest possible dose of OCS should be used to optimise asthma control. Patients who have multiple courses of OCS (>3/year) or on long-term steroids (>3 months) are at risk for steroid-related side effects including hypertension, diabetes mellitus, hyperlipidemia, osteoporosis, and cataracts. Patients requiring frequent short courses or maintenance prednisolone should have bone mineral density (BMD) measured and long-acting bisphosphonates prescribed if BMD is reduced.

Other Therapies

Anti-IgE (Omalizumab (Xolair®, Novartis, Switzerland))

Omalizumab is a recombinant humanized IgG1 non-complement fixing monoclonal antibody that binds to the high-affinity receptor binding domain (Cε3) on the Fc portion of free IgE. Omalizumab is absorbed slowly following subctaneous injection, reaching peak serum concentrations after seven to 8 days. Omalizumab is licensed for patient with serum IgE levels up to 1500 IU/ml and is administered subcutaneously every 2–4 weeks. Omalizumab is approved for use in patients with severe allergic asthma who have a documented positive skin prick test or *in vitro* test to an aero allergen, i.e. raised IgE level or positive radioallergosorbent testing (RAST), FEV1 < 80% predicted, frequent daytime symptoms or night-time awakenings, and multiple documented severe exacerbations despite regular high-dose ICS and LABA. Patients who are initiated on omalizumab treatment must be assessed at 16 weeks after the start of their treatment to examine its effectiveness, and should continue only if there is improvement in their asthma. Omalizumab's side effects include local injection site reactions and anaphylaxis presenting as bronchospasm, syncope, urticaria, and hypotension. In view of these risks, omalizumab should only be administered in a healthcare setting under direct medical supervision.

IL-5 Blocking Strategies

Eosinophilic inflammation is a distinguishing feature of asthmatic inflammation and IL-5 is a key cytokine that modulates eosinophil behaviour. IL-5 plays a central role in the production, mobilization, activation, recruitment, proliferation, survival, and suppression of apoptosis in eosinophils at the site of inflammation. Therefore antagonizing IL-5 is a promising target to attenuate eosinophil-mediated inflammation in patients with asthma. This has led to the development of humanized anti-IL-5 monoclonal antibodies (mAb), such as mepolizumab and reslizumab. Mepolizumab is now licensed for the treatment of severe eosinophilic asthma not controlled on maximal inhaled treatment. Patients are eligible if they have peripheral blood eosinophilia (>300/μL), and four or more exacerbations requiring oral steroids in the previous year, or require at least 5 mg maintenance prednisolone for the previous 6 months. The drug is administered by monthly subcutaneous injection, and side effects include headache, backache, local skin reactions, and occasionally anaphylaxis. Benralizumab, a mAb against the human IL-5 receptor (IL-5Rα), is in development.

Bronchial Thermoplasty

Bronchial thermoplasty involves delivery of controlled radio frequency energy to the airway wall to heat the tissue and thereby reducing the smooth muscle present in the airways. In patients with poorly controlled asthma despite maximal therapy, bronchial thermoplasty treatment has been shown to reduce the frequency of severe asthma attacks, emergency department visits, and days of lost work in the year after treatment. Assessment and treatment for bronchial thermoplasty is currently only undertaken in specialist centres where there is an expertise in the management of difficult-to-control asthma. The procedure is normally carried out with conscious sedation in three sessions, and common complications include mild exacerbations of asthma. The exact mechanism of improvement is currently unclear.

Devices and Drug Delivery

Choosing the correct inhaler can be a challenge. The main inhaler devices in asthma are pressurised metered-dose inhalers (pMDIs) and dry-powder inhalers (DPIs) and, more recently, the soft-mist inhaler. A slow (<60 L/min inspiratory pressure) and deep inhalation, as well as coordination, is essential for pMDIs translating into an inhalation lasting 2–5 s. A faster inhalation rate increases the likelihood of oropharyngeal deposition. A large proportion of patients prescribed pMDIs fail to inhale at the correct rate and hence get poor delivery of the drug to the lungs. Breath-actuated MDIs may be an alternative in patients finding difficulty in coordinating actuation and inhalation. The use of a spacer reduces oropharyngeal deposition and can as much as double lung deposition, though may not be the favoured option.

DPIs require a rapid and forceful inhalation (>30 L/min inspiratory pressure). It must be noted that the inspiratory flow may differ depending on the DPI considered. For each inhaler a minimum energy (inspiratory flow) is required to provide an efficient disaggregation of the formulation. It is important to remember that in the very young and elderly, and in patients experiencing a severe exacerbation, it may be challenging when using a DPI to generate sufficient turbulent energy to reach the lungs. The In-check Dial™ (Clement Clarke International) is a useful tool in identifying the patient's inspiratory capacity and choosing the appropriate inhaler for the patient. The soft-mist inhaler, like the pMDI, requires a slow, deep breath with a simultaneous depression of the dose-release button. It has a higher particle fraction then the aerosol cloud from pMDIs, attenuated oropharyngeal and good lung deposition, and with little dependence on inspiratory flow.

The use of nebulisers is limited mainly to patients who are unable to use inhalers due to dexterity, age (too young or old), disability, and during acute exacerbations of asthma. In the case of exacerbations, the nebulised medication is normally delivered with oxygen.

Management of Acute Severe Asthma

An asthma exacerbation is characterised by worsening of one or more of asthma symptoms leading to an increased use in reliever medications or hospitalisation, and usually associated with a decline in lung function (PEF and/or FEV1). Lessons from the national review of asthma deaths indicates that most deaths occur before admission to hospital [8]. Chronic severe asthma, inadequate treatment with ICS, OCS use, high use of β2 agonists, inadequate follow-up, and adverse psychosocial and behavioural factors contribute to asthma mortality. All patients with asthma should be provided with a written asthma management plan so they know how to recognize and respond to their exacerbation.

Acute severe asthma is suggested by a PEF of 30–50% predicted, respiratory rate >25/min, heart rate >110/min, and an inability to complete a sentence. Clinical signs of life-threatening asthma include altered consciousness, exhaustion, cardiac arrhythmias, hypotension, cyanosis, silent chest, and poor respiratory effort.

- Supplementary oxygen should be administered to maintain oxygen saturations of 94–98%.
- Administration of SABA (salbutamol and terbutaline) should be instituted to relieve bronchospasm. This could be done via a pMDI through a large-volume spacer or through a nebuliser. Patients not responding appropriately to initial treatment with SABAs may require continuous nebulisation. Intravenous β2 agonists are no more efficacious than nebulised drug and should be reserved for patients with acute asthma where the inhaled route cannot be reliably used. Signs of adrenergic toxicity may occur with intravenous or high-dose inhaled β-agonist therapy and include worsening tachycardia, tachypnoea, and metabolic (lactic) acidosis.
- Nebulised ipratropium bromide should be added to treatment if patients are not responding to initial treatment.

- Systemic corticosteroids in the form of prednisolone 40 mg by mouth or hydrocortisone 100 mg four times a day intravenously should be initiated. There is no difference in efficacy between prednisolone and hydrocortisone.
- Magnesium sulphate (2 g IV over 20 min) has bronchodilator effects and a single dose of magnesium sulphate can be considered in patients with acute severe asthma responding poorly to inhaled bronchodilator therapy.
- In acute asthma, intravenous aminophylline is unlikely to be useful when added to nebulised bronchodilators and systemic corticosteroids can cause arrhythmias and vomiting. Anecdotally, occasional patients with near-fatal or life-threatening asthma with a poor response to initial treatment seem to respond to aminophylline infusion (0.5–0.7 mg/kg/h. omitting the loading dose of 5 mg/kg if already on oral theophylline) but these cases are probably rare.
- The routine prescription of antibiotics is not indicated in an asthma exacerbation unless there is clear evidence of bacterial infection precipitating the exacerbation.

Worsening PEF, hypercapnia, persisting or worsening hypoxia, drowsiness, altered level of consciousness and respiratory arrest despite initial therapies are indications for admission to the intensive care unit. Non-invasive ventilation for acute severe asthma with hypercapnia has not been rigorously tested, so cannot be recommended, particularly as the mortality associated with invasive mechanical ventilation is so low. Patients with acute-on-chronic hypercapnia secondary to chronic asthma or ACOS behave more like patients with COPD and can be considered for NIV.

Special Populations

Asthma in Pregnancy

Asthma is the most common chronic condition associated with pregnancy, and asthma control worsens in one-third, improves in a third and remains stable in a third of patients. 10–15%

of pregnant asthmatics have at least one asthma exacerbation needing emergency treatment and, of those, two-thirds will require hospitalisation. Exacerbations are more common in the second trimester and are due to a combination of mechanical and hormonal changes. Poor symptom control and exacerbations are associated with maternal complications like pre-eclampsia, and poor foetal outcomes including low birth weight, pre-term delivery, and increased perinatal mortality. When asthma is well controlled there is no increase in adverse maternal or foetal outcomes.

The management of asthma during pregnancy is complicated by concerns with use of medications during pregnancy, however the advantages of active treatment far outweighs any risk of usual controller and reliever medications. No significant association has been demonstrated between adverse perinatal outcomes or congenital malformations and exposure to SABAs, LABAs, ICS, or theophyllines. OCS should be used normally during pregnancy during an asthma exacerbation. There is a concern that OCS may be associated with cleft lip, though the evidence is poor. Should a patient require LTRAs to achieve adequate control of their asthma, then they should be continued during pregnancy. Cromoglycate or nedocromil can be used normally during pregnancy but there are no clinical data on immunotherapy in pregnancy. The omalizumab pregnancy registry reports no apparent increased prevalence of birth defects.

The most common reasons for deterioration in asthma control during pregnancy are virally-induced exacerbations and non-compliance with regular asthma medications. Acute severe asthma during pregnancy should be managed actively, with close monitoring of the mother and foetus. Available evidence gives little cause for concern regarding treatment side effects, and maternal and foetal risks of uncontrolled asthma are much greater than the risks from using acute conventional asthma medications. Oxygen saturation should be maintained between 94 and 98% to avoid maternal or foetal hypoxia. If there are concerns, continuous foetal monitoring should be employed and drug therapy should be given as for a non-pregnant patient with acute asthma.

Close liaison between the respiratory and obstetrics teams and early referral to critical care are essential.

During labour, regular controller medications should be taken routinely, and relievers if needed. Acute exacerbations during labour are uncommon, perhaps due to endogenous steroid production. Prostaglandin E2 is safe for induction of labour, but prostaglandin F2α used for postpartum haemorrhage can induce bronchospasm. Similarly, bronchospasm can be associated with ergometrine but not with syntometrine (syntocinon).

Maternal smoking during pregnancy can lead to poor asthma control and an increased risk of infant wheezing, with adverse effects on infant lung function. There is insufficient evidence to recommend house dust mite allergen avoidance during pregnancy. One study reported FeNO-guided management algorithms were associated with fewer exacerbations and better foetal outcomes compared to ACQ-based algorithms. Given the evidence that asthma exacerbations can have significant effect on maternal and foetal outcomes, a low priority should be placed on stepping down treatment until after delivery. A pro-active approach with monitoring respiratory infections, patient education, self-management plan, and timely access to health care professional would significantly improve asthma care during pregnancy.

Exercise-Induced Asthma (EIA)

EIA (or exercise-induced bronchoconstriction) typically occurs within 15 min of exercise and usually resolves within an hour. It is usually seen after high-intensity aerobic exercise during which high minute volume ventilation leads to airway dehydration, increase in airway osmolarity, and mast cell activation, leading to mediator release. Increased exposure to allergens or airway irritants may exacerbate the bronchoconstriction. The reported incidence of EIA can vary between 10% and 50% in high-level athletes. The prevalence is high in both summer and winter sports, but is more common in the latter [9].

EIA can occur in children and adults ranging from recreational to elite competitors. Typical symptoms include breathlessness, wheeze, cough, and chest tightness during or after exercise. These symptoms can limit the sporting performance of individuals. Formal diagnosis of EIA would require direct airway challenges like mannitol or methacholine with a >12% fall in FEV1 being the threshold. Indirect challenges are preferable over direct challenges, as they replicate the physiology more accurately and include high-intensity exercise or eucapnic voluntary hyperpnoea. Exercise-induced VCD can mimic EIA but needs direct laryngoscopy to visualise paradoxical closure of the vocal cords during inspiration.

Patients with EIA should be treated in the same way as a regular asthmatic. Baseline therapy is anti-inflammatory with ICS. In athletes with rare episodes of EIA, prophylactic administration of SABA might suffice. If the use of SABA is more than twice a week, then regular anti-inflammatory therapy should be commenced. LABAs are not used as sole therapy for EIA/ EIB due to the potential risk of severe asthma and death. LTRAs cannot reverse bronchoconstriction but may prevent episodes if taken 2 h before exercise and the protection can last for 24 h. Prior to vigorous intensity training, a warmup procedure that includes continuous high-intensity activity or sprint interval bouts reduces the later fall in FEV1.

Asthma in the Elderly

Symptomatic asthma needing treatment affects between 3% and 7% of population over the age of 65 years. The mortality from asthma in this group has not declined, probably due to difficulties in diagnosis with sub-optimal use of spirometry and other diagnostic tests, under-treatment, atypical presentations, mis-classification as COPD, and the effect of co-morbidities. With age there is a decrease in elastic recoil and respiratory muscle strength. The former offsets the latter, so TLC is unchanged but VC declines and RV increases.

Dynamic airway narrowing means maximum expiratory flows decline reflected in a reduced FEV1/VC ratio. In addition, immunosenescence can compromise both innate and adaptive immunity, the clinical impact being an increased predisposition to microbial infection leading to asthma exacerbations.

The management of asthma in the elderly should follow the same rules as for younger patients. The main goals are to achieve asthma control and prevent exacerbations. Multiple patient factors lead to suboptimal disease control, including misunderstanding of asthma as a disease and the treatment regimen, poor adherence to treatment recommendations, memory problems, and socioeconomic challenges. Appropriate use of inhalers (ICS/LABA/LAMA) would depend upon cognition, manual dexterity, vision, and presence of co-morbidities like arthritis. The inhaler technique of older asthmatics should be checked regularly. Most patients with an MMSE <24 or AMT <7 are unable to learn inhaler technique. Some patients who learned to use an inhaler while their cognition was intact retain their ability in early dementia. Use of a spacer device can reduce the issues with timing of inhalation. While DPIs may be a solution to incorrect timing, these devices require higher inspiratory pressures. Drugs frequently prescribed for cardiovascular conditions such as β-blockers, even in the form of eye drops for glaucoma, can induce bronchoconstriction and their use should be reviewed and avoided in asthmatic patients. A few patients with advanced dementia would not be able to use inhaled medications, in which case medications can be given as nebulised solutions.

Aspirin-Induced Asthma

The triad of aspirin sensitivity, nasal polyps, and asthma (Samter's triad) encompasses aspirin-exacerbated respiratory disease (AERD). The classical feature of AERD is worsening respiratory symptoms after ingestion of cyclo-oxygenase-1 (COX-1) inhibitors like aspirin and NSAIDs [10]. The prevalence of AERD is approximately 7% in asthmatics, but this does double in patients with severe asthma. The disease tends to develop in adulthood, unlike atopic asthma, and is more common in females and occurs in patients with no history of atopy. The key pathophysiologic feature of AERD is dysregulation of pro- and anti-inflammatory mediators of the arachidonic acid pathway. The expression of COX-2 but not COX-1 is markedly reduced, and as COX-2 is functionally coupled with PGE2 (an anti-inflammatory prostaglandin), the level of PGE2 is reduced in AERD. PGE2 exerts its anti-inflammatory effects by impairing eosinophil activation and mast cell degranulation. Furthermore, the enzymes 5-lipoxygenase (5-LO) and leukotriene (LT) C4 synthase are upregulated with a resultant increase in the downstream lipid mediators LTC4, which is converted to LTD4 and LTE4, which causes bronchoconstriction. Levels of LTE4 are elevated in the urine and respiratory secretions in patients with AERD.

Clinical risk factors for AERD include age <40 years, poor sense of smell, and a history of previous reactions to aspirin/NSAIDs. The gold standard for diagnosing AERD remains an aspirin challenge, as there are no substitute in vitro diagnostic tests. A positive test occurs when an upper or lower respiratory reaction occur during the challenge tests.

In addition to standard asthma therapies like ICS, LABAs, and SABAs, the management of AERD includes leukotriene blockade. Leukotriene blockade involves two classes of medications—LTRAs like montelukast and zafirlukast and the 5-LO inhibitor, zileuton. While zileuton impairs all leukotriene synthesis, LTRAs selectively target cysteinyl leukotrienes. Aspirin desensitisation followed by continued daily ingestion of aspirin improves patients' quality of life, reduces symptoms, and slows the regrowth of nasal polyps in 70–80% of patients with AERD. The protocol is conducted by starting with small doses of aspirin and gradually achieving doses of 600–1300 mg/day. Subsequently, 300–1300 mg of aspirin daily is the recommended maintenance dose following desensitisation. Evidence for doses less than 100 mg/day is inconsistent. Current therapies focus on the leukotriene pathway, but future therapy with biologicals targeting IL-4 and IL-5 are being evaluated for this group of patients.

Asthma COPD Overlap Syndrome (ACOS)

In some adults the differentiation between asthma and COPD becomes difficult. These patients are older, have a history of smoking, diagnoses of both asthma and COPD, and chronic airflow limitation with some reversibility on spirometry. These patients have a significant risk of exacerbations, hospital admission, and healthcare utilisation. ACOS should not be used to define a disease entity but as a term encompassing this group [11]. Predictors for incomplete reversibility in patients with asthma include male sex, increasing age, childhood asthma diagnosis, hospital admission in infancy, increased duration of asthma, adult-onset asthma, atopy, early-onset asthma with blood eosinophilia, sputum eosinophilia, a history of smoking (even low pack-years), low baseline FEV1, AHR, low usage of ICS, and aspirin hypersensitivity. Whilst there are no clear diagnostic criteria, a Spanish consensus statement proposed that patients with COPD should be deemed to have "overlap phenotype COPD–asthma" if they satisfied two major criteria: ≥15% increase in FEV1 or >400 mL on bronchodilator reversibility, sputum eosinophilia, or a personal history of asthma, or one major and two minor criteria (high serum total IgE, personal history of atopy, or ≥12% increase in FEV1 or/and ≥200 mL on two or more occasions) [12].

In the absence of clear guidelines for the diagnosis, the treatment of ACOS currently involves drugs approved for asthma and COPD. The GINA-GOLD guidelines recommend a default towards treating for severe asthma as there is no evidence to support withholding ICS in patients with ACOS. With improved understanding of phenotyping and endotyping in this particular group, the future direction for ACOS treatment is likely to change.

Vocal Cord Dysfunction (VCD)

VCD can mimic or coexist with asthma, may be present in 10% of the difficult-to-treat population and, if not recognised, can lead to overtreatment with steroid toxicity and unnecessary intubation. The essential feature is paradoxical vocal cord motion (PVCM) with inspiratory adduction. It is commoner in females, athletes, and subjects with exercise-induced asthma, and may be associated with gastroesophageal reflux and upper respiratory infection. The complex innervation of the larynx and the association with stress has led to the belief that it is largely a conversion disorder, although in some, precipitation by exercise suggests a degree of laryngeal hyper-responsiveness. While the development of wheezy breathlessness and cough suggests asthma, there is often voice change, inspiratory wheeze, and very sudden onset "attacks." Flow volume loops may show inspiratory limitation, but it is unusual to obtain spirometry or confirm PVCM acutely. Speech therapy may be successful in the long-term management, but some cases are refractory.

Difficult Asthma/Severe Asthma

The definition of difficult-to-treat/severe asthma is unclear. The 2014 American Thoracic Society/European Respiratory Society Task Force report reserves the term *severe asthma* for patients in whom alternative diagnoses have been excluded, co-morbidities treated, trigger factors removed, and adherence confirmed, and who still have poor asthma control or frequent exacerbations despite high-intensity treatment [13]. Patients with severe asthma should be seen in a specialist centre with provision for confirming the diagnosis and identification of factors and mechanisms for persisting symptoms and assessment for adherence to therapy. This should be through a multi-disciplinary team approach. Before escalation of treatment it is imperative to identify patients who have poor control due to poor adherence to therapy, which could be improved by monitoring and educational interventions. Other co-morbidities like obesity, vocal cord dysfunction, dysfunctional breathing, psycho-social issues, persistence of triggers coexistent rhinitis, and gastro-oesophageal reflux disease (acid or non-acid) should be investigated in this sub-population of asthmatics to achieve optimum control.

Summary

Our understanding of asthma has changed significantly over the past two decades, however this has not translated to a similar degree in therapeutic benefit for patients on the severe end of the spectrum. Successful management of asthma relies on galvanising patients to have a better understanding of their condition to appropriately manage their asthma, and importantly, to be able to determine when they would need referral to a HCP. Improving adherence and enhancing treatment adherence would be a huge step forward to decrease asthma-related mortality and morbidity, which is clearly evident from the national review of asthma deaths. The role for biologicals for patients with severe asthma has been evident with the introduction of omalizumab and newer anti-IL-5 therapies. Modulation of IL-4, IL-13, and IL-17 are showing potential in clinical trials as future therapies for asthmatic patients with unmet needs.

Acknowledgements We would like to acknowledge Dr. Alex Hicks for critiquing the chapter.

References

1. Holt PG, Sly PD. Viral infections and atopy in asthma pathogenesis: new rationales for asthma prevention and treatment. Nat Med. 2012;18(5):726–35.
2. The global asthma report 2014. Available at: www.globalasthmareport.org.
3. Asthma UK. Available at: www.asthma.org.uk. Accessed 5 Mar 2015.
4. Asthma Statistics. British lung foundation. 2015. Available at: https://statistics.blf.org.uk/asthma.
5. Global initiative for asthma. Global strategy for asthma management and prevention. 2015. Available at: www.ginasthma.org.
6. BTS/SIGN guideline on the management of asthma. 2016. Available at: www.brit-thoracic.org.uk.

7. Surveillance of work-related and occupational respiratory disease (SWORD) 2013–2015. Work-related and occupational asthma in Great Britain 2016. Health and safety executive. Available at: http://www. hse.gov.uk/statistics/.

8. Royal college of physicians. Why asthma still kills: the National Review of Asthma Deaths (NRAD) Confidential Enquiry report. London: RCP; 2014.

9. Parsons JP, Hallstrand TS, Mastronarde JG, Kaminsky DA, Rundell KW, Hull JH, et al. An official American Thoracic Society clinical practice guideline: exercise-induced bronchoconstriction. Am J Respir Crit Care Med. 2013;187(9):1016–27.

10. Simon RA, Dazy KM, Waldram JD. Aspirin-exacerbated respiratory disease: characteristics and management strategies. Expert Rev Clin Immunol. 2015;11(7):805–17.

11. Bateman ED, Reddel HK, van Zyl-Smit RN, Agusti A. The asthma-COPD overlap syndrome: towards a revised taxonomy of chronic airways diseases? Lancet Respir Med. 2015;3(9):719–28.

12. Soler-Cataluna JJ, Cosio B, Izquierdo JL, Lopez-Campos JL, Marin JM, Aguero R, et al. Consensus document on the overlap phenotype COPD-asthma in COPD. Arch Bronconeumol. 2012;48(9):331–7.

13. Chung KF, Wenzel SE, Brozek JL, Bush A, Castro M, Sterk PJ, et al. International ERS/ATS guidelines on definition, evaluation and treatment of severe asthma. Eur Respir J. 2013;43(2):343–73.

COPD

4

Rod Lawson

COPD, Phenotypes, and Endotypes

Chronic obstructive pulmonary disease (COPD) is a problematic name. It has replaced earlier terms such as chronic obstructive airways disease (COAD) and chronic obstructive lung disease (COLD). In the United Kingdom, NICE (National Institute for Health and Care Excellence) guidelines use a lengthy definition which commences "COPD is characterised by airflow obstruction that is not fully reversible. The airflow obstruction does not change markedly over several months and is usually progressive in the long term. COPD is predominantly caused by smoking" [1]. This definition causes difficulty as it is based around a single physiological variable (airflow obstruction) which is common to other conditions such as asthma and bronchiectasis, and although it recognises smoking as a cause, only a minority of smokers develop the disease. Further, the full definition goes on to recognise the importance of inflammation as an underlying mechanism, but is only able to define this imprecisely and by its difference from asthma.

Some years ago, lumping together COPD as a single entity was a useful public relations exercise. Despite high prevalence and mortality, COPD was relatively neglected in public health terms. The unitary label allowed initiatives such as the Global Initiative for Chronic Obstructive Lung Disease (GOLD) to focus healthcare efforts worldwide [2]. However, COPD includes chronic bronchitis, emphysema, and small airways disease in varying amounts, giving differing clinical presentations.

Classically these were recognised as the "pink puffer" who was thin, normoxic, and breathless, with predominant emphysema, and the "blue bloater" who was obese, hypoxic, and less breathless, but with cor pulmonale. Though patients fitting these classical definitions are seen, this division fell into disrepute as the link between phenotype and underlying pathological abnormality was inconsistent and the distinction failed to offer different treatment options.

Later the concept of phenotypes resurfaced, with a wider recognition that COPD is associated with a range of different co-morbidities and clinical presentations, and the sense that new treatment might need to be developed and used selectively in differing patient groups [3]. For instance, principle component and cluster analysis has been used to define four phenotypes within a cohort, using eight clinical characteristics, [4] which the authors describe as:

Phenotype 1: young subjects with predominant severe to very severe respiratory disease
Phenotype 2: older subjects with mild airflow limitation, mild symptoms, and mild age-related comorbidities

R. Lawson
Sheffield Teaching Hospitals NHS Foundation Trust, Sheffield, UK
e-mail: Rod.lawson@sth.nhs.uk

© Springer International Publishing AG, part of Springer Nature 2018
S. Hart, M. Greenstone (eds.), *Foundations of Respiratory Medicine*,
https://doi.org/10.1007/978-3-319-94127-1_4

Phenotype 3: young subjects with moderate to severe airflow limitation, but few comorbidities and mild symptoms

Phenotype 4: older subjects with moderate to severe airflow limitation and severe symptoms ascribed, at least in part, to major comorbidities (e.g. chronic heart failure)

Importantly, each phenotypic cluster contains subjects with similar values of FEV_1. NICE uses a classification based purely on measures of FEV_1, (Table 4.1) [1].

The NICE guidelines note that its classification was originally in line with GOLD guidelines, though subsequently these have been adapted to use a bivariate classification acknowledging symptoms and "risk" (Fig. 4.1) [2]. It is clear

these limited, though pragmatic, classifications fail to address fully the diversity of phenotypes described and are likely to need to be revised in future, particularly as more targeted treatments for COPD are developed. An early instance is roflumilast, which seems to reduce exacerbations only in the COPD phenotype characterised by chronic sputum production [5].

More recently still, there has been a move beyond phenotypes. With the advent of proteomics it is recognised that a given phenotype may result from differing underlying mechanisms. A unitary underlying mechanism is defined as an endotype [6]. This has resulted in the uncomfortable realisation that traditional diagnostic boundaries between COPD and asthma may in fact be artificial, and that mechanistic understandings will make different distinctions allowing specific targeting of therapies [7]. Instead of the current practice of lumping COPD together, there is likely to be a splitting of airways disease according to mechanisms and treatable traits, for instance that associated with eosinophilic inflammation [8]. A number of large observational studies are currently in the process of reporting results, helping to forward understanding of phenotypes and

Table 4.1 Classification of COPD according to NICE (UK National Institute for Health and Care Excellence)

Stage	Classification	Range
1	Mild	FEV1 in the normal range (over 80%), but FEV1/FVC <0.7 (plus symptoms)
2	Moderate	FEV1 between 50% and 79%
3	Severe	FEV1 between 30% and 49%
4	Very severe	FEV1 under 30%

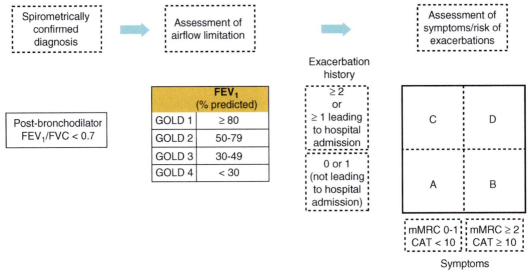

© 2017 Global Initiative for Chronic Obstructive Lung Disease

Fig. 4.1 GOLD classification of COPD. Used with permission from Global Initiative for Chronic Obstructive Lung Disease—GOLD

endotypes, with the promise of progress in the near future, with updated reports available on host websites [9].

History and Clinical Features

Chronic Lung Disease

The cardinal symptoms of COPD are breathlessness, cough (with or without sputum), with onset in middle or old age, usually in those with a significant smoking history. NICE guidelines suggest it should be considered in subjects aged over 35 years with a chronic cough and a smoking history [1]. It is important to be alert to the significance of these symptoms, which otherwise may be attributed to the effects of age, or dismissed as merely a "smoker's cough." Once COPD is established there is little short-term variation, but there is a progressive decline in the longer term (though the course may be punctuated by short-term exacerbations).

Breathlessness may be categorised by the MRC breathlessness scale (Table 4.2). Confusingly, the GOLD guidelines use a modified score, the mMRC. The categories are the same, but use a scale of 0–4 rather than 1–5.

Other clinical factors are determined largely by co-morbidity, but a key factor is that limitation of activity (in terms of ordinary daily activity as opposed to exercise) is curtailed even in Stage 1 disease. This reduction is independently linked to mortality. COPD also leads to a marked reduction in health-related quality of life, which is

rather loosely though statistically significantly linked to disease severity as scored by FEV_1.

In addition to smoking, a history of workplace exposure to dust and chemicals, for instance in the mining and steel industries, may make a significant contribution [10].

Exacerbations

According to NICE, "an exacerbation is a sustained worsening of the patient's symptoms from their usual stable state which is beyond normal day-to-day variations, and is acute in onset. Commonly reported symptoms are worsening breathlessness, cough, increased sputum production and change in sputum colour. The change in these symptoms often necessitates a change in medication" [1]. Whilst clinically what this means may be apparent on a day-to-day basis, the definition is imprecise; the change is a subjective difference from baseline. Further, a circular argument ensues if deciding whether an exacerbation requires treatment when the requirement for treatment is within the definition. Additionally, severity has traditionally been judged on criteria including the necessity for hospital admission, but with changing medical practice this alters with time, and is contingent on social as well as pathological factors. In order to define exacerbations more objectively, diaries such as ExactPro® have been developed. These have made it clear that in addition to traditionally recognised clearcut exacerbations, there are frequent selfterminating milder exacerbations, often not reported to healthcare professionals, and that these have an adverse overall impact on healthrelated quality of life.

The ECLIPSE (Evaluation of COPD Longitudinally to Identify Predictive Surrogate Endpoints) cohort hoped to identify predictive factors for exacerbation, but was somewhat disappointing. What it did establish was the "exacerbator phenotype." Whilst exacerbations became more frequent with increasing disease severity as judged by FEV_1, even in mild disease, exacerbations were found. Importantly, those who exacerbated in 1 year were likely to exacerbate the

Table 4.2 MRC and mMRC breathlessness scales

Scale Score	Scale Score	Description
MRC 1	mMRC 0	Excess breathlessness on marked exertion
MRC 2	mMRC 1	Breathlessness on hills
MRC 3	mMRC 2	Breathlessness limiting speed or necessitating stopping on the flat
MRC 4	mMRC 3	Exercise limited to 100–200 m on the flat
MRC 5	mMRC 4	Housebound or breathlessness on activities of daily living

next and *vice versa*. One of the few other predictors of exacerbations was the presence of gastro-oesophageal reflux [9].

Exacerbations may be caused by a variety of common respiratory viruses, by bacteria (particularly *Haemophilus influenza*, and also Moraxella and pneumococci, though occasionally Pseudomonas and other opportunistic pathogens are implicated), and by environmental triggers such as particulates and oxides of nitrogen and sulphur. Much of the economic burden of COPD is due to the cost of treating exacerbations. For patients, they cause not only increased symptoms and decreased quality of life, but also have an independent negative prognostic impact [11]. Indeed, for patients admitted to hospital with an acute exacerbation of COPD, all cause of mortality is higher than for those admitted with an acute myocardial infarction. Although median time to recovery of symptoms is 7 days, peak flow fails to recover to baseline in 7% of subjects at 91 days. This prolonged perturbation is also reflected in mortality figures, with excess mortality persisting after discharge in those admitted to hospital for an exacerbation. Formerly it was thought that exacerbations were "bad luck" events occurring largely by chance, but it has become clear they are in fact clustered; one exacerbation is often followed by another, with further long-term impact.

Co-morbidity

The fact that COPD presents in older smokers means it is no surprise to find evidence of other smoking-related diseases such as heart disease and cancer. However, it has become apparent that a number of conditions are present in patients with COPD above and beyond that expected when allowing for these shared risk factors. These diseases include ischaemic heart disease and heart failure, osteoporosis, renal disease, and diabetes. Two possible mechanisms have been suggested to account for this. Firstly, COPD is associated with uncontrolled inflammation within

the lung and it is suggested that this "spills over" from the lung, causing chronic systemic exposure to inflammatory mediators with passive bystander damage. Perhaps more likely is that there is a shared genetic predisposition to chronic and excessive inflammation at different sites. Only one-quarter to one-third of smokers develop COPD, suggesting a genetic background leading to "sensitive lungs" in which excessive and uncontrolled inflammation occur in response to the noxious stimulus of cigarette smoke. In this model an individual's genetic background will predispose to excess inflammatory response not only to cigarette smoke in the lungs, but also to lipid deposition in inflammatory atherosclerotic plaques with accelerated coronary artery disease, and so on through the body. The genetic background is highlighted in alpha-1 antitrypsin deficiency. Smokers who are homozygous for this autosomal recessive condition develop early emphysema and indeed, non-smoking subjects may develop emphysema. However, usually the predisposition is polygenetic, and efforts to characterise an individual's genetic risk have yet to be successful.

In assessing and treating individuals with COPD it is important to proactively seek co-morbidity and to treat it in its own right. This may cause important diagnostic challenges; for example the patient with ischaemic heart disease may have breathlessness and chest tightness, but both are common in COPD. Indeed, breathlessness is a cardinal feature of COPD, but exertional discomfort is common too, due to musculoskeletal pain from a hyperexpanded rib cage working at mechanical disadvantage. This is usually not absolutely exercise limiting, and lacks the characteristic radiation of cardiac pain, but tends to persist much longer after exercise (15–60 min). However, the distinction may be challenging clinically. The importance of assessing co-morbidity is emphasised by the TORCH study [12]. This failed to conclusively demonstrate a prognostic benefit from treatment with an inhaled steroid/LABA combination but did critically assess the cause of death in a large cohort of subjects with an FEV_1 less than half predicted during 3 years of follow-up. Here, only about a third of deaths were due to respiratory failure, with a similar number due to cardiac disease, and about a fifth due to cancers.

There are a number of particularly important extra-pulmonary complications. Whilst inactivity may promote obesity, a more common problem is weight loss, and in particular loss of fat-free mass. Best prognosis is found in those slightly overweight (BMI 25–30), with marked fall with a BMI lower than 20, which is dramatic with a BMI under 15. Recent weight loss is particularly important, whilst a loss of weight during an admission is a predictor of early re-admission.

Whilst in early COPD patients are normoxic, in more severe disease, chronic hypoxia may arise with its own complications. Respiratory failure is defined as a PaO_2 of <8 kPa on air, and is divided into type 1 respiratory failure in which the PaCO2 is normal or low, and type 2 with a high PaCO2.

Respiratory failure (particularly type 2) may give rise to *cor pulmonale* or "right-sided heart failure." Here there is fluid retention with oedema, ascites, and pleural effusions, and an elevated pulmonary artery pressure. Though referred to as "heart failure" the cardiac output is in fact well preserved unless there is co existent left ventricular systolic dysfunction. Although the pulmonary artery pressure is modestly elevated, it rarely exceeds systolic pressures greater than 40–50 mmHg. On the occasions it is substantially more than this, then the prognosis is poor.

Depression and anxiety are common accompaniments of COPD. Whilst it may appear no surprise that those with unpleasant symptoms and activity limitation develop these symptoms, subjects with high anxiety and depression levels have increased symptoms and decreased activity compared to others with similar physical disease, are less concordant with medications, and participate less well in pulmonary rehabilitation and self-management plans. Depression and anxiety are independently associated with poor prognosis.

Epidemiology and Natural History

The global burden of COPD is discussed in the GOLD guidelines, which note self-reported COPD (i.e. people report they have been given this diagnosis) in around 6% of the population in most countries. However, as COPD is often not diagnosed, particularly (but not exclusively) in milder cases, this is no doubt an underestimate. Careful studies in some countries (e.g. Montevideo, Uruguay) report an incidence approaching 20%. In 1990 COPD was thought to be the sixth ranked cause of death worldwide, and it is projected to rise to third with better control of other diseases alongside the expansion of tobacco use in the global south [2].

The definition of COPD used by NICE includes the statement that it is usually progressive [1]. However, recent studies show that it is less predictable [3]. A cohort followed for 3 years revealed that though some showed gradual deterioration (in terms of FEV_1), others deteriorated rapidly, whilst others remained stable or even improved. However, it has not proved possible to differentiate these groups prospectively. Likewise, as discussed earlier, there is a frequent exacerbator phenotype which is difficult to segregate other than by exacerbation history. Whilst in population terms mortality is high, individual survival may be prolonged, even with severe disease. In the TORCH study designed to look at the effect of treatment on mortality, the subjects had, on average, an FEV_1 of under a half predicted and yet 3-year survival was 85% [12]. In our own unpublished audit of 450 subjects commenced on long-term oxygen therapy for severe COPD with respiratory failure, median survival was about 3.5 years, with 15–20% showing prolonged survival, which is of the same order as many cancers treated with radical intent.

Examination

The cardinal feature of COPD is hyperexpansion of the chest, with an increase antero-posterior dimension apparent as a barrel-shaped chest. The hyoid cartilage is closer to the sternal notch and the area of hepatic dullness may be displaced downwards. The area of cardiac dullness may be diminished. The chest is hyper-resonant, and on auscultation there may be some expiratory wheezes. The term "poor air entry" should be avoided; breath sounds are often quiet, but this may reflect obesity or complications such as pneumothorax.

Hands may show signs of tar staining. Clubbing is not a feature of COPD and should prompt a search for neoplasia. There may be tachypnoea, tachycardia, and signs of CO_2 retention (a coarse flap and altered consciousness). *Cor pulmonale* and pulmonary hypertension may result in a raised JVP, peripheral oedema (and possibly ascites and/or pleural effusion), a right ventricular heave, and a loud P2 on cardiac auscultation. Cardiac signs may be masked by hyperexpanded lung interposed between the heart and the chest wall.

Pathology and Pathogenesis

As noted, COPD is an imprecise term for a collection of conditions, rather than being a unique disease. As such, its pathological appearance is varied [13].

Emphysema relates to destruction of lung parenchyma; the alveoli and respiratory bronchioles in the commoner centrilobular pattern, or more widespread in panacinar emphysema. Confluent areas of destruction may cause macroscopic bullae.

Bronchitis is characterised by submucosal bronchial gland enlargement and goblet cell metaplasia, with mucus hypersecretion. Bronchial glands are inflamed. There is airway epithelial squamous metaplasia, ciliary dysfunction, and hypertrophy of smooth muscle and connective tissue.

The involvement of the smaller airways (<2 mm) is crucial. They are involved early and represent the major site of airflow obstruction, with peribronchial fibrosis and airway narrowing and obliteration. There is inflammation with exudates, goblet cell proliferation, and squamous metaplasia.

The pulmonary vasculature exhibits intimal thickening and endothelial destruction, with later hypertrophy of vascular smooth muscle and collagen deposition, with progressive obliteration of the capillary bed.

Inflammatory changes are found in all these areas. The role of neutrophils has been emphasised mechanistically. In alpha-1-antitrypsin deficiency, neutrophil proteases are not opposed, with resultant tissue destruction and emphysema. However, analogous imbalances are usually difficult to demonstrate in COPD without such specific deficiency. Oxidant damage is important too, both directly and indirectly by modification of proteases and anti-proteases, the complex balance being crucial.

Traditionally, as well as the importance of neutrophils, the controlling role of macrophages and CD8 lymphocytes have been emphasised. This is contrasted with the eosinophilic inflammation and CD4 positive lymphocytes in asthma. However, there is increasing recognition that this is an oversimplification, and a subset of those with COPD may have eosinophilic inflammation too.

Investigations

Pulmonary Function Tests

Spirometry is central to the diagnosis of COPD. NICE [1] and GOLD [2] guidelines characterise airflow obstruction as being an essential component of the disease, requiring the FEV_1/ VC post bronchodilator ratio to be <0.7. However, this ratio is age-dependent and, in terms of symptoms, may overdiagnose the elderly and underdiagnose younger subjects. FEV_1 is also used to classify disease. In each case obstruction must be demonstrated. If the FEV_1 is >80% (with symptoms of disease) this is mild (stage 1). In stage 2 (moderate) it is 50–79% predicted, stage 3 (severe) 30–49%, and severe 29% or less. Classically acute reversibility testing may help differentiate COPD from asthma, with a threshold of a 400 ml improvement in FEV_1 taken as suggestive of asthma. However, there is no sharp cut-off in the degree of FEV_1 change between the two diseases, and reversibility may vary when tested on different days. A number of screening tests such as FEV_6 are available, but should always be backed up by definitive spirometry. Mid-expiratory flows may be affected early in disease, but measurements are poorly reproducible. Oscillometry and multiple-breath gas washout techniques are appealing, as they may selectively measure small airways disease thought to be important in early COPD, but are more complex and not widely used in routine clinical practice.

Fractional expired nitric oxide (FeNO) may help to demonstrate eosinophilic inflammation, but its utility is limited in active smokers.

Alveolar destruction and vascular changes result in poor $V/\dot{Q}$ matching, resulting in a low transfer factor and transfer coefficient (TL_{co} and K_{co}), particularly in emphysematous disease. Hyperexpansion is demonstrated by a large TLC, and gas trapping by a raised RV and RV/TLC. Normally tidal inspiratory and expiratory flow are considerably submaximal and occur at a relaxed lung volume.

With exercise, flow is easily increased, allowing both greater respiratory rate and tidal flow. In COPD there is loss of lung elasticity. Though the increase in intrathoracic pressure occurring during expiration tends to collapse the airways, the lung elasticity splints the airways open. The loss of elasticity in COPD means there is increased airways collapse and this may become flow-limiting at a given lung volume. Increased flow can only be obtained by moving up the flow volume curve to higher volumes, which increases work of breathing and is uncomfortable: a feature known as dynamic hyperexpansion [14]. Complex methodologies may be used in research contexts to study this, but most simply hyperexpansion can be tracked by a fall in inspiratory capacity (IC). This fall in IC (and its change with exercise) is one of the best correlates with decreased exercise capacity and symptoms in COPD. However, its measurement is exacting and is not used in routine clinical practice.

Transcutaneous pulse oximetry is a basic part of assessment of patients with COPD, particular during exacerbations. However, it gives no information on pH or $PaCO_2$, so a low reading requires measurement of blood gases. The gold standard is arterial blood gas measurement, though capillary blood gas measurement is less invasive and has increased patient acceptability, so may be preferred in non-critical situations.

Radiology

Plain chest radiographs may show increased lucency in areas of emphysema or bullae, or diaphragms that are low and flattened, hyperexpansion, and a narrow cardiac silhouette. None of these are pathognomonic and depend on technical factors and body habitus. The main utility of plain radiology in COPD is to identify other factors such as lung cancer, pneumonia, pneumothorax, and heart failure.

Computed tomography (CT) demonstrates areas of emphysema as areas with low Hounsfield units. This may be useful in diagnosis and in planning surgical treatment. Complications such as bronchiectasis and lung cancer can be identified.

Lung perfusion scans may be useful in planning either bulla or lung cancer surgery, identifying poorly perfused areas that can be safely sacrificed. Routine magnetic resonance imaging (MRI) produce poor lung images, as they are proton poor. Coils can instead be tuned to inhaled hyperpolarised inert gases, producing images of gas flow within the lungs, but this remains a research technique.

Blood Tests

Full blood counts may demonstrate anaemia as a cause of dyspnoea, or neutrophilia suggesting infection. A raised blood eosinophil count (for example, $\geq 2\%$, or above the upper quartile of the normal range) of the total leukocyte count may suggest steroid-responsive disease [8].

Alpha-1-antitrypsin levels may be depressed in this inherited disorder. They may be somewhat low in clinically insignificant heterozygous deficiency, or elevated as part of an acute phase response, so suspect levels should be confirmed by genotyping.

Sputum

Sputum tests may be useful in identifying pathogens in exacerbations, particularly if there has been a failure in treatment. They are not necessarily indicated for isolated exacerbations [1]. In stable disease the airways often contain bacteria. These may be regarded as colonising when there are no clinical signs of exacerbation such as sputum purulence and increased dyspnoea. Though such colonisation may be associated with poorer clinical outcomes, attempts to eradicate bacteria may prove futile, and careful clinical judgement is required.

Exercise Tests

Field exercise tests such as the incremental and endurance shuttle walking tests and the 6-minute walk may be useful in quantifying disability. They are relatively time consuming and other tests, such as sit-to-stand tests, are being investigated. Full cardiopulmonary exercise testing will more formally demonstrate exercise limitation and may occasionally be useful for differentiating cardiac and pulmonary causes of dyspnoea.

Quality of Life (QoL) Scores

Though spirometry is the mainstay of COPD diagnosis, the relationship of quality of life (QoL) scores with FEV_1 is poor (though statistically significant). Questionnaires such as the St. George's Respiratory Questionnaire and the Chronic Respiratory Questionnaire are too

cumbersome for routine clinical practice. The COPD Assessment Test (CAT) is a simple eight-question, self-fill questionnaire that is more practical and sensitive to change with exacerbations and interventions, and is reproducible. It forms a useful part of routine assessment.

Composite Scores

The recognition that COPD is a multi-component disease poorly described by FEV_1 alone has led to the development of a number of composite scores. The best known of these is the BODE score, which gives categorical scores which are then summed for body mass index (B), FEV_1 as a measure of obstruction (O), dyspnoea measured by the mMRC score (D), and 6-min walking distance as a measure of exercise capacity (E) (Table 4.3). In populations BODE score is a better mortality predictor than individual components, but for individuals the confidence intervals are broad. However, the predictive power of a change in BODE score in response to an intervention has not been demonstrated, and the accuracy may vary in different populations. As they are categorical, small clinical changes may produce a large change in BODE score and *vice versa*. Thus the utility of such composite scores for individuals is limited.

Table 4.3 BODE score: composite score for prognostic prediction in COPD

Score	0	1	2	3
FEV_1 (% predicted)	≥65	50–64	36–49	≤35
6 MWD	≥350	250–349	150–249	≤149
mMRC	0–1	2	3	4
BMI	>21	≤21		

BMI Body Mass Index (B—BMI), *FEV₁* FEV₁% predicted (O—Obstruction), *mMRC* modified MRC breathlessness score (D—Dyspnoea), *6 MWD* 6 min walking distance in metres (E—Exercise capacity)
Each component is scored, the result summed and the 4-year survival is given below:
0–2 Points: 80%
3–4 Points: 67%
5–6 Points: 57%
7–10 Points: 18%

Differential Diagnosis

Classically, the main differential diagnosis is from asthma. COPD is regarded as fixed airflow obstruction that is slowly progressive in time with little day-to-day or diurnal variation. It is without an allergic component, and whilst there is exercise limitation, post-exercise symptoms are not a feature. Asthma shows short-term and diurnal variation, including in response to short-term treatment or provocative changes (e.g. mannitol or methacholine). Nocturnal and post-exercise symptoms are characteristic. An allergic component is common. COPD tends to arise in the fifth decade or later in smokers, whilst asthma often arises earlier in life, often without any history of smoking. Whilst these distinctions appear clear cut in many text books and guidelines, in clinical practice there are many grey areas. ACOS (asthma/COPD overlap syndrome) is a term coined to cover such areas, but it is unclear whether this truly identifies a distinct group of patients or better guides clinical management. Pragmatically what matters is a diagnostic classification which will help predict treatment response and prognosis. As discussed in the introduction, the current classification does this poorly, and in the future diagnoses based on endotypes are likely to become more common.

Other causes of dyspnoea must be distinguished. Cardiac disease shares age and smoking as risk factors as well as being a disproportionately common co-morbidity. Orthopnoea may suggest cardiac disease but is often present in COPD. Ankle swelling may be part of *cor pulmonale* rather than left-sided heart disease. Exertional chest pain due to musculoskeletal factors resulting from hyperexpansion in COPD and to angina may be difficult to interpret. Exercise electrocardiograms may be non-diagnostic in the dyspnoeic patient of whatever cause, and radionuclide scans may be necessary to demonstrate ischaemia. Measurement of serum BNP may be useful, but may be elevated in left or right sided heart failure. Echocardiography may be limited by poor acoustic windows. Invasive diagnostic procedures may be required.

Some series suggest thromboembolic disease is particularly common in patients with COPD, and CT pulmonary angiography should be considered in patients with exacerbations failing to respond to treatment, especially in the absence of infective symptoms such as altered sputum.

Lung cancer also shares risk factors with COPD and is common. Haemoptysis or clubbing should prompt a search for neoplasia. Patients with COPD often lose weight. Judging when to investigate this separately is a difficult judgement, but a change in weight trajectory, especially with systemic malaise and anorexia, should be viewed with suspicion.

Patients with chronic sputum production and frequent infections should be investigated for bronchiectasis. Some minor degree of bronchiectasis is exceptionally common in COPD and not necessarily of separate significance, but definite bronchiectasis requires additional attention, including a search for underlying factors such as immune deficiency, aspergillus, atypical mycobacteria, rheumatoid arthritis etc. (see Chap. 11).

Interstitial lung disease is easy to overlook. Classically in obstructive lung disease, the FEV_1 is reduced but the VC is preserved. However, as the RV is often very high, this encroaches on VC, which may be relatively reduced. Further, subjects may be unable to breathe out long enough to reach VC, or the manoeuvre may be incomplete because of cough. Thus, it may be difficult to spot coexistent restriction. Patients with interstitial lung disease may be clubbed, have basal crackles on auscultation, and may have an abnormal chest radiograph, but if there is doubt, then extended lung function tests and computed tomography will be required. Some literature reports combined pulmonary fibrosis and emphysema as an entity. However, radiologically, pathologically, and physiologically, the abnormalities are as would be expected as the sum of each disease. As COPD is extremely common, it would be no surprise were some people with interstitial lung disease to have COPD too, and it is not clear this represents a truly distinct condition.

Treatments

Strategy and Guidelines

Space precludes full discussion of all treatments. This section provides a commentary to provide a framework and to understand the approach to therapy. Available clinical guidelines contain executive summaries which should be consulted in conjunction with this chapter [1, 2].

As lung damage in COPD is permanent and largely irreversible, management of COPD should always consider harm reduction first, with smoking cessation and vaccination. Pulmonary rehabilitation is more efficacious than drug treatment and should receive the highest priority, as should attention to diet, social care, and psychological well-being.

Guidelines contain quite extensive algorithms for the pharmacological treatment of COPD. In general, long-term drugs are used with two aims: to relieve symptoms of dyspnoea (and thus to increase activity and exercise capacity), and to prevent exacerbations. The NICE guidelines utilise a scheme based primarily on FEV_1 to do this. All patients are offered a short-acting bronchodilator. For those with an FEV_1 above 50% predicted, a long-acting bronchodilator is recommended if there are persistent symptoms and/or there are frequent exacerbations. For those with a lower FEV_1, long-acting bronchodilators are recommended for those with persistent dyspnoea despite short-acting bronchodilators. However, if there are frequent exacerbations, a combination long-acting beta-2 agonist and inhaled corticosteroid (LABA/ICS) is recommended. Other drug classes may be added if there is a failure of these additional recommendations.

GOLD guidelines attempt a more nuanced approach. In fact the differences between the two guidelines are often overemphasised, as most patients will receive similar treatment whichever guide is utilised. GOLD seeks to recognise that FEV_1 is not a full descriptor of disease, so stratifies patients into symptoms (using dyspnoea and/or CAT score) and "risk" (using exacerbation history and/or severity of airflow obstruction) (Fig. 4.1). Four groups are thus defined: low symptom/low risk (A), high symptom/low risk (B), low symptom/high risk (C) and high symptom/high risk (D). In practice there are rather few patients in group C, and there isn't a simple progression through groups as disease advances in the individual. The categories are less discriminating for prognosis compared to the classification using airflow obstruction alone, as in classification of disease severity by NICE. Nevertheless, this can provide a relatively simple guide to treatment (see guidelines).

Smoking Cessation

Any discussion of treatment of COPD must commence by addressing smoking. No other treatment has been shown to alter disease progression, so are of subsidiary importance. Smoking status should be checked at all reviews, with psychological and pharmacological support easily available.

Organisation of Care

Self-management

In chronic disease, the volume of the task for health care systems as well as patient advocacy has encouraged self-management strategies. In many cases (such as asthma) there is no doubt about the value of such approaches. It has proved much harder to prove self-management has a helpful impact in COPD, with contradictory evidence from available trials. Brief interventions seem futile; success in initiating self-management seems to require much more complex and prolonged education and support.

Strategies particularly focusing on patients having a reserve supply of steroids and antibiotics to initiate in the event of an exacerbation has become the standard of care. Limited evidence exists on the efficacy of this, showing such provision increases utilisation of steroids and antibiotics but without a decrease in use of health care resources or improvement of quality of life. Such provision needs ongoing active monitoring to ensure treatment is used appropriately.

Supported Discharge and Hospital at Home

Antibiotics, steroids and bronchodilators are easily and conveniently delivered in a domiciliary setting. This has encouraged the development of admissions avoidance/hospital at home/supported discharge services which have demonstrated that around a third of patients traditionally admitted to hospital for an exacerbation can be safely and effectively treated at home with adequate monitoring (though around 10% of these will require re-admission as a result of such monitoring). The ability to manage many patients at home depends as much on social support (the ability to cope with daily living) as strictly medical factors.

Telehealth

In many chronic diseases, the use of Telehealth has produced improvements in health. The evidence in COPD is much less secure. This may be because physiological changes do not necessarily antedate a change in symptoms during an exacerbation. If patients are unwell they know this without the need for technology to tell them. Calculations of cost per QALY suggest prohibitive expense. These calculations are based on older, more complex systems. More recent interest centres on far simpler ways of using technology to support self-management, and prompt and remind subjects of appropriate actions.

Non-pharmacological Treatments

Vaccinations

All patients should receive annual influenza vaccination. They should receive a single vaccination against pneumococci.

Pulmonary Rehabilitation

Pulmonary rehabilitation is secondary only to smoking cessation in treatment of COPD [15]. It is a clearly cost-effective treatment, producing impressive improvements in exercise capacity and quality of life, with a decrease in dyspnoea and decrease in anxiety. Inpatient bed days are reduced in the year after pulmonary rehabilita-

tion. The treatment is based on the premise that a decrease in exercise due to dyspnoea produces physical deconditioning, with a further decrease in exercise capacity, a downward spiral being established. A mix of aerobic and strength training reverses this, with classes taking place as a group for two or more sessions per week over 6–8 weeks. The socializing and re-integration of the group may have additional benefits that are difficult to quantify.

Pulmonary rehabilitation is conventionally considered in all with MRC3 breathlessness or worse, but should be offered to all who consider themselves functionally limited. A repeat course should be considered annually as routine. An acute exacerbation is likely to produce accelerated functional loss, so services should be organised to allow early rehabilitation afterwards.

The main limitation of pulmonary rehabilitation is that only two-thirds of those appropriately offered a course will accept it, with further patients dropping out during the course. Acceptance is promoted by positive presentation of benefits by the referring health care professional. It is reduced by transport and access problems, and by depression (though depression is alleviated in those who attend). There are few contraindications. Recent myocardial infarction and unstable cardiac disease are the most important. Musculoskeletal problems and problems working in groups are relative contraindications.

Pharmacological Treatments, Oxygen and Ventilatory Support

Beta₂ Agonists

Beta$_2$ agonists can be conveniently divided into short- (SABA) and long-acting agents (LABA). The former (which include salbutamol and terbutaline) are the workhorses of drug treatment in COPD. They provide rapid onset bronchodilation, relieving breathlessness within a few minutes, with an effect persisting for 4–6 h. However, they have no long-term action in terms of preventing exacerbations or altering natural history of disease. LABAs (including salmeterol, formoterol, indacaterol, olodaterol and vilanterol) not only produce broncho-dilation and relieve breathlessness, but also lead to improvement in overall quality of life and reduce exacerbation frequency. The first two are administered twice per day, the others daily. Salmeterol is a partial agonist with a slow onset of action and a dose-response curve which plateaus early, so it has a less favourable profile. All act via β_2 adrenergic receptors on bronchial smooth muscle cells, leading to a rise in intracellular cyclic AMP by activation of G protein-linked adenylyl cyclase. Vilanterol is only available as a combined product with fluticasone fumarate. NICE guidelines suggest LABAs are used to treat breathlessness that persists despite short-acting agents, or for the prevention of exacerbations in those with an FEV_1 greater than 50% predicted (or for exacerbators with poor lung function in the form of LABA/ICS) [1]. There has been concern about possible adverse effects of LABAs in asthma. They are clearly dangerous in asthma if used instead of ICS, but it remains unproven if there are detrimental effects above and beyond this. However, this concern resulted in vilanterol not being available as monotherapy. LABAs appear in practice to be very safe in COPD but may give tachycardia and tremor, and worsen angina, heart failure, and thyrotoxicosis.

Anticholinergics

Anticholinergics can also be divided into short-acting agents (SAMA) and long-acting agents (LAMA). The former are somewhat slower in onset of action than SABAs and act for 6–8 h. Like SABAs they have no appreciable long-term effects, but have useful short-term bronchodilator actions which relieve breathlessness. As their onset in action is slower than SABAs, they tend to be used regularly rather than on an "as required" basis. They act by blocking muscarinic receptors on bronchial smooth muscle myocytes, reducing the bronchoconstrictor action of the vagus nerve. In the case of the LAMAs, there is some selectivity for the M3 receptor, with less blockade of the pre-ganglionic M1 receptors, leaving negative feedback inhibition intact. All reduce exacerbations and improve indices of

quality of life, in addition to producing broncho-dilation and relieving breathlessness. Aclidinium is given twice per day, whereas tiotropium (the archetypal class member), glycopyrronium, and umeclidinium are given once daily. NICE guidelines suggest LAMA are used to treat breathlessness that persists despite short-acting agents, or for the prevention of exacerbation in those with an FEV1 greater than 50% predicted (or for exacerbators with poor lung function in whom LABA/ICS has failed to produce control, or in whom ICS cannot be used). NICE guidelines do not suggest a preference for LAMA or LABA, but the former are marginally more efficacious. Generally speaking, these are safe drugs, but trials have usually excluded those with a history of recent onset or unstable cardiac disease. Theoretically drugs could have a detrimental effect in these cases, and a safety notice mandates caution in such cases in the UK. Dual LAMA/LABA bronchodilator inhalers lead to 60–70% more bronchodilatation than either of the mono-components and have become a popular first-line therapy in COPD.

Steroids

With the appreciation that COPD involves ongoing inflammation, a number of trials of inhaled steroids were carried out to see if their anti-inflammatory action would reduce the rate of progression of lung disease (measured as FEV_1). These were uniformly negative. However, the reputation of inhaled steroids was rescued when the ISOLDE trial demonstrated that though the FEV_1 decline was not altered over time, the rate of decline of quality of life was reduced, and this was linked to a reduction in exacerbation frequency. This trial studied those with an FEV_1 of less than 50% predicted. On this basis, inhaled steroids are recommended by NICE guidelines for those with exacerbations and an FEV_1 of <50% [1]. Subsequent trials, however, have suggested benefit in those with better FEV_1. They appear synergistic with LABA and currently both GOLD and NICE guidelines advocate use of ICS only with LABA and not as sole maintenance therapy [1, 2, 12]. Similar research findings have validated the use of fluticasone/salmeterol, budesonide/formoterol, beclomethasone/formoterol, and fluticasone/vilanterol.

Whilst showing the efficacy of these drugs, recent trials have also revealed that although overall exacerbation frequency is reduced, there is an excess of pneumonias. These are more common in the elderly, those with severe disease, and those with a past history of pneumonia. Overall these seem mild and not associated with excess mortality (except with fluticasone/vilanterol in a dose higher than that licenced). In view of these concerns, the WISDOM trial took subjects with severe COPD treated with LABA/LAMA/ICS combination and carried out a staged withdrawal of ICS and showed no excess of exacerbations over a year (though a slight and perhaps insignificant decline in FEV_1). This has encouraged a reappraisal of the role of ICS. Recent reanalysis of seminal trials establishing the role of ICS suggest that the benefit of ICS may be confined to those with an eosinophil count of $\geq 2\%$ of peripheral blood leukocytes at the start of the trial. This is within what is usually regarded as the normal range and represents a significant proportion of COPD patients. Risk of exacerbation and steroid-responsiveness in COPD stratify with blood eosinophil count—those with low eosinophil counts (the majority of those with COPD) seem not to benefit from ICS treatment, whilst the most benefit is seen in those with the highest counts. Whilst there are few prospective interventional trials to support this conclusively, the available evidence is consistent and persuasive, but yet to be recognised in major guidelines. Eosinophilic inflammation and steroid response is traditionally associated with asthma, and this finding is one that lends support for the re-examination of disease categorisation aligned to disease endotypes in COPD.

Theophyllines

Theophyllines are adenosine antagonists and also inhibit phosphodiesterase, leading to an increase in intracellular cyclic AMP. They have fallen into disfavour, due to a high incidence of side effects (headache, nausea, diarrhoea, and dysrhythmias) and many drug interaction via the cytochrome P450 system. Their narrow therapeutic index necessitates monitoring of blood levels, adding to complexity. Histone deacetylase-2 (HDAC2) suppresses inflammatory gene activity but is reduced in smokers and patients with COPD, perhaps preventing corticosteroids from suppressing airway inflammation. *In vitro* theophyllines restore histone deacetylase (HDAC) activity. Clinical trials have failed to demonstrate that this theoretical benefit is useful clinically.

Phosphodiesterase Type 4 (PDE4) Inhibitors

PDE4 inhibitors target the phosphodiesterase in bronchial smooth muscle and inflammatory cells (macrophages and neutrophils) that are relevant to COPD. Their selectivity means they have a better therapeutic window compared to non-selective agents. Trials show they reduce exacerbation frequency, but only in those with chronic sputum production. However, they have no overall beneficial effect on QoL, meaning they have not been approved by NICE in the UK and are unfunded, though available elsewhere in the world. The main side effect is weight loss, though this appears to plateau, and fat-free mass is relatively well preserved.

Macrolides and Long-Term Antibiotics

Long-term antibiotics have been used in COPD in an effort to prevent exacerbations. However, little evidence supports this, and it risks development of resistance and it is not recommended. An exception to this is macrolides, where trials of erythromycin and azithromycin have shown clear reductions in exacerbation frequency (though subgroup analysis suggests this is not the case in continued smokers). The anti-inflammatory actions of macrolides are likely to be crucial to this effect, but there is again concern about widespread use leading to resistance. They are not recommended in current guidelines, though are being increasingly used in routine practice. Erythromycin is used at the low dose of 250 mg bd, which limits side effects, but drug interactions (particularly statins) may be an issue in patients requiring drug treatments for multiple comorbidities. In trials azithromycin has mostly been used at 250 mg daily, and this is associated with a significant incidence of high-frequency hearing loss. Macrolides prolong the QT interval, and caution is advised in patients predisposed by medication or risk factors for dysrhythmias.

Mucolytics

There is conflicting evidence on the use of mucolytics long term to reduce exacerbation frequency. They may provide symptomatic benefit by allowing ease of expectoration of mucus, and a therapeutic trial may be carried out.

Domiciliary Oxygen and Non-invasive Ventilation

Those with established hypoxaemia derive prognostic benefit from prolonged oxygen treatment. UK guidelines specify this should be provided for those with a $PaO_2 < 7.3$ kPa whilst stable and breathing air, on two occasions at least 2 weeks apart [16]. These criteria are relaxed to 8 kPa for those with signs of end organ damage such as cor pulmonale or secondary polycythaemia. Oxygen should be titrated to produce a PaO_2 of 8 kPa, and used for >15 h each day, usually including overnight use. It is provided by the use of an oxygen concentrator, with backup cylinders. On occasion adequate oxygenation cannot be produced without causing an unacceptable rise in pCO_2, and fall in pH. Patients with symptoms of nocturnal hypoventilation and persistent hypercapnia might be considered for a trial of domiciliary nocturnal positive pressure ventilation.

Oxygen therapy has not been shown to relieve breathlessness except in those with significant hypoxaemia. Ambulatory oxygen to abolish hypoxaemia on exercise may reduce symptoms and increase exercise capacity. Oxygen can be provided for those patients with exercise-induced hypoxaemia who improve exercise capacity and/or decrease symptoms in formal exercise tests, though precise thresholds are not specified and, indeed, short-term benefits have not been shown to correlate with longer term QoL benefits.

Opiates and Benzodiazepines

Despite optimisation of all other therapies, some patients may still have distressing breathlessness. Low-dose opiates (10–20 mg of slow-release morphine twice per day) or lorazepam (0.5 mg taken sublingually prn) may relieve the sensation of breathlessness. Whilst in subjects with low (or indeed normal) carbon dioxide levels these are very safe, they are respiratory depressants and some caution is required in those with type 2 respiratory failure. Some risk may be acceptable in those clearly approaching the end of life.

Investigational Treatments

Though there is a long list of treatments in COPD, there is a frustration that even with the best of these, while exacerbations are reduced, they still continue and there has been little if any impact on rate of decline of disease and prognosis. With the understanding of COPD as an inflammatory disease there is an interest in targeting underlying mechanisms, including endotypic targeting, and the use of these earlier in disease to prevent progression before damage is done. These include MAP kinase inhibitors, CXCR2 antagonists, eosinophil and IL-5 antagonists, and others. Whilst some show promise, to date there have been problems with toxicity which have thwarted their utility.

Interventional Treatments

Lung Volume Reduction Surgery (LVRS)

The lung in COPD loses elasticity. Resultant hyperexpansion and gas trapping gives a mechanical mismatch between the chest wall and the lungs. Volume reduction surgery aims to remove particularly damaged areas of the lung which contribute little useful function, with the diaphragm, other respiratory muscles, and the chest wall able to work at better mechanical advantage. The pivotal NETT trial compared optimal medical therapy with surgery (bilateral via sternotomy or thoracoscopy). The primary end point of the trial (prognostic benefit of surgery) was not met. However, exploratory analysis suggested a benefit in those with upper lobe predominant emphysema and poor exercise capacity and prognostic detriment where the opposite conditions pertained. Those with either poor exercise capacity or upper lobe predominant emphysema (but not both) derived a variable amount of symptomatic benefit.

Applicability of this technique is limited, as only a small subgroup of people with COPD are fit for major surgery. Even in carefully selected subjects there is an acute mortality rate of 2% or 3%, and though groups likely to benefit can be identified, individual success is variable.

Endoscopic Volume Reduction Surgery and Associated Techniques

Endobronchial valves aim to produce the same physiological effects as LVRS but utilising minimally invasive techniques. They are placed endoscopically in bronchi supplying target lung, allowing air to leave but not return, resulting in segmental or lobar collapse. Collateral ventila-

tion within the lung will cause this to fail, and may be predicted if there are incomplete fissures on CT scan, or directly measured by endobronchial catheter pressure/flow measurement using Chartis® (see Fig. 4.2 for research imaging of collateral ventilation). Target areas can be identified using CT to show areas of maximal emphysema, with perfusion scanning showing areas with poor blood supply. Physiologically, those with high TLC and RV are most likely to benefit.

A randomised control trial of treatment versus sham bronchoscopy shows good improvements of lung function and quality of life. However, scrutiny of individual results shows a subgroup little changed by treatment, whilst others gain a substantial improvement. It is unclear how to differentiate these in advance. However, this is a

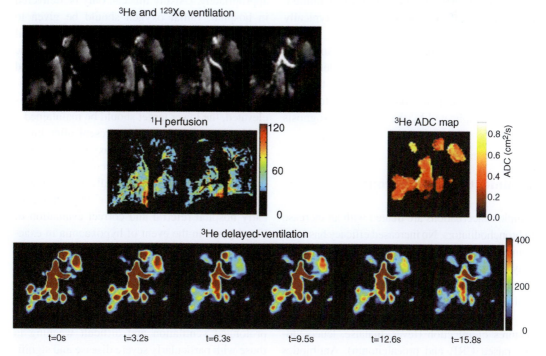

Fig. 4.2 Magnetic resonance lung imaging with demonstration of collateral ventilation (Images used with permission from Lawson RA, Wild J, and Marshall H. Sheffield, UK). *Upper panel*: Images of lung ventilation. ³He or ¹²⁹Xe are polarised and are imaged by a tuned coil to directly image gas in the lungs. The images show the patchy distribution of ventilation with large areas largely devoid of ventilation in a patient with COPD. *Middle panel*: gadolinium enhanced proton MRI (left), showing variable perfusion of lungs in a patient with

COPD. On the right is a map of the apparent diffusion coefficient (ADC). This measures the mean free path of gas molecules and hence relates to alveolar size; that is, to emphysema (though it can only assess areas of lung that are ventilated). *Bottom panel*: MRI images during a breath hold after inhalation of polarised He³. Time of acquisition of successive images is shown below in seconds. Maximum ventilation is reached early in most areas, but is delayed in the right upper zone, representing collateral ventilation

minimally invasive procedure which appears reasonably safe, and valves can, if necessary, be retrieved should problems ensue. The major acute side effect is pneumothorax, though subjects suffering this appear to do well long term. Most clinical trials are short term (less than a year) so long-term safety has yet to be fully established.

Endobronchial coils are also deployed bronchoscopically, acting as splints to open airways and combat lack of elasticity. Potentially, they may complement valves, as they are unaffected by collateral ventilation. As of 2015 the world literature reported about 150 procedures, of which a minority were treated in randomised, controlled trials. Publication of a completed large RCT is awaited.

Lung Transplantation

The utility of transplantation in COPD is limited, as the disease affects older subjects who typically have significant co-morbidity. However, it has a role in younger subjects with isolated lung disease. Historic series suggest only a modest prognostic benefit, but there may be significant quality of life advantage. Selection of appropriate candidates is complicated by the uncertain prognosis in COPD.

Treatment of Exacerbations

Simple exacerbations are treated with an increase in bronchodilators. No increased efficacy has been demonstrated for delivery by nebulisers, but this may be a convenient form to deliver larger doses. A proportion of exacerbations are associated with bacterial infection, which is suggested by the production of purulent sputum and systemic features of infection (fever, malaise, leucocytosis, raised CRP, and procalcitonin). Antibiotics should cover pneumococci, *Haemophilus influenzae*, and Moraxella. The choice should be guided by local policies, and may include doxycycline and co-amoxiclav. Oral steroids are frequently used, though have limited efficacy. Trials suggest they may speed recovery, lessening hospital stay by a day, but without affecting ultimate outcome. There is no benefit from prolonged courses beyond 5–7 days, though if courses have been so frequent as to cause adrenal suppression, they may need to be reduced gradually. Given their wide range of side effects, they should not be considered essential for mild exacerbations. A recent trial suggested only those patients with higher eosinophil counts derived benefit.

As discussed, many exacerbations can be managed in the domiciliary setting, supplemented by home monitoring as needed. The development of hypoxaemia is more complex. Patients with COPD are at risk of CO_2 retention, so oxygen can only be safely delivered with the ability to measure blood gases and titrate oxygen appropriately. Usually this can only be delivered in hospital. Initial oxygen should be given to achieve an oxygen saturation of 88–92% until blood gases have been measured [17]. If the pCO_2 is normal or low, the target can be revised to 94–98% (unless there are known to be previous episodes of type 2 failure). If the pCO_2 is elevated, the lower target should be maintained.

If respiratory acidosis is present after initial treatment despite appropriate oxygen saturation, ventilatory support should be considered. Non-invasive ventilation is potentially life-saving in this situation, emphasising the importance of early hospital referral and correct evaluation of blood gases in the event of hypoxaemia in exacerbations. However, it is also true that this can be a difficult and unpleasant treatment, and may not be appropriate for those clearly approaching the end of life. Sometimes invasive ventilation may be appropriate, though there is a concern about prolonged ventilation and difficult weaning in those with particularly severe disease and significant co-morbidity. Ideally there should be advanced consideration of the appropriate ceiling of intervention involving the patient and family, and the multi-disciplinary clinical team.

Summary

Management of COPD stands at a crossroads. Extensive guidelines should be consulted for current standards of care. However, it is a collection of poorly confined conditions with multiple subtypes. Coming years are likely to lead to increased mechanistic understanding with a need for greater diagnostic clarity. The goal of therapies able to modify disease trajectory may yet be achieved, and diagnostic categorisation allowing more usefully targeted treatment selection is very likely to change clinical practice significantly.

References

1. NICE. Chronic obstructive pulmonary disease in over 16s: diagnosis and management. 2010. http://www.nice.org.uk/guidance/cg101/chapter/1-Guidance. Accessed 20 Dec 2015.
2. GOLD. Global iniative for chronic obstructive lung disease. 2015. http://www.goldcopd.org/uploads/users/files/GOLD_Report_2015.pdf. Accessed 20 Dec 2015.
3. Han MK, Agusti A, Calverley PM, Celli BR, Criner G, Curtis JL, et al. Chronic obstructive pulmonary disease phenotypes: the future of COPD. Am J Respir Crit Care Med. 2010;182(5):598–604.
4. Burgel PR, Paillasseur JL, Caillaud D, Tillie-Leblond I, Chanez P, Escamilla R, et al. Clinical COPD phenotypes: a novel approach using principal component and cluster analyses. Eur Respir J. 2010;36(3):531–9.
5. Rennard SI, Calverley PM, Goehring UM, Bredenbroker D, Martinez FJ. Reduction of exacerbations by the PDE4 inhibitor roflumilast–the importance of defining different subsets of patients with COPD. Respir Res. 2011;27:12–8.
6. O'Neill SE, Lundback B, Lotvall J. Proteomics in asthma and COPD phenotypes and endotypes for biomarker discovery and improved understanding of disease entities. J Proteome. 2011;75(1):192–201.
7. Vanfleteren LE, Kocks JW, Stone IS, Breyer-Kohansai R, Greulich T, Lacedonia D, et al. Moving from the Oslerian paradigm to the post-genomic era: are asthma and COPD outdated terms? Thorax. 2014;69(1):72–9.
8. Siva R, Green R, Brightling C, Shelley M, Hargadon B, McKenna S, et al. Eosinophilic airway inflammation and exacerbations of COPD: a randomised controlled trial. Eur Respir J. 2007;29(5):906–13.
9. ECLIPSE. Recent updates. 2015. http://www.eclipse-copd.com/. Accessed 18 Dec 2015.
10. Darby AC, Waterhouse JC, Stevens V, Billings CG, Burton CM, Young C, et al. Chronic obstructive pulmonary disease among residents of an historically industrialised area. Thorax. 2012;67(10):901–7.
11. Wedzicha JA, Donaldson GC. Exacerbations of chronic obstructive pulmonary disease. Respir Care. 2003;48(12):1204–13.
12. Calverley PM, Anderson JA, Celli B, Ferguson JT, Jenkins C, Jones PW, et al. Salmeterol and fluticasone propionate and survival in chronic obstructive pulmonary disease. N Engl J Med. 2007;356(8):775–89.
13. MacNee W. ABC of chronic obstructive pulmonary disease: pathology, pathogenesis, and pathophysiology. BMJ. 2006;332:1202–4.
14. Puente-Maestu L, Stringer WW. Hyperinflation and its management in COPD. Int J Chron Obstruct Pulmon Dis. 2006;1(4):381–400.
15. Bolton CE, Bevan-Smith EF, Blakey JD, Crowe P, Elkin SI, Garrod R, et al. British Thoracic Society guideline on pulmonary rehabilitation in adults. Thorax. 2013;68(Suppl 2):ii1–30.
16. Hardinge M, Annandale J, Bourne S, Cooper B, Evans A, Freeman D, et al. British Thoracic Society guidelines for home oxygen use in adults. Thorax. 2015;70(Suppl 1):i1–43.
17. O'Driscoll BR, Howard LS, Davison AG. BTS guideline for emergency oxygen use in adult patients. Thorax. 2008;63(Suppl VI):vi1–68.

Acute and Chronic Cough

5

Alyn H. Morice and Helen Fowles

Introduction

A cough is recognised by its characteristic sound, produced by a forced expulsive manoeuvre against a closed glottis. The cough reflex is a protective mechanism in humans and other vertebrates, aimed at protecting the airway from foreign matter and clearing the mucus produced by the airways. It is normal to cough, on average, about 20 times a day. When coughing becomes more frequent than this, patients may seek treatment or advice from their healthcare provider, who is frequently unable to provide any evidence-based management.

Despite sub-specialisation within the respiratory field, chronic cough is one of the most common presentations to general respiratory clinics. This suggests that whilst the pathophysiology and treatment of chronic cough is often poorly understood, the respiratory practitioner needs to have a reliable protocol for managing such patients.

Whilst research in the area of cough and its treatment has greatly increased over the last few decades, there is still a paucity of data from clinical trials. As a result, much of the guidance on the management of chronic cough is dated, based on consensus opinion, and sometimes controversial.

Acute Cough

Epidemiology

Acute cough is arbitrarily defined as a cough which lasts less than 2 weeks. It is the commonest new symptom with which patients present to their GP, accounting for approximately 12 million presentations a year in the UK. Clearly this represents only a fraction of the morbidity caused by this condition, since many patients either self-medicate with over-the-counter (OTC) products or use home remedies. The overwhelming majority of cases of an acute cough are due to viral upper respiratory tract infection caused by a myriad of highly adapted pathogens. It is normally benign and self-limiting, but if it lasts longer than 3 weeks it is usually termed "post-viral" cough. In this phase of the illness the afferent sensory nerves remain hypersensitive even though the infection has disappeared. Patients are exquisitely sensitive to external stimuli such as a change in atmosphere, smoke, or strong smells. Why the hypersensitivity persists in some patients is unknown, but may be due to persistent low-grade inflammation.

Upper respiratory tract infections (URTI) are commoner in young children than adults, with

A. H. Morice (✉)
Respiratory Research Group, Hull York Medical School/University of Hull, Castle Hill Hospital, Cottingham, UK
e-mail: A.H.Morice@hull.ac.uk

H. Fowles
Respiratory Research Group, Hull York Medical School, Castle Hill Hospital, Cottingham, UK

© Springer International Publishing AG, part of Springer Nature 2018
S. Hart, M. Greenstone (eds.), *Foundations of Respiratory Medicine*,
https://doi.org/10.1007/978-3-319-94127-1_5

about five episodes per year, as opposed to one to two episodes in the normal adult population. About 50% of URTI have cough as a symptom, and in the evolution of the illness, cough follows the coryzal symptoms by about 2 days.

Nearly a billion pounds is spent annually in the UK on OTC remedies for acute cough. However, as an estimate of the impact on the economy, this does not include loss of productivity and healthcare utilisation [1].

Clinical Assessment

In acute cough, advice regarding preventing spread of viral infection is recommended and may include avoidance of social contact. Since viral transmission is both by the aerosol route and by hand, handwashing should be encouraged. Simple home remedies such as honey and lemon are sufficient and are thought to have a demulcent effect, reducing cough reflex sensitivity through an as-yet undefined mechanism.

Occasionally acute cough is part of the presentation of a serious condition. Symptoms which indicate the need for further investigation such as a chest radiograph are haemoptysis, breathlessness, fever, chest pain, and weight loss. Pneumonia often presents with cough as a predominant symptom and should be suspected on examination of the chest by localised findings of dullness on percussion, bronchial breathing, and crackles [1].

Many adverts for OTC antitussive medication focus on whether a patient's cough is dry and tickly or "mucous" and chesty. Recently this classification, beloved of pharmacists, has been called into question, and indeed the classification of medicines into expectorants, antitussives and mucolytics is now regarded by many as obsolete. Clinically, in acute cough, there is little evidence that this should alter management.

Treatment

Benefit from OTC medications in acute cough has been questioned. Simple remedies provide much of the antitussive efficacy seen with OTC cough syrups. Over-the-counter medications are often targeted at control of other symptoms of upper respiratory tract infections and may thus contain several active ingredients [1].

The evidence for dextromethorphan as an antitussive is probably the strongest. Dextromethorphan, although derived from opiates, has few, if any, characteristic opiate effects and is thus non-sedating. Recommended doses may be sub-optimal to suppress cough efficiently, and concern exists over its recreational use as a hallucinogen. It is estimated that 60 mg once daily provides additional cough suppressant activity of about 15% over the demulcent effect of the linctus. A number of currently licensed OTC medications in the UK contain dextromethorphan.

When inhaled, menthol has been found to produce a short-lived suppression of cough. This may be of benefit acutely, when administered via menthol crystals dissolved in steam, although many OTC linctuses also contain this as an active ingredient. Recent work has suggested that the antitussive activity is from the vapour acting on nasal afferents rather than within the airways.

First-generation antihistamines such as chlorpheniramine suppress cough but can also cause drowsiness. They may be suitable for a nocturnal cough. Until recently there was no evidence to support the use of second-generation antihistamines in the treatment of acute cough. However, a recent randomised, controlled trial demonstrated significant reduction in cough severity and a more rapid resolution of symptoms using a preparation containing diphenhydramine.

Codeine and pholcodine are not recommended in the treatment of acute cough. Their cough suppression effect is no greater than that of morphine, for which they are pro-drugs. A particular problem is their variable metabolism within the liver, giving no effect in some patients, whereas others have a high degree of sedation. Following deaths in children, the regulatory authorities have banned their sale for use in children under age 12. There is no evidence that antibiotics or steroids are effective in acute cough, and their prescription should be avoided [1].

Chronic Cough

A chronic cough is usually defined as a cough that persists for more than 8 weeks. This is, however, an arbitrary definition, which whilst agreed in both the American and European guidelines, does vary somewhat in cough research literature. Most cases of chronic cough referred to secondary care in the UK have persisted for much longer than 8 weeks [1–3].

Epidemiology

The prevalence of chronic cough is difficult to estimate, and suggested figures vary from 3% to 40%. This wide range probably reflects the variation in the specific question asked in different prevalence studies. A recent comprehensive literature review of 90 studies found the overall global prevalence of chronic cough to be 9.6%. The most common time definition used was greater than 3 months, rather than the guideline [1] stated time of more than 8 weeks. There were regional differences in chronic cough, with prevalence being higher in Australasia, Europe, and America, and lower in Asia and Africa. The authors speculate that this may be due to environmental factors or comorbidities, such as obesity, but recognise that the majority of the studies considered were carried out in Europe [4].

Chronic cough seems to be twice as common in women as men, and more prevalent in postmenopausal women. Cough frequency is also higher in female healthy volunteers and respiratory patients. Women have been shown to have increased sensitivity of their cough reflex, and functional MRI studies suggest that their "sensory cough centre" is more pronounced [5].

Tobacco smokers have a higher prevalence of chronic cough than non-smokers, and this effect is dose-related. Smokers, however, seem to be less likely to present to healthcare providers complaining of cough, which may be due to a cultural acceptance that smoking causes cough. Interestingly, nicotine delivered either by cigarette or by e-cigarette has been shown to suppress the cough reflex, and smokers have a lower cough sensitivity than normal subjects. Smoking cessation removes this inhibition and explains the frequent observation of patients complaining of increased cough in the month or two after quitting.

Obesity has been shown to be a risk factor for cough, and the rising prevalence of obesity in the United States and Europe may account for the increased prevalence in these areas. With rising levels of obesity in the United Kingdom, chronic cough is predicted to become an even greater cause of morbidity.

Other risk factors for chronic cough include an underlying diagnosis of asthma, living in an area with higher particulate matter and pollution, symptoms of gastro-oesophageal reflux, and irritable bowel syndrome.

The Cough Reflex

Like any other reflex in the body, the cough reflex is made up of an afferent arc (the vagus nerve) and an efferent arc—the nerves supplying the inspiratory and expiratory respiratory muscles (Fig. 5.1).

The nerves that appear to be implicated in the afferent limb of the cough reflex are myelinated A-delta fibres (sometimes also referred to as rapidly activated receptors or RARs); and myelinated C-fibres of the vagus nerve. The involvement of these nerves in cough is better established in animals than in humans, although recent studies suggest that similar entities do exist in humans [6, 7].

The receptors involved in signalling at these afferent nerve endings are of interest as targets for therapies for cough. The TRPV1 receptors were the first to be described as potential "cough receptors". They respond to heat and irritant substances such as capsaicin and acids. TRPV1 receptors form ion channels which respond to external stimuli and open to cause depolarisation of the cell they are located on.

Inhalation of capsaicin provokes a reliable cough response, which has been utilised experimentally as a cough challenge. Another

Fig. 5.1 Sensory receptors and inflammatory pathways in chronic cough. Stimulation of sensory pathways, including rapidly adapting receptors (RARs), C-fibres, and slowly adapting stretch receptors (SARs), and cough receptors TRPV1, TRPV4, TRPA1, ASIC, signal via the vagus nerve to the cough centre in the medulla of the brain. Efferent signals are then transmitted to inspiratory and expiratory muscles that mediate cough. Factors that sensitise cough receptors and lead to cough hypersensitivity are shown. *LTD4* leukotriene D4, *ATP* adenosine triphosphate, *PGE2* prostaglandin E2, *TNF* tumour necrosis factor, *TRPV* transient receptor potential vanilloid, *TRPA* transient receptor potential ankyrin, *ASIC* acid sensing ion channel (by kind permission of Mahboobeh H. Sadeghi)

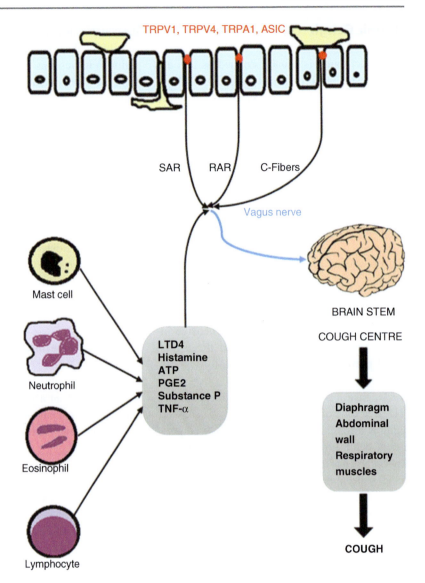

commonly used cough challenge substance is citric acid. Whilst TRPV1 seems to respond to citric acid, there also seems to be a cough response to citric acid even when TRPV1 is blocked, suggesting the presence of other acid-sensing channels.

Experimentation *in vitro* and *in vivo* in humans and guinea pigs has shown that the TRPA1 receptors are involved in the cough reflex and that TRPA1 agonists stimulate vagal nerves; indeed a wide variety of substances are known to stimulate TRPA1 receptors, including the aromatic compounds contained in perfumes, oxidising agents such as bleach, and even tear gas. The TRPA1 agonist cinnamaldehyde provokes a

cough response in healthy volunteers and appears to do so independently of other cough challenge stimuli. The many other substances which stimulate TRPA1 receptors *in vitro* have yet to be studied in man. These include a number of substances that patients commonly describe as provoking their cough, such as smoke, perfumes, and other strong smells, indicating that TRPA1 may be the main sensory receptor involved in the cough reflex and its hypersensitivity.

TRPM8 receptors respond to cold temperatures and menthol, and have been implicated in the cough response, perhaps explaining the antitussive effects of menthol. All of the above-mentioned TRP receptors are also sensitive to change in temperature. The archetypal TRPV1 is a "hot" receptor, explaining why capsaicin-containing chili peppers taste hot and why patients frequently complain of their cough being precipitated by a change in ambient temperature.

Purinergic receptors which respond to adenosine triphosphate (ATP) have more recently become implicated in the physiology of cough, and inhalation of ATP induces cough in healthy volunteers and chronic cough patients.

There are many other receptors which appear to be implicated in the cough response, including voltage-gated sodium channels, acid-sensing receptors, and other TRP classes such as TRPV4.

Whilst coughing is often unavoidable when certain stimuli are introduced, the cough reflex in humans is under a considerable degree of voluntary control. Simply instructing patients with an acute cough not to cough can reduce their coughing levels. This cortical influence leads to a high placebo effect in antitussive trials, making study of antitussives difficult. In addition, it means that some therapies which show good effect in animal studies show very little effect in human trials. It would be incorrect, however, to suggest that chronic cough is "all in the mind." Psychogenic cough (a form of Tourette's syndrome) is very rare in adults.

Whilst chronic cough is a condition often referred to the respiratory physician, it is worth remembering that cough is often caused by, or associated with, pathology throughout the vagal nerve radiation, such as oesophageal dysfunction and irritable bowel syndrome.

Disease Patterns and Subsets

Key to an understanding of both acute and chronic cough is the concept of cough hypersensitivity. Objective testing in a wide range of cough syndromes has demonstrated increased sensitivity when the aforementioned receptors are challenged by inhalation of protussive agents. Thus virtually all patients with excessive cough are provoked by minimal stimulation, which in the normal subject would not lead to the urge to cough. It is clear that this hypersensitivity does not arise purely from the upregulation of cough receptors, since specific drugs blocking these receptors have no important effect in clinical cough. Recently, mediators such as ATP have been suggested to "irritate" the afferent nerves, leading to a syndrome of cough hypersensitivity akin to that of neuropathic pain.

The concept of cough hypersensitivity syndrome helps to explain why some patients with other respiratory conditions present with a cough which is resistant to therapies for that condition. The cough thus represents a separate disease of cough hypersensitivity, which is associated with, rather than directly caused by, for example, asthma.

Patients who are referred to specialist cough clinics with persistent cough are typically middle-aged female non-smokers who have no apparent underlying respiratory disease. In these cases, traditionally the causes of cough considered have been gastro-oesophageal reflux disease (GORD), cough variant asthma, and postnasal drip. However, more recently Cough Hypersensitivity Syndrome (CHS) has been agreed as the unifying concept [8].

Reflux

Gastro-oesophageal reflux disease (GORD) is a widely accepted cause of chronic cough. It accounts for between 5% and 41% of chronic cough. This wide variation in reported incidence is probably due to the lack of recognition of its existence as a cause of cough in non-specialist clinics, highlighting again the importance of thinking "outside the lung" when managing chronic cough.

More recently it has become clear that GORD is merely the tip of the reflux iceberg, and that many patients do not have features such as heartburn and indigestion typical of acid-related liquid reflux. This was first recognised by ear, nose and throat (ENT) specialists where the term *laryngopharyngeal reflux* was coined. Others prefer the term *airway reflux* to describe this phenomenon.

Patients often provide a classical history with coughing occurring at peak times of reflux and

Within the last Month, how did the following problems affect you? 0 = no problem and 5 = severe/frequent problem						
Hoarseness or a problem with your voice	0	1	2	3	4	5
Clearing your throat	0	1	2	3	4	5
The feeling of something dripping down the back of your nose or throat	0	1	2	3	4	5
Retching or vomiting when you cough	0	1	2	3	4	5
Cough on first lying down or bending over	0	1	2	3	4	5
Chest tightness or wheeze when coughing	0	1	2	3	4	5
Heartburn, indigestion, stomach acid coming up (or do you take medication for this, if yes score 5)	0	1	2	3	4	5
A tickle in your throat, or a lump in your throat	0	1	2	3	4	5
Cough with eating (during or soon after meals)	0	1	2	3	4	5
Cough with certain foods	0	1	2	3	4	5
Cough with you get out of bed in the morning	0	1	2	3	4	5
Cough brought on by singing or speaking (for example, on the telephone)	0	1	2	3	4	5
Coughing more when awake rather than asleep	0	1	2	3	4	5
A strange taste in your mouth	0	1	2	3	4	5

TOTAL SCORE _____ /70

Fig. 5.2 Hull cough hypersensitivity questionnaire. Symptoms are each scored 0–5, and added to provide the total score. Normal people score an average 4/70. The upper limit of normal is 13/70. Higher scores indicate a strong likelihood of Cough Hypersensitivity Syndrome. The most common cause for this is airway reflux

lower oesophageal sphincter relaxation (after meals, on rising from bed, on bending over). A validated questionnaire (Fig. 5.2) is available at: http://www.issc.info in a wide variety of languages.

There are two proposed mechanisms whereby this "non-acid" reflux precipitates coughing. Firstly that micro-aspiration of oesophageal contents into the larynx and lungs occurs, leading to irritation of vagus nerve endings in these areas. Secondly, reflux into the oesophagus itself stimulates a vagal reflex which leads to cough. A further mechanism has been postulated in that, because of the hypersensitivity, spasm or dysmotility of the oesophagus may lead to the urge to cough via an aberrant or "referred" sensation. Thus reflux may not be a prerequisite for production of the symptom by the oesophageal sensory nerves.

Table 5.1 Features of the "Asthma-like" cough syndromes

	Variable airflow obstruction	Airway hyper-responsiveness	Capsaicin cough hyper-responsiveness	Sputum Eosinophilia
Asthma	Yes	Yes	Sometimes	Yes
Cough variant asthma	Sometimes	Yes	Sometimes	Yes
Eosinophilic bronchitis	No	No	Yes	Yes–by definition
Atopic cough	No	No	No	Yes

Eosinophilic Cough Syndromes

A number of patients with chronic cough appear to have cough that is responsive to steroid treatment. The cough shares some features with asthma, namely nocturnal cough, airway hyper-responsiveness on methacholine challenge testing, and positive markers of eosinophilic airways inflammation (blood eosinophilia, sputum eosinophilia or raised exhaled nitric oxide). Patients vary in their degree of airways hyper-responsiveness, leading to a variety of diagnostic labels being applied including cough variant asthma, atopic cough and eosinophilic bronchitis (Table 5.1). More recently it has been posited that these are all variations on a single clinical syndrome, which can be expressed in lay terms as "asthmatic cough." Thus classic asthma includes variable bronchoconstriction, bronchial hyper-responsiveness, and sputum eosinophilia; cough variant asthma does not exhibit bronchoconstriction; and eosinophilic bronchitis is only characterised by sputum eosinophilia. All respond to steroid treatment, although perhaps less well than in classic asthma. The "asthma-like" cough syndromes account for about 20% of referrals to cough clinics.

Recent evidence provides an explanation for the diverse nature of these asthmatic cough syndromes. Unlike the classic asthma of childhood, which is mediated through allergic adaptive immunity and IgE, the main trigger in the older coughing patient may be mediated by a non-allergic mechanism involving the innate immune system. This hypothesis proposes epithelial injury (for example, caused by reflux, infection, or air pollution) causes release of interleukin 33, activation of innate lymphocyte type 2 cells, and

release of IL-5 and IL-13, leading to eosinophil recruitment.

Postnasal Drip (Upper Airways Cough Syndrome)

Whilst widely described as a cause of cough, postnasal drip has been the subject of some debate. The prevalence of postnasal drip also appears to vary, with much higher incidence in the United States, suggesting a possible cultural aspect. This also means that it features much more heavily in the United States guidelines than the European ones. The U.S. guidelines now refer to the existence of nasal stuffiness, sinusitis, or the sensation of secretions draining into the posterior pharynx from the nose or sinuses in association with cough as the "Upper Airways Cough Syndrome" (UACS). In our opinion whilst rhinitis is associated with chronic cough, there are many patients who have rhinitis, postnasal drip, or sinus disease without cough, and the association remains dubious. Reflux of gaseous non-acid refluxate throughout the airways, including the nose, seems an equally plausible explanation.

ACE-Inhibitor-Induced Cough

The association between ACE-inhibitors and cough is well recognised, as these drugs increase cough sensitivity. In some patients this sensitivity is sufficient to reveal a previously occult cough hypersensitivity syndrome (of diverse cause) to produce a clinically noticeable persistent cough. Stopping the ACE-inhibitor usually leads to resolution of the cough, although this may require many months for the cough sensitivity to reset.

Auricular Nerve Stimulation

Irritation of the auricular branch of the vagal nerve by a substance in the external acoustic meatus can stimulate cough. Removal of the irritant (cerumen, foreign body, or a hair) should have an effect within a few days.

Other Clinical Conditions Associated with Isolated Chronic Cough

Patients with a congenital tracheo-oesophageal fistula (TOF)/oesophageal atresia with subsequent repair are often left with a dysfunctional oesophagus. These patients often present with a typical cough or bronchiectasis due to recurrent aspiration—the "TOF cough" [9].

Associations between chronic cough and various neurological conditions have been described. These include motor, sensory, and autonomic neuropathies such as Holmes-Adie Syndrome and Hereditary Sensory Neuropathy 1. These associations support the role of an abnormality in the autonomic nervous system as a cause of chronic cough [10].

History

A detailed history of chronic cough is aimed at eliciting risk factors, excluding any differential diagnosis, and determining where to target treatment. It may negate the need for further investigation.

A cough of very sudden onset may be associated with aspiration of a foreign body. Many patients associate the onset of chronic cough with symptoms indicative of an upper respiratory tract infection such as a sore throat. Whilst it is useful to be aware of how long a cough has been present, there is no association between any particular condition and the length of the cough.

Production of excessive amounts of purulent or mucopurulent sputum on a daily basis may point to a diagnosis of bronchiectasis or other underlying pulmonary pathology, which should then be investigated and managed in the usual way. However, patients with CHS may not always describe a dry cough, and many complain of the sensation of persistent mucus at the back of their throat, with difficulty expectorating it from their larynx, often only producing very small quantities of sputum. Patients with reflux may typically describe production of moderate volumes of watery secretions after a coughing bout.

Diurnal variation in cough may prove helpful in determining cause. Using cough-counting technology, the marked reduction of cough seen at night is, however, seen in all forms of cough, including asthmatic cough. It is important to carefully tease out exactly what is meant by reports of "waking with a cough" and "coughing more at night." Patients with reflux-associated cough are rarely woken from sleep by cough, as the lower oesophageal sphincter usually remains closed during sleep. They often report coughing shortly after rising from bed, due to relaxation of the lower oesophageal sphincter at this time to allow release of the stomach gases which have collected overnight. They also frequently cough on first lying down. These symptoms should be carefully distinguished from the classical early morning wakening with breathlessness and wheeze as described by asthmatics.

Some patients describe severe coughing spasms and paroxysms which can lead to retching, vomiting, pre-syncope, or even syncope.

Patients often describe certain triggers and aggravants of their cough—these tend to be common irritants such as scented sprays, and are probably not clinically helpful. Equally, eliciting the location of the irritant sensation within the respiratory tract is unlikely to be of diagnostic value, although some patients can be highly specific about exactly where they feel the tickle in their throat.

A full drug history can sometimes elicit a medication which may be responsible for increased cough sensitivity, in particular ACE-inhibitors. The effect of these medications can take several months to resolve after stopping treatment. It is also useful to know if the patient has already trialled any therapies for their cough and whether they gained any benefit from these.

Other drugs associated with coughing are prostaglandin eye drops, which descend into the throat through the lacrimal duct, and drugs which precipitate reflux through their effect on the lower oesophageal sphincter, such as calcium channel antagonists and high-dose salbutamol.

Certain features in the history may suggest one or other of the three widely accepted causes of cough. Whilst UACS-related cough rarely exists without the presence of one of the classical symptoms suggestive of rhinitis or sinusitis, cough due to reflux or one of the "asthma"- like syndromes often exist without the classically recognised features of these conditions. However, careful history taking and a knowledge of the physiology of the lower oesophageal sphincter often elicit features which suggest reflux-related cough. Some clinical features show a degree of overlap between the different diagnoses, and their presence or absence should not lead to exclusion of the possibility of reflux or eosinophilic airways disease as a cause of the cough.

The presence of wheeze, shortness of breath, and chest tightness may suggest asthma, but are equally as likely with a non-eosinophilic aspiration event and can occur during a bout of coughing from any cause. Their presence is therefore more significant if they are occurring independently of coughing bouts.

Features of "classical" reflux symptoms such as heartburn or indigestion may be present in patients with reflux-related cough, but their absence does not exclude it. Features which point towards a reflux-associated cough include exacerbation of coughing shortly after meal times and association with certain types of food, such as chocolate or curry. Coughing also characteristically occurs during times of diaphragmatic relaxation such as speech, singing, or laughing, particularly when seated such as when driving or talking on the telephone. Movement of the diaphragm disrupts the lower oesophageal sphincter because part of the sphincter is accounted for by the crural diaphragm. Symptoms of airway reflux are also often described and include a hoarse voice, globus (the sensation of a lump in the throat), throat clearing, and an odd taste.

A thorough history of chronic cough should include an occupational history. Occupational sensitizers to cough include hot acid in bottle factories and chili peppers.

Past medical history should include other respiratory conditions, including previous pertussis infection, other atopic disease, and organ-specific auto-immune disease. There is evidence that patients with these conditions are more at risk of developing chronic cough.

Family history may establish a familial tendency to chronic cough, perhaps through the mechanism of atopy. Reflux also seems to have familial tendencies, although this may be more attributable to commonality of diet. An inherited autonomic sensory neuropathy (vagal) associated with chronic cough has been described.

Assessment of patients with chronic cough in clinic should include an assessment of cough severity. Validated tools include the visual analogue score and the Leicester Cough Questionnaire. However, in practice, simply asking the patient to score their cough out of 10 is a simple and accurate measure.

Examination

Examination of the patient with chronic cough should focus on the afferent sites most commonly associated with cough.

A respiratory examination is more useful to exclude respiratory disease such as bronchiectasis and interstitial lung disease (ILD) than providing any specific diagnostic benefit in chronic cough. A chronic cough associated with finger clubbing or signs consistent with a pleural effusion or lobar collapse should be investigated accordingly.

Examination of the nose may reveal nasal polyps or inflamed turbinates. Secretions trickling down the posterior pharynx or tonsillar enlargement may be visible on throat examination. Laryngoscopy can show irritation of the larynx and pharynx consistent with laryngopharyngeal reflux. However, scoring systems have shown this to be inaccurate as a diagnostic test, and we use laryngoscopy only in the presence of stridor.

If a family history of cough is present, neurological examination of the legs may suggest familial neuropathy.

Investigations

A chest radiograph and spirometry are essential in any patient presenting with chronic cough.

Airway reversibility testing is useful to screen for patients with one of the eosinophilic cough syndromes, although the absence of reversibility does not preclude the diagnosis. Other investigations which may aid with the diagnosis include exhaled nitric oxide measurement to detect eosinophilic airways inflammation. The blood eosinophil count is often overlooked but has been shown to correlate with the presence of airways eosinophilia. Identification of sputum eosinophilia is useful but not widely available.

Bronchoscopy is indicated in the initial investigation of chronic cough if the history suggests foreign body inhalation. In the absence of a suggestive history, bronchoscopy in cases of chronic cough rarely provides a diagnosis, although should be considered in treatment-resistant cough. A persistent productive cough should prompt investigations for possible bronchiectasis.

Other investigations should be targeted depending on patient history. It is often appropriate and more cost effective to trial treatment targeted at likely contributors to chronic cough prior to carrying out expensive and invasive testing.

A trial of treatment for GORD is usually suggested prior to further investigation of the upper GI tract. Given the lack of evidence that acid suppression improves cough, and because positive 24-h pH monitoring does not predict treatment response, oesophageal pH monitoring is unlikely to be helpful, particularly if non-acid reflux is causing the cough. As there is no effective test for non-acid reflux currently available, oesophageal function testing in the form of high-resolution oesophageal manometry is probably the most accurate indication of oesophageal disease. However, the interpretation needs to be viewed in the light of cough rather than some other oesophageal pathology. Since therapeutic trials provide a quicker and cheaper relief as well as a diagnosis, manometry is best reserved for patients in whom surgical options such as Nissen's fundoplication are being considered.

Upper airway investigations of the sinuses such as plain radiography or CT imaging may be suggested by ENT examination. The American guidelines suggest a trial of treatment if UACS is suspected before further imaging is carried out.

Cough provocation testing by cough challenges such as citric acid and capsaicin shows a wide variation of cough sensitivity within a normal population. Therefore it has no role in the diagnosis of chronic cough, and its usefulness is confined to clinical research.

The partial correlation between subjective symptom scores and objective measurement (such as cough recording) suggests that objective assessment of cough may be useful in clinical practice. In addition, it is suggested that there is a difference in the cough sound produced by different disease mechanisms. Measurement and monitoring of cough by ambulatory cough monitors would therefore be a viable way of objective cough monitoring. However, currently their use remains essentially limited to clinical trials.

Differential Diagnosis

In a patient who presents with a chronic cough, a careful history, examination, and initial investigations, particularly a chest X-ray, are usually sufficient to exclude other respiratory conditions such as lung cancer, bronchiectasis, ILD, COPD, and tuberculosis.

Course, Prognosis, and Outcome

Cough hypersensitivity has considerable impact on quality of life. Patients with a persistent cough have been shown to have worse levels of depression than those with other chronic conditions such as COPD. Some patients may have to cease employment due to their cough, particularly those who rely on talking. Many patients will report that they avoid public gatherings such as concerts and the theatre for fear of having a coughing attack. The fact that coughing is culturally associated with a risk of infection also tends to limit patients' activities.

With targeted treatment, many patients see improvement in their cough. However, in a small group of patients, no treatment appears to be successful, and the cough may be lifelong.

Cough Syncope

Syncopal episodes precipitated by coughing are likely to be due to the elevated intrathoracic pressures caused by a coughing bout. Typical patients who report episodes of cough syncope are males in their middle ages who are overweight, with obstructive airways disease. Elimination of cough will resolve the syncopal episodes. Patients should be made aware of the DVLA guidelines on cough syncope. These state that with a Group 1 car or motorcycle license, driving must cease for 6 months after a single episode of cough syncope. This cessation is increased to 12 months if multiple attacks have occurred. Group 2 license holders who drive lorries or buses must cease driving for 5 years from the last attack. Reapplication may be considered at an earlier time for both types of license if certain criteria are confirmed by a specialist. These are that any underlying chronic respiratory condition is well controlled, the driver has stopped smoking, has achieved a BMI of under 30, and any GORD is treated.

Other Complications of Chronic Cough

Urinary incontinence amongst patients with chronic cough is frequent, particularly in women. Uterine prolapse is also seen in chronic cough patients. Severe coughing bouts often lead to musculoskeletal chest wall pain, or even rib fractures.

Assessment of Chronic Cough

A recommended pathway for assessment in the cough clinic is shown in Fig. 5.3.

Fig. 5.3 Recommended pathway for assessment in the cough clinic

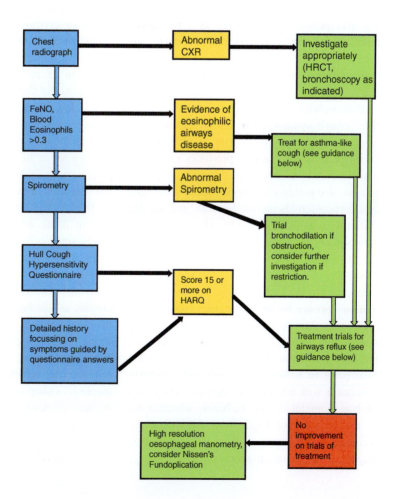

Treatment

Randomised clinical trials of treatments for isolated chronic cough are limited. The choice of treatment should be guided by the history. Any underlying respiratory pathology should be treated according to treatment guidelines for that condition. Despite these measures, chronic cough often persists and is dismissed as idiopathic. In reality it is often the failure to appreciate the true diagnosis, particularly non-acid reflux, or a failure to understand the differences in treatment required for cough arising from the diagnosis. Treatment specifically targeted at the cough reflex may be required when specific therapy has been ineffective.

Most guidelines recommend establishing a diagnosis by therapeutic trials. Some guidelines suggest that prolonged therapeutic trials are required. Given the relapsing remitting course of some patients with cough, then it is likely that any therapeutic success from such prolonged treatment is more likely to be due to spontaneous remission. We suggest that a month is sufficient to decide whether a particular drug is effective or not.

Patients with evidence of one of the "asthma-like" cough syndromes typically respond to a course of oral steroids. A trial of treatment of 20 mg prednisolone usually produces a response within a few days. Cessation of treatment leads to relapse, also within a few days. Clearly prolonged oral corticosteroids are inadvisable, and inhaled corticosteroids (ICS) should be substituted. There is no specific evidence regarding doses of ICS in cough, and it is recommended that the asthma guidelines are utilised. ICS may be less effective than they are in classic asthma because inflammation appears to be more deep-rooted, with mast cells having been located near airway nerves. Since most asthmatic cough patients do not have prominent bronchoconstriction, there is little point in adding long-acting beta agonists. Treatment with leukotriene receptor antagonists such as montelukast may be highly effective due to the presence of high levels of leukotriene receptors on the innate lymphoid cells controlling the eosinophilic inflammation.

For the large numbers of patients in whom reflux is the precipitant, the first thing to consider is the deleterious effects of concomitant medication. Many patients are on therapies which can worsen reflux, and eliminating these can lead to significant improvement in cough. These include bisphosphonates, nitrates, calcium channel blockers, theophylline, and progesterones.

Reflux leading to cough tends to be predominantly non-acid and often does not respond to gastric acid-suppressing therapies such as proton pump inhibitors or H2 receptor antagonists such as ranitidine. However, a therapeutic trial of these agents remains recommended by most cough guidelines, and they may be of clinical benefit in patients who do have co-existing symptoms of typical acid reflux. Pro-motility agents such as metoclopramide or domperidone seem to be more effective in treating the cough, presumably by reducing non-acid reflux and improving oesophageal motility. Macrolides such as azithromycin or erythromycin also act as pro-motility agents through their action as motilin agonists and are well established in paediatric practice for treatment of reflux in children. Baclofen may also be useful through its role in increasing tone of the lower oesophageal sphincter as well as having a non-specific effect on the cough reflex through the $GABA_B$ receptor. None of these medications seem to have a universal effect in all patients with GORD-related cough, and a sequential trial is recommended.

There is some evidence to suggest that weight loss in those who are overweight will reduce cough severity scores [11]. Treating co-existing sleep apnoea is also advised [12]. There is little evidence supporting other lifestyle measures aimed at reducing GORD lead to improvement in chronic cough, but some experts suggest that they may be of benefit. Advice includes adapting diet to include no more than 45 g of fat in 24 h and excluding coffee, tea, fizzy drinks, chocolate, mints, citrus products (including tomatoes), and alcohol. Other suggested lifestyle measures include smoking cessation and limiting vigorous exercise that increases abdominal pressure. Elevation of the head end of the bed again has little supporting evidence, but patients at high risk of aspiration, such as those with co-existent COPD, may do this automatically.

Speech and language therapy has been shown in randomised controlled trials to reduce cough both objectively and subjectively. The technique is a very specific, however, and the protocol developed by Anne Vertigan and colleagues from Newcastle Australia requires experience and skill. Recently it has been combined with prega-balin in a multidisciplinary approach to chronic cough.

Surgical intervention for reflux may be con-sidered, however, its success rates in controlling chronic cough appear to be less than in control-ling symptoms such as heartburn or indigestion. There are no specific identifying markers for those who are more likely to benefit. However, it may be a more acceptable treatment option to both the patient and the surgeon if there is clear evidence of reflux on investigations, particularly if there are indications of recurrent aspiration. If abnormal oesophageal motility is identified, there may be less satisfactory surgical outcomes. Careful discussion with the patient regarding risks and benefits needs to be undertaken before pursuing surgical treatment.

Given the concept that chronic cough caused by all of these mechanisms is due to a hypersen-sitivity of vagal afferent neural pathways, the ideal treatment would appear to be one which reduces this hypersensitivity. Current therapies are likely to have a more centrally acting effect, and therefore can have an unacceptable side effect profile. A recent trial of gabapentin sug-gested some benefit to patients with chronic cough [13]. Side effects were prominent, and in our experience, outweigh any beneficial effects seen. In some patients there appears to be an ini-tial effect, with this ceasing to be of benefit after a few weeks, suggesting perhaps an initial down regulation in the hypersensitivity but followed by reversion to hypersensitivity.

Low doses of morphine sulphate (5–10 mg) have been shown to be of benefit. In about a third of patients it appears to act like a switch to turn off their cough. There is no evidence that higher doses are of added benefit, and at these low doses the only significant side effect appears to be constipation [14]. Dexbrompheniramine and other first-generation antihistamines also seem to reduce cough hypersensitivity in some patients. However, its lack of availability in the UK limits use, and other first-generation antihistamines such as chlorpheniramine may be tried. The effi-cacy of these drugs has led to the recommenda-tion of treatment of UACS in the U.S. guidelines, however, efficacy does not seem to be limited to this syndrome and may represent a central cough-suppressing activity.

The paucity of available treatments and clini-cal trial data for existing treatments in chronic cough make it a viable target for future research. As better understanding is gained of the mecha-nisms involved in the cough reflex, future targets for therapies are identified. Clinical trials with TRP agonists have so far proved unfruitful, how-ever current work suggests that purinergic recep-tor antagonists such as AF 219 hold promise.

References

1. Morice AH, McGarvey L, Pavord I. Recom-mendations for the management of cough in adults. Thorax. 2006;61(Suppl 1):i1–24.
2. Morice AH, Fontana GA, Sovijarvi AR, Pistolesi M, Chung KF, Widdicombe J, et al. The diagnosis and management of chronic cough. Eur Respir J. 2004;24(3):481–92.
3. Irwin RS, Baumann MH, Bolser DC, Boulet LP, Braman SS, Brightling CE, et al. Diagnosis and management of cough executive summary: ACCP evidence-based clinical practice guidelines. Chest. 2006;129(1 Suppl):1s–23s.
4. Song WJ, Chang YS, Faruqi S, Kim JY, Kang MG, Kim S, et al. The global epidemiology of chronic cough in adults: a systematic review and meta-analysis. Eur Respir J. 2015;45(5):1479–81.
5. Morice AH, Jakes AD, Faruqi S, Birring SS, McGarvey L, Canning B, et al. A worldwide survey of chronic cough: a manifestation of enhanced somato-sensory response. Eur Respir J. 2014;44(5):1149–55.
6. Widdicombe JG. Neurophysiology of the cough reflex. Eur Respir J. 1995;8(7):1193–202.
7. West PW, Canning BJ, Merlo-Pich E, Woodcock AA, Smith JA. Morphological characterization of nerves in whole mount airway biopsies. Am J Respir Crit Care Med. 2015;192(1):30–9.
8. Morice AH, Millqvist E, Belvisi MG, Bieksiene K, Birring SS, Chung KF, et al. Expert opinion on the cough hypersensitivity syndrome in respiratory medi-cine. Eur Respir J. 2014;44(5):1132–48.

9. Love C, Morice AH. After repair of tracheo-oesophageal atresia. BMJ. 2012;344:e3517.
10. Karur PS, Morjaria JB, Wright C, Morice AH. Neurological conditions presenting as airway reflux cough. Eur Respir Rev. 2012;21(125):257–9.
11. Smith JE, Morjaria JB, Morice AH. Dietary intervention in the treatment of patients with cough and symptoms suggestive of airways reflux as determined by Hull Airways Reflux Questionnaire. Cough (London, Engl). 2013;9(1):27.
12. Faruqi S, Fahim A, Morice AH. Chronic cough and obstructive sleep apnoea: reflux-associated cough hypersensitivity? Eur Respir J. 2012;40(4):1049–50.
13. Ryan NM, Birring SS, Gibson PG. Gabapentin for refractory chronic cough: a randomised, double-blind, placebo-controlled trial. Lancet. 2012;380(9853):1583–9.
14. Morice AH, Menon MS, Mulrennan SA, Everett CF, Wright C, Jackson J, et al. Opiate therapy in chronic cough. Am J Respir Crit Care Med. 2007;175(4):312–5.

Lung Cancer

6

Seamus Grundy, Rachael Barton, Anne Campbell, Michael Cowen, and Michael Lind

Aetiology and Epidemiology

Lung cancer accounts for more than 90% of primary lung malignancies and is a leading cause of cancer mortality in men and women. Ninety percent of cases are caused by smoking, with 965,500 lung cancer deaths attributable to smoking worldwide in 2010. Changes in lung cancer incidence and mortality have paralleled past trends in cigarette smoking. Whilst tobacco had been widely used throughout the world for centuries, the marked increase in incidence and mortality observed in the twentieth century followed the introduction of manufactured cigarettes with

addictive properties, which resulted in a new pattern of sustained exposure of the lung to inhaled carcinogens. Lung cancer incidence in developed countries peaked in the late 1980s/early 1990s, decreasing in men since the mid 1980s but continuing to increase amongst females through the late 1990s. The male-to-female incidence rate ratio for lung cancer overall is now 1.3 (squamous cell carcinoma 2.1, small cell carcinoma 1.2, and adenocarcinoma 1.1). Evidence suggests that the increase in adenocarcinoma relative to other subtypes of lung cancer since the 1960s has resulted from changes in the design and composition of cigarettes since the 1950s, such as ventilated filters and increased levels of tobacco-specific nitrosamines. The risk of lung cancer among cigarette smokers increases with the duration of smoking and the number of cigarettes smoked per day (in one study men aged 60–69 who smoked 20 cigarettes per day for 30 years had an age-specific mortality rate of 224.3, whereas if they smoked for 40 years, this increased to 486.8) and progressively declines following smoking cessation so that after 15 years the relative risk reduces to 1.6.

The risks from passive smoking have been increasingly recognised in recent years, with a relative risk of 1.25 (equivalent to smoking one cigarette per day).

Other causes of lung cancer include:

Occupational Exposure The proportion of lung cancers related to occupational exposure differs

S. Grundy (✉)
Thoracic Medicine, University Hospital Aintree, Liverpool, UK
e-mail: Seamus.grundy@nhs.net

R. Barton
Queen's Centre for Oncology and Haematology, Hull and East Yorkshire Hospitals NHS Trust, Castle Hill Hospital, Cottingham, UK

A. Campbell
Cellular Pathology, Hull and East Yorkshire Hospitals NHS Trust, Hull Royal Infirmary, Hull, UK

M. Cowen
Cardiothoracic Surgery Department, Hull and East Yorkshire Hospitals NHS Trust, Castle Hill Hospital, Cottingham, UK

M. Lind
Queen's Centre for Oncology and Haematology, Hull York Medical School, Castle Hill Hospital, Cottingham, UK

© Springer International Publishing AG, part of Springer Nature 2018
S. Hart, M. Greenstone (eds.), *Foundations of Respiratory Medicine*,
https://doi.org/10.1007/978-3-319-94127-1_6

between populations, but on average is around 10%. Occupational exposure occurs to carcinogens such as radon (mining), arsenic (glass, metals, and pesticides), asbestos (insulation, filters, textiles), chromates (pigments, metal industry, chrome plating), chloromethyl ethers (chemical intermediates), nickel (metallurgy, alloy, catalyst), and polycyclic aromatic hydrocarbons.

Environmental Radon Radon is an inert gas that is produced naturally from radium in the decay series of uranium. It is naturally occurring in soil and rocks. The highest levels in the UK are in Cornwall. Once inhaled, radon continues to decay and emit alpha particles. Environmental radon accounts for approximately 1000 premature deaths per year in the UK (compared with 28,000 for smokers). Occupations with a slight increase in risk include air crew and nuclear fuel plant and power station workers.

Outdoor and Indoor Air Pollution In developed countries the two indoor pollutants that most strongly increase the risk of lung cancer are passive smoking and radon. In developing countries the greatest risk is from the use of unprocessed solid fuels for cooking and space heating.

Underlying Chronic Lung Disease and Infections Pulmonary fibrosis, chronic obstructive pulmonary disease, tuberculosis, and HIV are all associated with an increased risk of developing lung cancer.

Family History A positive family history of lung cancer is a clinically useful risk factor.

Smoking interacts with many of these risk factors in an additive or synergistic fashion. For example, heavily exposed asbestos workers have a fivefold and smokers an 11-fold increase in risk, whereas asbestos workers who are also smokers have a 53-fold increase.

Pathology

Lung Cancer Carcinogenesis

The properties of a malignant neoplasm such as excessive growth, local invasiveness, and ability to form metastases are acquired in a stepwise fashion corresponding at the molecular level due to accumulation of genetic lesions. The actions of a carcinogenic substance may be either direct or indirect via the induction of chronic inflammation, hyperplasia and metaplasia (Fig. 6.1a, b). Cigarette smoke is a powerful mutagen and contains at least 43 known carcinogens. Some, such as polycyclic aromatic hydrocarbons, tobacco-specific nitrosamines, and polonium 210, are organ-specific. Carcinogenic metals present within cigarette smoke include arsenic, nickel, cadmium, and chromium. Acetaldehyde and phenol are potential promoters. Chemicals such as nitrogen dioxide and formaldehyde act as irritants, and hydrogen cyanide is toxic to cilia.

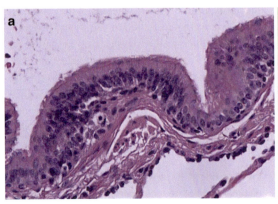
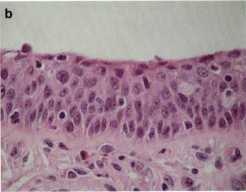
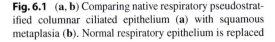

Fig. 6.1 (**a**, **b**) Comparing native respiratory pseudostratified columnar ciliated epithelium (**a**) with squamous metaplasia (**b**). Normal respiratory epithelium is replaced by squamous cells but the changes are considered reversible and are distinct from premalignant dysplasias

Carcinomas of the lung contain many genetic abnormalities but only some ("driver mutations") are essential for tumour cell survival. Whilst many genetic abnormalities are common to all lung cancer subtypes, there are also significant differences between them.

Adenocarcinoma

Driver gene alterations in adenocarcinoma include EGFR, ALK, KRAS, BRAF, ERBB2/HER2, ROS1, RET, NTRK1, and NRG1. EGFR mutations (commoner in women and non-smokers) are mutually exclusive, with the other major lung cancer driver genes such as KRAS (commoner in smokers) presumably because these all converge on the same intracellular signalling pathways. EGFR and ALK are the most clinically relevant of these gene alterations, as targeted drugs are available for those patients whose tumours have these genetic abnormalities. Drugs targeting other mutations including KRAS, ROS1, RET, and HER2 are currently being studied in lung cancer.

Squamous Cell Carcinoma

Squamous cell carcinoma is strongly associated with smoking and has 3–10 times more mutations per megabase than other common cancers. The most frequent gene mutation is TP53.

Small Cell Carcinoma

Small cell carcinoma is driven by inactivating mutations in the TP53 and RB1 genes. These high-grade tumours contain the characteristic tobacco carcinogen associated molecular signature common to all lung cancers, but inactivating RB1 mutations are a hallmark of small cell carcinoma.

Cytological and Histological Diagnosis

Traditionally the histological classification of carcinoma of the lung has been divided into small cell carcinoma (SCC) and non-small cell carcinoma (NSCLC). Within NSCLC, squamous carcinomas have become less common and adenocarcinomas are now the commonest subtype. The most recent UK data [1] apportions histological subtypes as follows: small cell (11%) and carcinoid (1%); and of the remaining 88% NSCLCs adenocarcinoma (36%), squamous (22%), other including large cell, sarcomatoid carcinoma, and some tumours not otherwise specified (11%); and no histological diagnosis in 31%. With the advent of modern oncological treatments, subtyping of NSCLC and molecular testing have become crucial for deciding the most appropriate treatment for individual patients.

Cytological diagnosis entails looking at preparations of individual cells obtained by brushing, washing/lavage or fine-needle aspiration (FNA) at bronchoscopy and endoscopic or endobronchial ultrasound (EUS and EBUS respectively). Diagnoses of lung cancer may also be made from other specimens such as pleural effusions or FNA of skin nodules or cervical lymph nodes. Diagnosis is based on recognising malignant characteristics of the tumour cells such as loss of cell cohesion, high nuclear-cytoplasmic ratios, nuclear pleomorphism (variation in shape and size), and hyperchromasia and mitotic activity. Features such as keratinisation or gland formation and/or presence of intracytoplasmic vacuoles may indicate the tumour sub-type (squamous cell carcinoma and adenocarcinoma respectively). Crucially, tissue architecture cannot be assessed by cytology.

Histological diagnosis entails microscopic examination of thin tissue sections prepared from specimens taken at procedures including bronchoscopy, image-guided biopsy, and surgery. Because architectural features of the tissue can be assessed, information can be gained not simply of tumour type, but also of factors important for staging such as lymphovascular invasion, lymph node involvement, tumour size, and extent of tumour spread.

Histological (and to a lesser extent cytological) diagnosis and subtyping of lung cancer is currently made using a combination of morphological and immunohistochemical features as summarised in Table 6.1.

Table 6.1 Morphological and immunohistochemical characteristics of the commonest histological types of lung cancer

Tumour type	Morphological features	Positive immunohistochemical markers
Adenocarcinoma	Gland formation and/or mucin production	TTF-1
Squamous cell carcinoma	Keratinisation, intercellular bridges	P40 (or P63, or CK5/6)
Small cell carcinoma	Small to intermediate sized cells with scanty cytoplasm, hyperchromatic nuclei and finely granular or glassy nuclear chromatin	CD56, TTF-1, Chromogranin A, synaptophysin

Following histological diagnosis, biopsy or cytology specimens may be sent for molecular testing, e.g. in adenocarcinoma the biopsy or cytology specimen can be tested for EGFR mutations and ALK gene rearrangements using techniques such as immunohistochemistry, PCR and Fluorescent In Situ Hybridisation (FISH). Expression of PD-L1 is also performed using immunohistochemistry to evaluate suitability for immunotherapy. As more genetically targeted drugs become available, and with the introduction of immunotherapy, the list of required tests is increasing.

Diagnosis and Staging

Presentation

In primary care the frequent presenting symptoms which trigger an urgent referral to rule out lung cancer include haemoptysis, cough (lasting longer than 6 weeks), breathlessness, weight loss, and pain. Most patients referred for assessment for possible lung cancer have multiple symptoms. However, the symptoms with which lung cancer presents are non-specific and are commonly associated with other lung diseases.

Haemoptysis Coughing up blood is the only presenting symptom which is statistically associated with a cancer diagnosis in those referred for assessment for possible lung cancer [2]. Haemoptysis can vary from streaks of blood mixed in with sputum through to expectorating clots. Rarely, lung cancer can present with massive haemoptysis.

Cough Differentiating cough caused by malignancy from cough caused by the myriad other aetiologies is very difficult. There are no specific cough features which accurately suggest malignancy. Smokers with a persistent cough, or where the nature of their cough has changed, particularly if associated with other red flag symptoms, require further evaluation, initially with a chest X-ray.

Breathlessness Breathlessness is another non-specific symptom which can be caused by lung cancer. Small peripheral tumours do not cause breathlessness. In order to cause dyspnoea the tumour needs to narrow an airway, cause atelectasis, or be associated with a pleural effusion.

Weight Loss Weight loss is commonly reported by patients as a presenting symptom associated with lung cancer. However, it is rarely the only symptom, and is non-specific. Significant weight loss commonly triggers the initial interaction with healthcare professionals, as the public recognise unexplained weight loss as a serious symptom.

Pain Pain caused by lung cancer is due to either local invasion into the parietal pleura or chest wall, bulky mediastinal nodal involvement, or due to metastatic disease, in particular bone metastases. Liver metastases can also cause pain as a presenting symptom.

Lethargy Symptoms of malaise and lack of energy are common but non-specific.

Symptoms Associated with Metastatic Disease Unfortunately, presentation with symptoms from metastatic disease is common. The commonest sites of metastatic disease which lead to presentation are bone (pain, pathological fracture, hypercalcaemia, spinal cord compression), brain (headache, seizures, focal neurological signs/symptoms), and liver (capsule pain, jaundice, nausea). Rarely, lung cancer can present with adrenal insufficiency due to bilateral adrenal metastases [3].

Aside from unexplained haemoptysis, the common symptoms with which lung cancer first presents are all non-specific, and frequently associated with other smoking related diseases such as COPD. Furthermore, symptoms become increasingly common with more advanced lung cancer. Indeed, many early stage lung cancers are incidental findings rather than "classical" presentations. Paraneoplastic syndromes are not uncommonly due to lung cancer and can present to the endocrinologist, neurologist, or general physician. Some of the commoner presentations are shown below.

Syndrome	Comment
Clubbing, hypertrophic osteoarthropathy (HPOA)	HPOA usually associated with NSCLC
Inappropriate ADH secretion	SCLC usually
Cushing's syndrome	Ectopic ACTH secretion. Biochemical abnormalities (hypokalaemic alkalosis, hypercortisolaemia) rather than clinical CS
Humoral hypercalcaemia	Parathyroid hormone-related peptide secreted by tumour (usually squamous)
Thrombophilia	Venous thromboembolism, may be in unusual site
Subacute sensory neuropathy	Commonest neurological syndrome
Polymyositis/ Dermatomyositis	Gottron's papules, periorbital rash and oedematous eyelids
Eaton-Lambert myasthenic syndrome	Weak legs, autonomic dysfunction, ocular movements preserved. Anti-voltage-gated calcium channel antibody
Cerebellar degeneration	Anti-Yo and anti-Hu antibodies
Limbic encephalitis	Anti-Hu antibody
Glomerulopathy	Usually membranous

Physical signs on examination in patients with lung cancer can include finger clubbing, supraclavicular/cervical lymphadenopathy, hoarse voice due to vocal cord palsy, fixed monophonic wheeze, signs consistent with pleural effusion or lobar atelectasis and, rarely, hypertrophic pulmonary osteoarthropathy.

A chest X-ray should be the first investigation of choice in patients presenting with symptoms suggesting the possibility of lung cancer [4]. However, chest X-ray is significantly less sensitive at detecting lung cancer than CT scanning [5] and so a normal chest X-ray should not be considered entirely reassuring as a method of excluding a diagnosis of lung cancer.

Emergency Presentations

Emergency presentation of lung cancer warrants specific focus, as it is a major challenge for those diagnosing and treating lung cancer, and is associated with significantly worse outcomes compared to patients who are referred as outpatients [6]. In the United Kingdom approximately 35% of lung cancers are diagnosed during an emergency presentation. These patients frequently are older, have later stage disease, and worse performance status. However, even when these factors are corrected for, emergency presentation is associated with a 51% higher 12-month mortality [7]. The factors driving such high rates of emergency presentation are complex, and include cultural factors, the non-specific nature of early symptoms associated with lung cancer, and the fact that most patients with lung cancer have significant co-morbidities. The UK continues to have worse outcomes for lung cancer compared to many other countries in the European Union [8].

NICE Recommendations for Investigation and Referral of Patients with Suspicion of Lung Cancer [4]

Refer people using a suspected cancer pathway referral (for an appointment within 2 weeks) for lung cancer if they:

- Have chest X-ray findings that suggest lung cancer *or*
- Are aged 40 and over with unexplained haemoptysis

Offer an urgent chest X-ray (to be performed within 2 weeks) to assess for lung cancer in people aged 40 and over if they have two or more of the following unexplained symptoms, *or* if they have ever smoked and have one or more of the following unexplained symptoms

- Cough
- Fatigue
- Shortness of breath
- Chest pain
- Weight loss
- Appetite loss

Consider an urgent chest X-ray (to be performed within 2 weeks) to assess for lung cancer in people aged 40 and over with any of the following

- Persistent or recurrent chest infection
- Finger clubbing
- Supraclavicular lymphadenopathy or persistent cervical lymphadenopathy
- Chest signs consistent with lung cancer

Approach to Diagnostic Testing

When assessing a patient with suspected lung cancer, the clinician must take a systematic approach to first confirm or refute the diagnosis, and then to stage and gain histology. The aim should be to achieve diagnosis and staging with the least possible tests in the shortest feasible time. Firstly ask: Which test(s) can best confirm or rule out lung cancer? Then, if after initial testing lung cancer is either confirmed or still suspected, ask a further two questions in parallel:

1. What is the best way to get a histological diagnosis?
2. Which tests will most accurately stage the cancer?

It is also essential that the clinicians ask themselves "Are these tests going to offer valuable information which will alter the patient's treatment options?". In patients with poor performance status for whom treatment will be limited to best supportive care, it is not necessary to fully stage and tissue type cancers.

Staging CT Scan

For all patients with either a chest X-ray suspicious for lung cancer or a normal chest X-ray and ongoing clinical concern for cancer, a contrast-enhanced CT scan of the thorax and upper abdomen, including the liver and adrenal glands, should be performed. The sensitivity and specificity of CT scan to detect lung cancer are 94% and 73% respectively [5].

The staging CT scan gives initial information about both the presence of lung cancer and its stage, and should guide further diagnostic decision-making with the aim of performing a single diagnostic test to give both pathological diagnosis and TNM staging.

Specifically, the CT scan gives important information about mediastinal staging. The most commonly accepted definition of pathological lymphadenopathy on CT criteria is lymph nodes with a short axis diameter of ≥ 1 cm. However, CT scanning in isolation carries significant false positive and negative rates, with a sensitivity of 55% and specificity of 84% for detecting malignant mediastinal lymph nodes [9].

Investigations Beyond the Staging CT Scan

Following CT further tests to accurately diagnose and stage lung cancer may include positron-emitting tomography combined with CT (PET-CT), bronchoscopy, EBUS, EUS, CT-guided biopsy, and image-guided sampling of extra-thoracic disease such as liver metastases or supraclavicular lymph nodes.

PET-CT

PET-CT combines a PET scan after administration of the radio-labelled glucose analogue fluoro-2-deoxy-d-glucose (FDG) with a non-contrast enhanced CT. Malignant cells demonstrate high uptake of glucose (and its analogues) and so FDG accumulates within malignant tissue. This is then detected by a PET scan. The PET scan images are overlaid onto a CT scan to give more detailed anatomical information.

PET-CT more accurately stages lung cancer compared to CT scanning alone. It detects previously unrecognised distant metastases in between 6% and 37% of cases and has better sensitivity and specificity for detecting malignant mediastinal lymph nodes (80% and 88% respectively) [9]. However, it is by no means a perfect test. Nonmalignant tissue, particularly inflammatory processes such as infection or granulomatous disease, display increased PET avidity, and certain tumours such as slow growing well-differentiated adenocarcinoma (particularly of lepidic-predominant type) and typical carcinoid can frequently display normal PET avidity. The investigation of innocent incidental findings, such as within the bowel, may cause a delay in decision-making [10].

EBUS

EBUS has partly replaced surgical mediastinoscopy as a diagnostic/staging investigation in recent years. There are two types of EBUS: convex probe EBUS, which is used to image and sample mediastinal lymph nodes and central parenchymal lesions; and radial probe EBUS, which can sample peripheral lung lesions that are either inaccessible or high risk for CT-guided biopsy, but it is not widely available.

EBUS can access mediastinal lymph node stations 2, 4, 7, 10, and 11 (Fig. 6.2). In experienced hands, EBUS has sensitivity of 89% for detecting malignant mediastinal lymph nodes and a negative predictive value of 91% [9]. For patients with radiologically suspected malignant mediastinal lymph nodes but negative EBUS, surgical mediastinoscopy prior to resection should be considered. Using PET avidity and ultrasonographic heterogeneity, a risk stratification model can be used to determine the need for further staging procedures prior to resection with a negative predictive value of 98% [11].

EBUS can provide both accurate mediastinal staging and a tissue diagnosis in a single procedure, and should be performed as the first test if mediastinal staging is required.

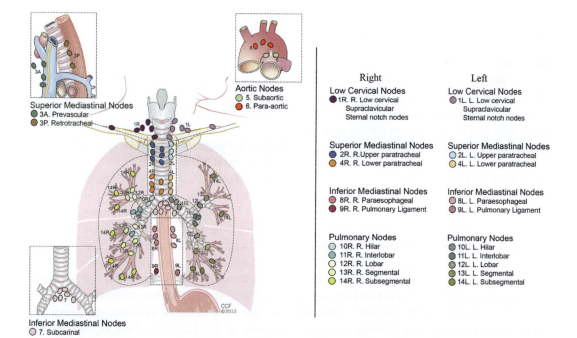

Fig. 6.2 International Association for the Study of Lung Cancer (IASLC) lymph node map. From El-Sherief AH, Lau CT, Wu CC, et al. International Association for the Study of Lung Cancer (IASLC) lymph node map: Radiologic review with CT illustration. RadioGraphics 2014;34:1680–91. With permission from RSNA—Radiological Society of North America

EUS

Endoscopic ultrasound guided needle aspiration is similar in principal to EBUS but involves intubating the oesophagus rather than the trachea. EUS can access the left-sided paratracheal nodes (2L, 4L), station 7, and stations below the diaphragm (station 8 and 9). It can also be used to sample possible adrenal metastases. Technically, it is easier to access 4L using EUS than EBUS. In cases with a pathological appearance on PET-CT or CT, EUS has a sensitivity of 89% and negative predictive value of 86% [9].

Combining EBUS with EUS at the same sitting allows access to almost the entire mediastinum. This approach offers a sensitivity of 91% and negative predictive value of 96% [9].

Image-Guided Trans-Thoracic Lung Biopsy

Most centres in the UK utilise CT for image-guided lung biopsy but fluoroscopy, ultrasound, and electromagnetic navigation can also be used. This technique is useful for peripheral lung lesions for which a histological diagnosis is required and in whom mediastinal staging is not required to guide management. This includes patients with metastatic disease for whom only a tissue diagnosis is required, and patients with peripheral tumours with no evidence of mediastinal or metastatic disease on CT and PET-CT. This procedure carries a risk of approximately 15% for pneumothorax and 1% significant haemorrhage.

Surgical Mediastinoscopy

Mediastinoscopy is a surgical procedure performed under general anaesthetic. A mediastinoscope is inserted through an incision above the suprasternal notch. Mediastinoscopy is historically the gold standard technique for pre-operative staging of the mediastinum. It is possible to access stations 2 and 4 on both sides, station 3 anterior to vessels, and not accessible by EBUS, and anterior station 7. Mediastinoscopy has a sensitivity of 78% for detecting mediastinal malignant nodes and negative predictive value of 91% [9]. This relatively low sensitivity is primarily due to some stations not being easily accessible. The decision regarding whether to proceed to surgical mediastinal staging if EBUS/EUS is negative depends on the level of suspicion of malignancy stratified according to PET findings and EBUS evidence of ultrasonographic heterogeneity.

Supraclavicular Ultrasound-Guided FNA

Lung cancer frequently metastasises to the supraclavicular lymph nodes. In patients with supraclavicular lymph nodes larger than 5 mm, ultrasound-guided assessment and fine-needle aspiration of suspicious nodes has been shown to detect malignancy in 45% of cases [12]. However, this study did not include PET-CT analysis. Current standard would be to perform ultrasound guided FNA for all neck/supraclavicular nodes which are ≥1 cm in diameter or display significant PET avidity.

Which Investigations to Choose Based on CT Findings

Based on the findings of the initial staging CT scan, patients can be broadly divided into five groups. The approach to diagnosis and staging of each of these groups is different.

Group 1: Peripheral Tumour with Normal Mediastinal Lymph Nodes

The most important next test for this group of patients is PET-CT, whilst simultaneously assessing fitness for radical treatment. Initially this is with full pulmonary function tests and consideration of co-morbidities. In the absence of mediastinal lymphadenopathy on CT and PET-CT, and no evidence of distant metastases, the false negative rate for this group of patients is 4% [13, 14]. This is deemed an acceptable level to make mediastinal staging unnecessary.

Group 2: Lung Tumour with Discrete Enlarged Mediastinal Lymph Nodes

These patients require PET-CT and mediastinal staging. The preferred method for mediastinal staging is dependent on local expertise/resource and the anatomical location of lymphadenopathy, but in general this would be EBUS ± EUS. When using EBUS there are two possible approaches to lymph node sampling, either systematic sampling of all stations from N3 to N2 to N1 or targeted sampling of the pathological stations based on radiology. A pragmatic approach is to perform targetted sampling in patients with N3 disease and multi-station N2 disease, but to perform systematic nodal sampling in patients with N1 disease and single station N2 disease according to radiology. These patients can potentially be treated radically.

Group 3: Lung Tumour Directly Invading the Mediastinum Without Metastases

These patients are not operable, and so gaining a tissue diagnosis is the priority. Choice of method between bronchoscopy, EBUS, or image-guided biopsy is dependent on the test most likely to give a positive diagnosis, availability of investigations, and patient choice. PET-CT should also be performed in these patients in order to detect distant metastatic disease not detected by CT scan if radical treatment is being considered.

Group 4: Central Tumour or N1 Disease

These patients all require a PET-CT acknowledging that the false negative rate for N2 may be as high as 25% [9]. EBUS can sample the most stations accurately with good sensitivity as described above. There is no published literature focusing specifically on the role of combined EBUS/EUS for this group. The question of whether to proceed to surgical mediastinoscopy if EBUS is negative depends on local availability of surgical mediastinoscopy, thoroughness of EBUS sampling, and awareness of local false negative rates.

Group 5: Lung Tumour with Metastatic Disease

These patients generally only require a histological diagnosis. Biopsy by the safest and most readily available technique is appropriate if the patient is fit enough for chemotherapy. In frail patients where no oncological treatment is planned, and where survival is likely to be only a few weeks, then histology is unnecessary. PET-CT should be reserved for patients with oligometastatic disease in whom radical treatment might be considered.

Lung Cancer Staging

There are two complementary staging systems for lung cancer; tumour, node, metastasis (TNM) as per the International Association for the Study of Lung Cancer, and Group stage [15]. The individual T, N, and M definitions are based on the fact that each descriptor has prognostic significance (Table 6.2).

The tumour (T) descriptor is based on both the size of the primary tumour and whether it is invading surrounding structures. The node (N) descriptor is based on the anatomical location of pathological nodes in respect to the primary tumour with increasing N status with more distant spread. The metastases (M) descriptor is based on the presence and distribution of metastases. The most recent (Eighth Edition) Lung Cancer Stage Classification was adopted in the UK in January 2018.

Group Staging and Survival

Group staging combines different TNM stages which have similar prognoses and are treated similarly (Fig. 6.3).

Lung cancer survival is critically dependent on staging, and many patients present late with stage 3 or 4 disease. Overall, 1- and 5-year survival in the UK is approximately 38% and 9% respectively [1]. By stage, 5-year survival is 35% (stage 1), 21% (stage 2), 6% (stage 3), and negligible for stage 4. These figures are significantly worse than the 5-year survival figures from a global database, shown in Table 6.3. The cause of

Table 6.2 International Association for the Study of Lung Cancer TNM staging criteria

Descriptor	Definition
T	*Primary tumour*
T0	No primary tumour
T1	Tumour ≤3 cm
T1a	Tumour ≤1 cm
T1b	Tumour >1 cm but ≤2 cm
T1c	Tumour >2 cm, but ≤3 cm
T2	Tumour >3 cm but ≤5 cm or tumour with any of the following: • Involves main bronchus but not carina • Invades visceral pleura • Associated with atelectasis or obstructive pneumonitis extending to the hilar region
T2a	Tumour >3 cm but ≤4 cm
T2b	Tumour >4 cm but ≤5 cm
T3	Tumour >5 cm but ≤7 cm or any of the following: • Directly invading chest wall, phrenic nerve, or parietal pericardium, • Separate tumour nodules in same lobe
T4	Tumour >7 cm or any size with • Invasion of diaphragm, mediastinum, heart, great vessels, trachea, recurrent laryngeal nerve, oesophagus, vertebral body, carina. • Tumour nodules in different ipsilateral lobe
N	*Regional lymph nodes*
N0	No regional lymph node metastasis
N1	Metastasis in ipsilateral peribronchial, ipsilateral hilar and intrapulmonary nodes
N2	Metastasis in ipsilateral mediastinal and/or subcarinal nodes
N3	Matastasis in contralateral mediastinal, contralateral hilar, any scalene or supraclavicular nodes
M	*Distant metastasis*
M0	No distant metastasis
M1	Distant metastasis
M1a	Separate tumour nodule(s) in contralateral lobe, tumour with pleural or pericardial nodules, malignant pleural or pericardial effusion
M1b	Single extrathoracic metastasis in a single organ
M1c	Multiple extrathoracic metastases in one or several organs

From: Peter Goldstraw, Kari Chansky, Johnn Crowley, Ramon Rami-Porta, Hisao Asamura, Wilfired EE Eberhardt, et al. The IASLC Lung Cancer Staging Project: Proposals for Revision of the TNM Stage Groupings in the Forthcoming (Eighth) Edition of the TNM Classification for Lung Cancer. J Thoracic Oncol. 2016; 39–51. With permission of Elsevier

this discrepancy is multifactorial and complex, but the UK data set is considered robust and more closely reflects everyday clinical practice.

Small cell lung cancer is staged as limited or extensive stage. Limited stage lung cancer is disease which is unilateral and can be encompassed in a radiation field. Extensive stage small cell lung cancer is defined by metastasis to contralateral lung or lymph nodes or distant metastasis.

Performance Status

The performance status scale was developed by researchers from the Eastern Cooperative Oncology Group (ECOG) to take into account a patient's level of functioning when planning trials of cancer treatments. It is often used in clinical practice when considering if a patient is fit enough for treatment such as radiotherapy or chemotherapy.

Fig. 6.3 Group staging of lung cancer. See Table 6.2 for explanation of abbreviations

T/M	Label	N0	N1	N2	N3
T1	T1a ≤1	IA1	IIB	IIIA	IIIB
	T1b >1-2	IA2	IIB	IIIA	IIIB
	T1c >2-3	IA3	IIB	IIIA	IIIB
T2	T2a Cent, Visc Pl	IB	IIB	IIIA	IIIB
	T2a >3-4	IB	IIB	IIIA	IIIB
	T2b >4-5	IIA	IIB	IIIA	IIIB
T3	T3 >5-7	IIB	IIIA	IIIB	IIIC
	T3 Inv	IIB	IIIA	IIIB	IIIC
	T3 Satell	IIB	IIIA	IIIB	IIIC
T4	T4 >7	IIIA	IIIA	IIIB	IIIC
	T4 Inv	IIIA	IIIA	IIIB	IIIC
	T4 Ipsi Nod	IIIA	IIIA	IIIB	IIIC
M1	M1a Contr Nod	IVA	IVA	IVA	IVA
	M1a Pl Dissem	IVA	IVA	IVA	IVA
	M1b Single	IVA	IVA	IVA	IVA
	M1c Multi	IVB	IVB	IVB	IVB

Table 6.3 Survival of patients from the International Association for the Study of Lung Cancer database diagnosed between 1999 and 2010

Clinical stage	5-year survival (%)
1A[a]	83
1B	68
2A	60
2B	53
3A	36
3B	26
4A	10
4B	0

[a]Stage IA refers to patients with 1–2 cm tumours. Survival figures for tumours <1 cm and 2–3 cm are 92% and 77% respectively [16]

Grade	Activity
0	Fully active, able to carry out all pre-disease activities without restriction
1	Restricted in physically strenuous activity but capable of light work
2	Ambulatory, capable of selfcare but unable to carry out any work. Up and about >50% of waking hours
3	Limited selfcare, confined to bed or chair >50% of waking hours
4	Completely disabled. Incapable of any selfcare. Confined to bed or chair

Lung Cancer Screening

Lung cancer frequently presents with advanced disease. The prognosis of stage 3 and 4 disease is poor, and treatment options are limited, with little impact on overall survival rates over the last two decades despite multidisciplinary working, thoracoscopic surgery, and more aggressive chemoradiotherapy regimes.

The aim of lung cancer screening is to detect lung cancer in high-risk individuals before it has reached the advanced stages and would allow radical treatments with improvement in mortality. Historically chest X-ray and sputum cytology have been studied as means of screening, but they were shown to be ineffective [17]. The development of CT technology has allowed high quality images to be obtained with excellent sensitivity for detecting lung cancer using low dose protocols. A low-dose CT (LDCT) protocol exposes the patient to approximately one-fifth of the radiation of a standard CT scan, equivalent to approximately 6 months' background radiation. Initial studies evaluating the efficacy of LDCT in screening high-risk, asymptomatic individuals showed that LDCT detects more cancers than chest X-ray and that the cancers detected were frequently stage 1. The U.S. National Lung Cancer Screening Trial recruited 53,454 individuals, either current smokers or ex-smokers within 15 years, with at least 30 pack years history, aged between 55 and 74 years. They were randomized to annual LDCT or CXR for 3 years, with further clinical follow-up for the next 3.5 years. Throughout the study period, 1060 lung cancers were detected in the LDCT group and 941 in the CXR group. Significantly higher numbers of detected cancers were stage 1 in the LDCT group. The trial reported a 20% relative risk reduction of lung cancer-related mortality in the group undergoing LDCT (absolute numbers of cancer related deaths 356 and 443 respectively) [18]. These results have led to the recommendation that lung cancer screening should be offered to high-risk individuals between the ages of 55 and 80 years in the USA.

There remain unanswered questions about the applicability of this to a European population/health care service. Important research questions include:

1. What is the optimal interval between scans?
2. What age range should be screened?
3. How best to engage high-risk, hard-to-engage populations?
4. Are there biomarkers which can help define high-risk individuals for CT screening?

Another issue is the false positive rate of LDCT because of detection of indeterminate lung nodules. The vast majority of these are benign, but a small proportion turn out to be malignant [19]. Consequently, they require ongoing CT follow-up, leading to anxiety, expense, and radiation exposure to individuals which otherwise would not have occurred. The psychosocial impact of this needs studying carefully to inform on the potential negative impacts of a lung cancer screening programme [20].

The cumulative radiation risk is negatively associated with age, and higher for females than males due to the risk of breast cancer. It is estimated that lung cancer screening will cause one to three cancers per 10,000 individuals screened [21].

Management of Lung Cancer

Management of Complications

Airways Compromise

Lung cancer commonly affects the central airways and can cause significant dyspnoea due to endobronchial disease or airway compression. As well as standard therapies such as chemotherapy and radiotherapy, endobronchial therapies can be useful in symptom relief or as a bridge to allow time for systemic treatments to work. For endobronchial disease which requires debulking there are a number of options including Nd:YAG laser, cryotherapy, or endobronchial stents. There is no evidence supporting these interventions as anything other than palliative.

Superior Vena Cava Obstuction

Thoracic malignancies can cause direct compression and symptomatic obstruction of the superior vena cava (SVC). The SVC syndrome occurs in 4% of non-small cell lung cancers and 10% of small cell lung cancers. It presents with signs of raised venous pressure, including facial and upper limb oedema, and congested chest wall veins. Oedema of the larynx can cause dyspnoea, cough, and rarely stridor.

Initial treatment with oral steroids and possibly diuretics is common practice, but not evidence-based. With severe symptoms, intravascular stenting of the SVC should be considered, which leads to rapid relief of symptoms. If the symptoms are not severe, time can be taken to treat the underlying disease.

Paraneoplastic Syndromes

Paraneoplastic syndromes present with signs and symptoms in association with the presence of lung cancer, but not caused directly by the physical effects of the tumour. They are present in approximately 10% of cases of lung cancer [22]. Paraneoplastic syndromes can cause endocrine, neurological, dermatological, and rheumatological effects. The specific neoplastic syndromes tend to associate with certain types of lung cancer with the syndrome of inappropriate antidiuretic hormone secretion (SIADH) being most commonly associated with small cell lung cancer, and humoral hypercalcaemia of malignancy being most commonly associated with squamous cell cancer. In general, the approach to managing paraneoplastic syndromes should focus on treatment of the underlying malignancy where possible. However, paraneoplastic syndromes can be refractory to treatment. Specific treatments are available, including demeclocycline or oral vaspressin antagonists for SIADH which is refractory to fluid restriction, and intravenous bisphosponates for symptomatic hypercalcaemia.

Surgery

Introduction

Until the development of radical radiotherapy, surgery offered the only chance of cure for non-small cell lung cancer. Radical surgery with curative intent is recommended for most early-stage disease and can be considered for higher staged tumours.

The Role of the Surgeon

The role of the thoracic surgeon in cancer management has evolved to include diagnosis, staging, and palliative care, as well as surgical resection. Rigid bronchoscopy for diagnosis is used when patients cannot tolerate fiberoptic bronchoscopy under sedation, or in patients with suspected carcinoid tumours at risk of bleeding. For peripheral tumours where biopsy has failed or is not safe a surgical biopsy, excision biopsy or frozen section can be performed at open thoracotomy or VAT (video-assisted thoracoscopy). There also remains a growing group of patients where the diagnosis is not known prior to resection and the diagnosis is only made post-operatively (up to 15% of cases of VATS resections reported from some units).

Cervical mediastinoscopy and video-assisted mediastinoscopy remain the gold standard for pre-operative mediastinal staging. Stations 2, 3, 4, and 10 (hilar nodes) can be accessed. Stations

5 and 6 are more routinely accessed by left anterior mediastinotomy. VATS can access most of the stations in the mediastinum but is rarely used as a staging procedure.

Surgical excision can be the only treatment for some cancers, and for many patients is the most important treatment giving the best chance of cure. A successful resection requires removal of the entire tumour with a clear resection margin leaving no residual disease (R0). This must be achieved safely without significantly compromising organ function or quality of life. As such, radical intention to treat with surgery is defined as treatment to significantly improve survival. When considering radical treatment with surgery, the patient needs to be assessed for resectability (the ability to achieve a R0 resection) and operability (that the patient is medically fit to undergo the lung resection surgery and will not be left disabled after the surgery because of the lung resection).

Radical surgery can be considered for all patients with early-stage disease (T1-3 N0-1) dependent on medical fitness. Surgery can also be considered in selected patients with T4 N0-1 disease where the tumour invades the carina, great vessels, and mediastinum. Surgery for N2 disease remains controversial. Single station N2 disease can be considered for radical resection, with a reported survival of up to 30% [23]. Survival is poor in multi-station N2 disease and should not be considered for radical surgery outside of a multi-modality clinical trial [24].

Fitness for Surgery

Patients with lung cancer are highly likely to suffer from other smoking-related cardio-respiratory diseases. Assessment is made using a tripartite risk assessment outlined in the BTS Guidelines on the Radical Management of Patients with Lung Cancer [24]. Other resources include NICE guidance [25] and the American College of Chest Physicians (ACCP) guidelines for assessing pre-operative patients with lung comorbidities [26]. A careful assessment of the patient's fitness is made to judge the degree of risk to the patient and assess whether surgery should be performed. Risk-scoring models are advised to assess peri-operative mortality, including the Thoracoscore model, [27] a logistic regression-derived model utilising nine variables. Although extensively used in Europe, there is evidence it may not be accurate in real world practice [28].

The risk of cardiac death or non-fatal myocardial infarction is 1–5% during lung resection. Cardiac risk factors include atrial fibrillation, hypertension, valvular disease, and a history of heart failure or ischaemic heart disease. Guidelines advise avoidance of surgery within 30 days of a myocardial infarction. It is safe to proceed with surgery if the patient has two or less cardiac risk factors and good functional cardiac capacity. However, if patients have an active cardiac condition, three or more cardiac risk factors, or poor cardiac functional capacity, they should be referred for a cardiological opinion. Other factors which need to be considered because of their effect on perioperative morbidity and mortality are the presence of cerebrovascular disease, diabetes requiring insulin therapy, and a raised serum creatinine level.

Anti-ischaemic medication should be continued in the peri-operative period. Where patients have stable chronic angina or other conventional indications for revascularisation, this should be considered before lung resection. If a patient has a coronary stent, antiplatelet therapy should be discussed with a cardiologist prior to surgery.

The risk of post-operative dyspnoea is calculated pre-operatively. Standard spirometry and gas transfer with segment counting can be used to estimate predicted postoperative (PPO) lung function. A PPO FEV1 and DLCO >60% predict a low risk of postoperative breathlessness, whereas a PPO FEV1 and DLCO <30% predict a high risk.

Further assessment measuring maximal oxygen uptake (VO2 max) with a cardio-pulmonary exercise test (CPET) is useful for borderline cases: VO2max of 10–15 ml/kg/min indicates an increased surgical risk, whereas a VO2max <10 ml/kg/min predicts a high risk of perioperative death.

Radical Surgery

Surgical procedures for curative resection include wedge resection, segmentectomy, lobectomy, bi-lobectomy, and pneumonectomy. Since the findings of the Lung Cancer Study Group in 1995, [29] lobectomy has been the gold standard operation for lung cancer confined to a lobe. Lobectomy had better outcomes than segmentectomy and wedge resection for all tumours over 1 cm in size. However, there is increasing interest in lung conservation, and segmentectomy can be indicated for tumours up to 2 cm provided there can be a good margin to the resection and the tumour is staged accurately with an appropriate lymph node dissection. Pneumonectomy is a major operation carrying increased operative risk and causing major physiological disturbance, especially in the older patient (>80 years). There has consequently been a significant decline in the number of pneumonectomies performed because of the wider utilization of sleeve resection.

Over the past 25 years VATS has had an increased role, especially in the treatment of early-stage lung cancer, with now over 30% of resections in many units performed by VATS. Non-randomised trials have shown the procedure to be safe and may allow as complete a cancer-clearing operation as at thoracotomy with lymph node sampling/resection. VATS appears to be associated with less post-operative pain, fewer complications, shorter post-operative stay, and faster recovery, factors which may well increase the uptake of adjuvant chemotherapy in a timely fashion. Overall, the reported series show survival is at least equivalent to open surgery [30]. Early results from robotic surgery are encouraging, with reports of considerable lower pain scores and quicker recovery.

Surgery may be considered for locally advanced T4 tumours or advanced oligometastatic disease where the metastasis can be treated radically. Evidence is confined mainly to small reported series, and surgery should only be considered offered following full discussion at the MDT and accurate disclosure to the patient.

Outcomes for Surgery

Despite the increasing resection rate, including higher risk patients, peri-operative 30-day mortality remains relatively constant at 2–2.5% for lobectomy and 5.8% for pneumonectomy [1]. There is further attrition, particularly in patients with more advanced tumours, with a 90-day mortality, which is double the 30-day mortality [31]. Adjuvant (post-operative) chemotherapy was found to be detrimental in stage 1a disease, but offers benefit in higher stage disease.

Radiotherapy for Lung Cancer

Radical and Palliative Treatment for Lung Cancer

The current gold-standard radical treatment for non-small cell lung cancer (NSCLC) is complete surgical resection with adjuvant chemotherapy for those at high risk of recurrence. However, the majority of patients with NSCLC present with disease which is too advanced for surgical resection. Patients with small-cell lung cancer (SCLC) rarely undergo radical resection, as their disease is usually locally advanced within the thorax and frequently overtly metastatic at the time of presentation. Most lung cancers managed with radical intent therefore undergo non-surgical treatment, comprising radiotherapy alone or a combination of radiotherapy and chemotherapy. Recently, advances have allowed the development of radical stereotactic radiotherapy techniques for patients with early-stage, non-small cell lung cancer who are medically unfit for surgical resection.

Palliative treatment for lung cancer is aimed at improving the symptoms of incurable disease and where possible, extending life expectancy. So far only palliative chemotherapy has been shown to improve length of life, but there is good evidence to support the use of radiotherapy in the palliative setting for symptomatic benefit.

Principles of Radiotherapy

Radiotherapy (RT) uses ionising radiation to treat cancers and is usually given as high-energy photons produced in a linear accelerator. Less commonly, RT is given as electron treatment for superficially situated cancers, and more rarely, as proton beam therapy. A fraction of radiotherapy refers to the dose of radiation, expressed in Grays (Gy), given at a single exposure, which is usually delivered once each day on consecutive working days. Fractions of RT can be given more often than once per day (hyperfractionation) or less frequently than once per day (hypofractionation), and can be given as a single exposure in the palliative setting. A course of RT refers to the sum of the fractions delivered, and is expressed as the total dose of radiation delivered in a given number of fractions over a specified period of time.

Radical RT can eradicate localised cancers if given in a way which maximises damage to malignant cells while allowing repair mechanisms to operate and restore the function of normal cell populations. Radiotherapy causes damage to DNA, in particular double strand breaks which are difficult to repair accurately. In normal dividing cell populations, DNA repair mechanisms and cell cycle controls are intact, DNA damage from RT is detected, and the cell cycle is halted until repair is complete or a terminally damaged cell is diverted along a cell death pathway. In malignant cells, mutations are frequent and can occur in genes which code for cell cycle control mechanisms and DNA repair enzymes. Damage to DNA by radiotherapy may therefore fail to induce the normal damage repair mechanisms, resulting in continuation of the cell cycle and abnormal mitosis with death of the daughter cells. It must be remembered that an inherent limitation of radiotherapy, and indeed chemotherapy, stems from the fact that a cancer consists of many varied populations of cells which have accumulated mutations and hence have different phenotypes, including their susceptibility to anti-cancer treatments. Conventional radical RT exploits the difference in the potential of malignant and normal populations of cells to repair radiation damage by splitting the total dose of RT into many small fractions delivered over several weeks. A typical radical dose for non-small cell lung cancer would deliver 66 Gy in 33 fractions over 6½ weeks. This allows time between fractions for normal cells to undergo more recovery than the malignant population. The difference in survival of the normal and malignant cells is manifest as the RT course continues, although as there is damage to both populations, cure can only be achieved if the malignant cells can be eradicated without irreparable damage to normal cells. To maximise this therapeutic differential and avoid dose-limiting normal tissue toxicity, it is important to deliver a high dose of RT to the cancer while minimising the dose to surrounding normal tissues. This is achieved by conforming the radiotherapy beams to the shape of the cancer mass, and by using accurate imaging to ensure that the target is covered by the beam at each fraction. These techniques are described below.

Risks of Radiotherapy

Toxicity from radiotherapy is usually divided into "early" and "late" with an arbitrary cut-off at 6 months after completion of RT. Early reacting tissues are those with a rapid turnover of cells such as the bone marrow, skin, and mucosal surfaces. These lose integrity because of radiation damage during the course of RT, and this may continue for several weeks after the end of treatment. Recovery from acute side effects occurs gradually over the weeks after RT is complete, and the severity of the toxicity depends more on the total dose delivered than the dose per fraction. Late reacting tissues are usually those with a slow turnover of cells, such as fibrous tissue, muscle, bone, glia, and blood vessels. Late damage usually causes changes such as fibrosis, necrosis, and telangiectasia, and may cause complications many years after the RT has finished. In general, late reacting tissues are more sensitive to the dose per fraction than the total dose. Thus in the development of dose and fractionation reg-

imens, it is important to balance the chances of cure of the cancer with the risks of both early and late side effects. Palliative RT uses the same photon energies and delivery mechanisms as radical RT, but as the aim is not cure but relief of symptoms, dose and fractionation regimens are designed to achieve maximal symptomatic benefit while minimising toxicity.

In the treatment of lung cancers with radiotherapy, the organs most at risk of damage—and therefore those which limit treatment dose and volume—are the lungs, oesophagus, heart, and spinal cord. Care must be taken when planning RT to the chest, as the length of oesophagus taken to high dose is linked to the severity of the acute radiation toxicity or late fibrosis and stricture. In the acute phase of radiation oesophagitis, patients may struggle to maintain their hydration and nutrition, and this should be anticipated and actively managed with help from dieticians and with the liberal use of analgesics. Oesophageal stricture is rare, and recurrent cancer should be ruled out in patients with a previously treated lung cancer who present with dysphagia. Endoscopic dilatation may be required and often needs to be repeated. The spinal cord is outlined during the planning process and the beams are carefully arranged to avoid overdose, which can lead to the late effect of radiation myelitis. If the cancer lies too close to the spine, particularly if the vertebral body is invaded, radical treatment may not be possible.

The lungs are also carefully delineated, and the percentage volume of lung outside the high-dose region which receives more than 20 Gy must be kept below a maximum of 35%. As many patients with lung cancer have co-existing chronic obstructive pulmonary disease, full lung function tests, including transfer factor, may be required to ensure that patents with poor respiratory reserve can be safely treated. Acute radiation damage ("radiation pneumonitis") usually presents as breathlessness and cough, which may be accompanied by a fever. It is difficult to distinguish from infection, and management usually comprises symptomatic measures plus steroids and antibiotics. Radiation pneumonitis is usually self-limiting, but the late side effect of radiation fibrosis may affect lung function if the volume is large, and therefore stringent pre-treatment assessment and careful radiotherapy planning are essential.

Planning and Delivery of Radiotherapy for Lung Cancer

In its early days, radical RT was delivered essentially as a "box" encompassing the lung cancer and surrounding tissues as defined by the available imaging. With more recent advances in radiotherapy and radiology, it has been possible to conform the radiotherapy volume to the shape of the cancer to be treated, excluding as much normal tissue as possible while still treating the cancer to high dose.

The planning of conventional three-dimensional conformal radiotherapy (3D CRT) for both non-small cell and small-cell lung cancer involves the careful delineation of the cancer and involved lymph nodes, usually with the help of CT or PET/CT images. The patient undergoes a radiotherapy planning CT scan, usually performed without contrast, lying supine on a flat bed with their arms supported above the head to allow for beam entry through the lateral chest wall (Fig. 6.4). Patients who are too breathless to lie in this way cannot, realistically, undergo radical RT unless their breathing can be improved by other interventions. Technology is available to allow RT planning using a PET/CT scan, and some UK departments are moving to adopt this for lung cancer, which should speed up the RT planning process, avoid an additional visit to hospital, and improve the ability of the clinical oncologist to define the target tissues. The planning CT scan is carried out after careful alignment of the patient with orthogonal lasers in the CT suite which are replicated in the treatment rooms. Small tattoos made on the skin along the laser lines ensure that the position of the patient during RT planning can be reproduced on each treatment day. The planning CT scan is viewed by the clinical oncologist using RT planning software, and the cancer and involved nodes are outlined in three dimensions with a margin added to take the uncertainties

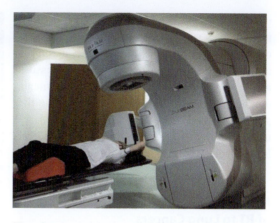

Fig. 6.4 Demonstration of the treatment position required for radical radiotherapy to the chest. The linear accelerator has side arms to allow cone-beam CT imaging

of microscopic spread, tumour movement, and patient positioning into account. RT beams are arranged by a team of specialist dosimetrists and physicists using RT planning computer software to maximise the dose to the cancer and minimise the dose to normal structures. The planning process takes 10–14 days and at each stage, stringent checks are put in place to ensure that the planned treatment volume is accurate and safe to deliver. Once treatment begins, the patient and their skin tattoos are aligned with the treatment room lasers on each day, and treatment is delivered with imaging checks for positioning as described below. The treatment should continue as prescribed without any unplanned breaks, although treatment is not given at the weekends in conventionally fractionated RT. Occasionally weekend treatments or an additional fraction at the end of the RT course may be required to account for planned departmental holidays, and occasionally for unscheduled interruptions, such as machine breakdown or patient illness.

Palliative RT is planned in a similar way, but the patient usually does not need to lie with their arms above their head unless the area to be treated lies laterally in the chest. Patient positioning can be more flexible according to the site to be treated, to take into account bony pain or breathlessness. Any available imaging, e.g. PET/CT, MRI, or isotope bone scan, can be used to assist in the definition of the treatment volume, which includes the area to be treated plus an adequate margin. This is usually covered by a single field or two opposing fields to provide a simple arrangement. Dose constraints to normal tissues are not usually of concern in palliative treatments unless there has been high-dose treatment in the same area in the past. Palliative treatments are usually carried out over fewer days than radical RT, typically in one to five fractions.

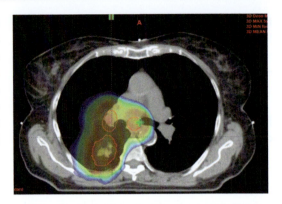

Fig. 6.5 A patient with a T2N2 non-small cell cancer of the right lower lobe was treated with radical radiotherapy using IMRT. The high-dose volume can be seen to conform to the volume containing the cancer and nodes while avoiding the spinal cord

Methods of Improving the Delivery of RT to Lung Cancers

Intensity-Modulated Radiotherapy

In order to deliver high doses of RT to a lung cancer while avoiding dose-limiting toxicity to surrounding normal structures, it is important to be able to conform the high-dose volume as closely as possible to the structure to be treated. Intensity-modulated radiotherapy (IMRT) describes a method of radiotherapy planning using sophisticated "inverse treatment planning" computer algorithms to achieve this [32]. Whereas standard RT planning for 3D CRT uses established field arrangements for localised lung cancers, adjusting the parameters of the field size, shape, angle, and weighting to generate a "best fit," IMRT uses clinician-defined high-dose regions in conjunction with dose constraints to organs at risk of toxicity (OARs). Planning algorithms generate a conformal RT "dose map" with each beam varying not only in shape, but also in intensity across the beam. For example, it is possible using IMRT to treat a high-dose volume close to the spinal cord, without exceeding the strict dose constraints required to avoid late toxicity to the spine (Fig. 6.5). IMRT is delivered using the same photon energies and the same linear accelerators as conventional 3D CRT, though recent developments have allowed the use of "arc" therapy. This involves the linear accelerator head moving axially around the patient while delivering IMRT, the shape and intensity of the beam being modulated as it travels to deliver a more uniform dose than previously possible. Technological developments are continuing with the aim of further improving the accuracy and specificity of RT delivery, maxi-

mising the chance of local control while minimising toxicity to surrounding structures. RT departments in the UK are rapidly moving towards the adoption of IMRT as the standard for radical RT treatment of non-small cell lung cancer.

The Clinical Application of RT for Lung Cancer

Radiotherapy Alone for NSCLC

Several factors limit the ability of radical radiotherapy alone to effect a cure for stage I–III non-small cell lung cancer: (1) the presence of metastatic disease, which is undetectable by current techniques; (2) the inherent radio-resistance of a proportion of the cancer cells; and (3) the propensity of malignant cells to repopulate at an increased rate once cell death is induced. Repopulation may in part be overcome by shortening the overall duration of a course of radiotherapy, thus reducing the time available for the cells to repopulate. Taking this to its maximal extent, the regimen of continuous hyperfractionated accelerated radiotherapy (CHART) was developed. The results of CHART compared to conventional RT have been encouraging, with a 9% absolute improvement in 2-year survival, from 20% to 29%, with a 14% improvement seen in patients with squamous cell lung cancer [33]. However, CHART remains difficult for many departments to implement, owing to the limitations of staffing. In addition, criticism of the CHART study has highlighted the dose of RT in the standard arm which, at 60 Gy, would be considered lower than the currently recommended dose of 66 Gy.

Radiotherapy in Combination with Chemotherapy

For patients with non-small cell lung cancer and involved mediastinal nodes, the results of radiotherapy alone are poor in terms of local control and long-term survival. Chemotherapy can be combined with radiotherapy to improve the measured outcomes, and may be given either sequentially (chemotherapy followed by RT to the residual mass) or concurrently with RT. The use of concurrent chemotherapy probably has a dual effect as a local radiosensitiser and also through its ability to target distant metastatic disease. In clinical trials, the benefits of concurrent treatment over sequential are clearly seen, with an absolute survival benefit of 8% at 2 years and an improvement in overall survival at 5 years of 4.5% (15.1% vs 10.6%) [34, 35] making concurrent chemoradiotherapy the gold-standard. However, normal tissue constraints may make sequential treatment preferable if the cancer is large, as concurrent treatment is more toxic in the acute phase than sequential, with a higher rate of neutropenia and radiation-induced grade 3–4 oesophagitis (18% vs 4%). Radiotherapy is planned and delivered in the same way as described above, a typical combination comprising two cycles of platinum doublet chemotherapy administered concurrently with the radical radiotherapy, and a further two cycles given in the adjuvant setting once RT is complete.

Stereotactic Ablative Body Radiotherapy

Stereotactic ablative body radiotherapy (SABR) is a method of administering high doses of radical RT to an accurately defined, small, extracranial volume, and is named to distinguish it from stereotactic radiotherapy or radiosurgery used to treat lesions in the brain. It has been developed as an alternative to surgical resection for patients

with T1-T2a node negative tumours who are not fit for surgery for medical reasons, including poor lung function or cardiac co-morbidities. SABR uses either multiple fixed beams or arc therapy to deliver ablative doses of RT well above those used for radical RT given by 3D-CRT or IMRT. SABR is planned using the same techniques as IMRT with a 4D-CT scan, PET/CT imaging, and inverse planning algorithms (Figs. 6.6 and 6.7). The margins around the cancer are small and cone-beam CT images taken before treatment and, if necessary, during and after each fraction, are critical to ensure that the target lies in the high-dose volume and that doses to surrounding normal structures are limited. Owing to the very high doses used, normal tissue constraints are strict: the high-dose volume cannot lie within 2 cm of the proximal bronchial tree or distal trachea; treatable cancers are limited to 5 cm diameter; and if the high-dose volume includes the chest wall, a smaller dose per fraction is used to reduce the late side effect of rib necrosis, fracture, and pain.

Current use of SABR is limited to patients who cannot undergo surgery, as it has not been tested in a randomised clinical trial against surgical resection, but initial results are promising. Analysis of the first 273 patients treated in the inaugural UK SABR centre showed a median survival of 27.3 months, with an overall survival of 78, 55,

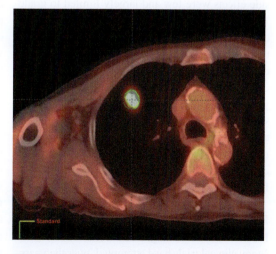

Fig. 6.6 PET-CT scan with pseudo colour. The right upper lobe T1N0 cancer is easily seen. The volume to be treated with SABR to high dose has been outlined

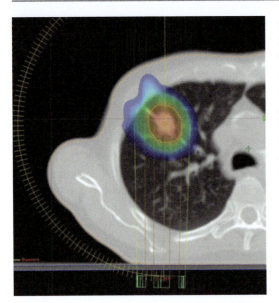

Fig. 6.7 Same patient as in Fig. 6.6. The small right upper lobe cancer is being treated with SABR to 54 Gy in three fractions. The colour overlay shows a range from 50% (dark blue) to 115% (pink) of the prescription dose. The curved hatched line around the patient's right chest represents the path of one of the two arc radiotherapy beams

and 39% at 1, 2 and 3 years, respectively [36]. Histological confirmation was obtained in only 35% of cases, reflecting the poor lung function and substantial comorbidities which precluded surgery in this medically inoperable cohort. Acute side effects were few and largely limited to grade 1–2 cough, shortness of breath, pneumonitis, chest pain, fatigue, oesophagitis, and skin reactions. Grade 3 toxicities beyond 12 weeks were rare, comprising breathlessness, fatigue, and chest pain, the latter affecting three patients at a year post-treatment. Although matched comparisons suggest that SABR provides survival results comparable to those of surgery, selection bias is unavoidable. Unfortunately, a planned randomised controlled trial comparing SABR with surgery failed to recruit adequately and was closed.

Post-operative Radiotherapy for Non-small Cell Lung Cancer

Many clinical trials have attempted, over the years, to define the role of post-operative RT (PORT) in completely resected non-small cell lung cancer. A

meta-analysis, first published in 1998 and updated in 2005, showed a detrimental effect on survival equivalent to an 18% relative increase in the risk of death, reducing overall survival at 5 years by 5%, from 58% to 53% [37]. Sub-group analysis suggests that this effect is most marked in stage I and II disease (N0 and N1), whereas for stage III, N2 disease, there is no evidence of either benefit or detriment, PORT possibly contributing to local control but not affecting overall survival. The studies contributing to these meta-analyses were largely conducted in the 1960s and 1970s, before modern linear accelerators were developed, and using what would now be considered unsatisfactory techniques and large volumes, planned without CT or PET/CT staging. It is possible that the increased risk of death stemmed from greater cardiac and lung toxicity. If so, the use of more modern RT techniques could conceivably overcome this and confer a survival benefit in stage III disease. A retrospective analysis of 4483 patients with completely resected stage IIIA non-small cell lung cancer compared overall survival with and without PORT and found a slight improvement in median and 5-year overall survival with the addition of PORT to adjuvant chemotherapy, although the 95% confidence intervals overlapped [38]. In order to answer this question, a phase III study, lungART, is underway, randomising patients with completely resected non-small cell lung cancer and mediastinal nodal involvement (N2) between two arms: post-operative conformal radiotherapy vs no post-operative radiotherapy (LungART protocol) and where the primary end point is disease-free survival. Until this study reports, PORT for completely resected stage III NSCLC remains controversial.

In contrast, in spite of a paucity of evidence, PORT is recommended in most lung cancer guidelines for the treatment of patients with positive margins or macroscopic residual disease following radical surgery for NSCLC. Retrospective analyses suggest that including the positive resection margin or residual disease and treating with 3D CRT or IMRT to a dose of 50–55 Gy reduces the risk of local recurrence [39]. Recent data suggest that there may be an influence on overall survival, but confirmation will require a randomised clinical trial.

Small-Cell Lung Cancer

Small-cell lung cancer (SCLC) is an extremely chemotherapy-sensitive cancer, which tends to metastasise early in its development and frequently before a diagnosis is made. Cure rates range from 10 to 15%, with a median survival of 16–24 months in limited stage disease, which can be defined in practical terms as cancer confined to one hemithorax, including supraclavicular nodes which can be encompassed within a radical radiotherapy field.

RT for Limited-Stage SCLC

For limited-stage SCLC, the combination of systemic chemotherapy and involved-field thoracic radiotherapy, given without elective irradiation of uninvolved intrathoracic lymph nodes, results in better overall survival rates than chemotherapy alone [40]. As with NSCLC, concurrent chemoradiotherapy is superior to sequential treatment, [41] particularly if the RT commences early, with the first or second cycle of chemotherapy [42]. However, large cancers are often not treatable concurrently in view of the volume to be encompassed within the radiotherapy field, and sequential treatment may be considered safer, particularly in patients with poor performance status and suboptimal lung function. Chemotherapy usually comprises a two-drug combination of a platinum agent with etoposide delivered as four to six cycles. As carboplatin is more likely to exacerbate the toxicity of radiotherapy than cisplatin, the latter is usually given in conjunction with radiotherapy.

Prophylactic Cranial Irradiation

Brain metastases are common in small-cell lung cancer, with at least 18% of patients having brain metastases at diagnosis, with the proportion approaching 80% in patients alive 2 years later. The brain has often been considered a sanctuary site for metastatic disease, with systemic chemotherapy penetrating less well because of the blood-brain barrier, and salvage treatment with chemotherapy or radiotherapy often proving

unsatisfactory. Meta-analysis has shown that the addition of prophylactic cranial irradiation (PCI) to the whole brain following a complete response to chemotherapy for limited-stage small-cell lung cancer improves overall survival. The proportion still alive 3 years from randomisation was shown to increase from 15.3% without PCI to 20.7% in the treatment group [34]. PCI decreased the risk of developing brain metastases, with an absolute reduction of 25% in the cumulative incidence at 3 years, from 58.6% in the control group to 33.3% in the treatment group. Standard management of patients with limited stage SCLC therefore includes PCI, usually given in the UK as 25 Gy in 10 fractions over 2 weeks. A study of 286 patients with extensive stage SCLC and a performance status of 0–2 who had achieved a response to chemotherapy compared either no further therapy or PCI delivered as one of several RT regimens [43]. At 1 year, the incidence of extracranial progression was similar in the two groups, but patients in the PCI arm had a median progression-free survival (PFS) of 14.7 weeks and a median overall survival (OS) of 6.7 months, compared to those in the arm receiving standard care, who had a median PFS of 12 weeks and OS of 5.4 months. Symptomatic brain metastases occurred in 16.8% of the group receiving PCI and 41.3% of the control group, corresponding to a risk of symptomatic brain metastases at 6 months of 4.4% in the PCI group and 32.0% in the control group. The main side effects of treatment were hair loss and fatigue, but there were no detectable differences in global health-related quality of life measures. PCI has therefore been adopted as standard treatment in the UK to be offered to patients with extensive stage SCLC who have achieved a response to chemotherapy and who maintain a performance status of 0–2. As the overall survival of these patients remains poor, radiotherapy regimens are usually limited to 1–2 weeks.

PCI in the acute phase may cause total, though temporary, alopecia, nausea, headache, skin erythema, and intense fatigue. Occasionally, patients will suffer a somnolence syndrome with lethargy and sleepiness, typically manifesting some weeks after RT is complete. This distressing side effect may be partially helped by steroids and gradually resolves, sometimes over months. Of more concern are the historical reports of a significant decline in cognitive function seen in patients who have had radiotherapy to the whole brain.

Thoracic Radiotherapy for Extensive-Stage SCLC

Involved field thoracic radiotherapy also confers a benefit for selected patients with extensive, incurable disease. An international study randomised 498 patients of performance status 0–2 with extensive stage SCLC who had achieved any response to chemotherapy and had thoracic disease considered treatable with an acceptable radiotherapy field [44]. All patients underwent prophylactic cranial irradiation. Consolidative RT reduced intrathoracic recurrence but did not confer any survival advantage at 1 year (the primary endpoint), although post-hoc analysis of a small subgroup of 2-year survivors suggested there may be a long-term survival benefit. On the basis of these unconfirmed findings, thoracic consolidation with RT may be recommended for patients with extensive stage SCLC who respond to chemotherapy, are of adequate performance status, and who have disease which can be encompassed within an acceptable RT field.

Palliative Radiotherapy

Intra-Thoracic Disease

Palliative radiotherapy for lung cancer of both small-cell and non-small cell types aims to relieve symptoms, but there is no good evidence that it extends survival. RT is usually given to local disease within the chest for troublesome symptoms such as cough, pain, haemoptysis, and breathlessness. Fourteen randomised clinical trials of 19 different radiotherapy regimens for symptomatic non-small cell lung cancer were analysed by meta-analysis [45]. A lack of consensus on criteria for reporting a response to RT

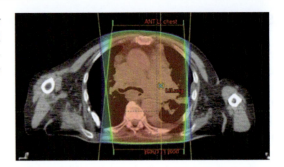

Fig. 6.8 A patient with locally advanced small-cell lung cancer and large airways narrowing treated with palliative intent using a large field to the mediastinum and 20 Gy in five fractions over a week

means that useful comparison between trials is probably not meaningful. All the studies showed that palliative RT improved local chest symptoms, though there was great variation between studies in the extent, duration, and speed of onset of symptom relief. Commonly quoted rates of symptom improvement are 50% for cough and 75% for chest pain and haemoptysis. RT regimens used frequently in the UK include 36 Gy in 12 fractions, 20 Gy in 5 fractions (Fig. 6.8), 16–17 Gy in 2 fractions delivered a week apart, and a 10 Gy single fraction. The shorter courses tend to be prescribed for patients with a poor performance, and there is good evidence that a single fraction of 10 Gy can provide good, rapid relief of symptoms without the disruption of a longer course of treatment.

Endobronchial RT is occasionally used to palliate obstructive symptoms of lung cancer. A meta-analysis of the small number of available trials has suggested that endobronchial radiotherapy is less effective that external beam RT in palliating symptoms [46]. There may be a role for endobronchial treatment in selected patients where prior external beam RT precludes further treatment by this modality.

Extra-Thoracic Sites

Bony metastases are common in lung cancer. A meta-analysis concluded that a single fraction of RT is as effective as multiple fractions in the treatment of painful bony metastases [47]. Dose-finding studies support a dose of 8 Gy as the optimal dose for a single fraction [48]. The caveat to this conclusion is that patients treated with a single fraction of RT seem to have a higher rate of retreatment than those treated with multiple fractions, although the time to recurrence of pain is not any shorter. This suggests that it may be the clinician's reluctance to treat a second time after a higher initial dose which leads to this finding. In the UK, the majority of uncomplicated bone metastases should be treated with a single fraction of RT. Metastases in long bones, especially the femur, are at particular risk of fracture and may require either prophylactic pinning or surgical fixation. Stratification of this risk is conveniently made using the Mirels score (see Table 6.4 below) where a score of 9 or greater is regarded as high risk and prophylactic fixation usually recommended. Most centres in the UK offer postoperatively RT in an attempt to prevent progression of the metastasis and failure at the surgical site, although there is no evidence to support this practice.

Other extra-thoracic metastatic sites commonly seen in patients with lung cancer include the liver, adrenal glands, and brain. Radiotherapy is rarely used in the treatment of metastatic disease to the adrenal glands unless they are very large and causing pain; toxicity from RT to the liver far outweighs any potential benefit, even if the metastasis is solitary.

Brain metastases are very common in both small-cell and non-small cell lung cancer. Brain metastases from SCLC are usually a marker of widespread disease, and although they are often sensitive to systemic chemotherapy and whole brain radiotherapy, results are disappointing, with patients having only a short life expectancy. For a patient with NSCLC, solitary metastases occurring in patients with a good performance status and limited extracranial disease will often be resected or treated with stereotactic RT (STRT). Several regional centres within the UK are now commissioned to deliver STRT to brain metastases using a technique similar to SABR, although the metastases are usually treated with a single large fraction. Until recently, whole brain RT (WBRT) was considered standard treatment for patients with multiple brain metastases from non-small cell lung cancer. In the QUARTZ trial, 538 patients with NSCLC and brain metastases which were not considered suitable for either surgical resection or stereotactic RT were randomised to receive whole brain radiotherapy to a dose of 20 Gy in 5 fractions or no radiotherapy [49]. Analysis of the results has shown no significant difference in the primary endpoint of quality adjusted life years, taking both survival and patient-rated quality of life into account. In addition, no significant difference was demonstrated in the secondary endpoint of overall survival. Median survival was 9.4 weeks (95% CI 7.7–11.0) in the group receiving steroids plus RT, and 8.1 weeks (95% CI 7.6–9.0) in the arm receiving steroids alone, underlining the poor prognosis of patients with unresectable brain metastases from NSCLC. Although no benefit from WBRT was seen in the QUARTZ trial, neither was there any evidence of detriment. Stereotactic radiotherapy or surgical excision is well established in the treatment of low-volume brain metastases in patients with NSCLC and a good performance status. Similarly, patients with small-volume extracranial metastatic disease limited to no more than three sites (termed oligometastatic disease) can be considered to have a better prognosis than most patients with metastatic non-small cell lung cancer. There are case reports and case series of patients who have had a prolonged survival following surgery or SABR to residual metastatic disease following a good response to systemic therapy, but randomised clinical trials are needed to define the potential benefit and selection criteria for treatment.

Table 6.4 Mirels score for stratifying fracture risk in patients with long bone metastases

Score	1	2	3
Site	Upper limb	Lower limb	Peritrochanteric
Pain	Mild	Moderate	Functional
Lesion	Blastic	Mixed	Lytic
Size (amount of cortex)	<1/3	1/3–2/3	>2/3

Chemotherapy

Whilst in the management of lung cancer, surgery and radiotherapy can successfully control local disease, many lung cancer deaths are due to metastatic disease. Hence systemic anti-cancer therapy (SACT) has been frequently used with varying degrees of success to treat this condition. Conventional cytotoxic agents have been the mainstay of SACT treatments for the last three decades, but are often limited by toxicity and relative lack of effectiveness. The increase in our understanding of the biology of lung cancer has led to the development of targeted treatments which may well supplant conventional cytotoxic chemotherapy in the future. SACT is used in the following stages and indications for lung cancer.

Palliative

- Stage IIIb and IV non-small cell lung cancer (NSCLC)
- Most small-cell lung cancer patients (SCLC)

Adjuvant

- Stage I and II resected NSCLC with tumours >4 cm or N1 disease
- Resected SCLC

Combined with Radiotherapy (Usually Concomitant)

- Stage IIIa and some IIIb NSCLC
- Limited SCLC patients of good performance status (0–2)

Neoadjuvant Chemotherapy

Neoadjuvant chemotherapy with or without radiotherapy has been used to downstage patients with N2 disease so they can be operated on. However, a recent meta-analysis of over 1000

patients has shown no survival benefit with this approach [50].

The Role of Chemotherapy as Palliative Treatment for Advanced Lung Cancer

Given the very poor prognosis of NSCLC patients, many have reasonably questioned the utility of subjecting patients to toxic chemotherapy. Early studies generally demonstrated a small survival advantage for platinum-based chemotherapy in advanced non-small cell lung cancer, and that this benefit was confined to patients with a performance status (PS) of 0–2 [51]. These findings have been confirmed by a large meta-analysis [52]. Furthermore, there does not appear to be any adverse effect on quality of life with such treatment. Over 50% of lung cancer patients are over the age of 70 years, and the usefulness of cytotoxic chemotherapy in elderly patients with advanced non-small cell lung cancer is debated. Early studies utilizing single-agent vinorelbine versus best supportive care demonstrated a survival advantage. A recent Cochrane systematic review has shown the elderly may benefit from platinum-based combination chemotherapy over single-agent therapy, but at the expense of higher toxicity, and so non-platinum-based chemotherapy for elderly patients with co-morbidities was recommended, although further studies are needed. For small-cell lung cancer not amenable to treatment with curative intent, platinum-based chemotherapy remains the best form of palliation.

The Role of Cytotoxic Chemotherapy in the Adjuvant Treatment of Resected Lung Cancer

Although surgery remains the best modality to cure patients with early stage lung cancer, nearly 50% will die from recurrent disease, and many of those will have distant metastases. A meta-analysis in 1995 suggested a non-significant improvement in survival by the addition of chemotherapy to surgery [53]. Since that time, a number of large randomised trials have demonstrated varying degrees of survival advantage to the use of platinum doublet chemotherapy postoperatively in non-small cell lung cancer. The LACE meta-analysis confirmed the efficacy of this approach except in Stage IA patients. A subgroup analysis suggested that the benefit of adjuvant chemotherapy in stage Ib patients was confined to tumours >4 cm.

Whilst patients with small-cell lung cancer rarely present with operable disease, if they do they should be offered surgery followed by adjuvant chemotherapy/radiotherapy.

Conventional Cytotoxic Treatment

Non-small Cell Lung Cancer

Single Agent Versus Doublet Chemotherapy

A number of single agents have been demonstrated to have activity in NSCLC, but cisplatin has been shown to be the most active agent. Subsequently it was shown that cisplatin/etoposide was superior to single-agent cisplatin and since that time, platinum doublets have become the norm in treatment of this condition. In the late 1990s several randomised trials were performed comparing cisplatin doublets with etoposide and vinorelbine with platinum doublets with docetaxel, paclitaxel, and gemcitabine. These results tend to show the third-generation doublets do slightly better, but that there are no real differences between individual third generation doublets [54]. Adding a third drug to a platinum doublet improves response rates, but not survival, and increases the toxicity. A recent meta-analysis of four randomised trials comparing six cycles of platinum doublet chemotherapy with fewer cycles showed there was no advantage to giving more than three or four cycles.

Cell-Type Specific Chemotherapy

It has been well known for many years that as well as pathological differences existing between squamous and non-squamous cancer, there are biological and clinical differences. A subset analysis of a large phase III trial comparing cisplatin/gemcitabine versus cisplatin/pemetrexed revealed the superiority of cisplatin/pemetrexed in non-squamous histologies.

Maintenance Therapy

Maintenance therapy is defined as continuation of usually a single drug to maintain remission following induction by a platinum doublet. This may be by a drug already used in the induction doublet (continuous maintenance) or a different drug (switch maintenance). A meta-analysis indicated that patients with adenocarcinoma (but not squamous cancer) and those with good PS (0–1) appear to derive most benefit from maintenance chemotherapy [55]. Long-term analysis of data from the PARAMOUNT study shows pemetrexed is well tolerated, with no adverse effects on quality of life, barring low-grade impairment of renal function and anaemia.

Second-Line Treatment with Cytotoxic Chemotherapy

Following relapse and/or progression with first-line chemotherapy, the life expectancy can generally be measured in weeks to months, and the maintenance of quality of life for these patients is paramount. Two drugs (docetaxel and pemetrexed) have been shown to improve survival by a very short amount. Comparison of docetaxel with pemetrexed as second-line treatment shows the two drugs were equivalent in terms of efficacy, but pemetrexed was less toxic.

Chemotherapy for Small-Cell Lung Cancer

Platinum (either cisplatin or carboplatin) and etoposide remain the mainstay for chemotherapy for this disease. Despite the inherent chemosensitivity of this disease, the vast majority of these patients relapse and die of their disease. Patients who have a reasonable disease-free interval following initial therapy may respond to rechallenge with the same chemotherapy regimen. The topoisomerase I inhibitor, topotecan, is the only drug to show meaningful second-line activity in this disease.

Targeted Treatments in Lung Cancer

Over the past 30 years conventional cytotoxic chemotherapy has resulted in modest gains in survival for patients with lung cancer. Greater understanding of the molecular events involved in the pathogenesis of this disease has resulted in the development of targeted therapies that appear to be more efficacious and less toxic, and can be tailored to the specific genetic makeup of a patient's tumour that may be amenable to therapeutic inhibition either by monoclonal antibodies or small molecule inhibitors. Three therapeutic areas appear promising:

- tyrosine kinase inhibitors
- anti-angiogenic agents
- immune checkpoint inhibitors

Tyrosine Kinase Inhibitors

Cellular functions such as proliferation and survival are controlled by extracellular growth factors which bind and activate cell surface receptors leading to phosphorylation of tyrosine residues on the intracellular domain of the receptor. This activates intracellular signalling pathways, resulting in transcription of genes involved in cell proliferation and survival. In cancer cells these processes are deranged, allowing cells to escape normal controls of proliferation and programmed cell death (apoptosis). One such system is the epidermal growth factor receptor (EGFR) pathway.

Two different classes of EGFR inhibitors are used clinically:

1. Monoclonal antibody–Cetuximab.
2. Receptor tyrosine kinase inhibitors (RTKI):
   - Gefitinib
   - Erlotinib
   - Afatanib

Initial studies in advanced non-small cell lung cancer—either in a first-line setting combined with chemotherapy or as a single agent in a second- and third-line setting—were disappointing, with no survival advantage with the RTKI. However, a subsequent trial of erlotinib versus best supportive care in the second- and third-line setting did show a small survival advantage. Analysis of the tumours of those patients who responded well to gefitinib in previous trials demonstrated that patients who harboured mutations consisting of deletions of exon 19 or a point mutation in exon 21 (L858R) responded very well to these agents. Such patients tended to be never smokers, of Asian descent, or have adenocarcinoma histology. A secondary acquired mutation at residue 790 of the EGFR resulting in a substitution of a methionine for a threonine (T790M) is thought to be an important mechanism by which NSCLC becomes resistant to RTKIs.

A number of prospective randomised studies have shown that response rates, progression-free survival, and toxicity favour the use of an RTKI as first-line therapy for NSCLCs that have EGFR-sensitising mutations. Overall survival does not seem to be prolonged with RTKI, probably due to patients on the chemotherapy arms being subsequently crossed over to RTKIs.

RTKIs can cause rash, diarrhoea, elevated liver enzymes, sore throat, hair and nail changes, and interstitial lung disease. There may be slight difference in the toxicity profiles between the different agents, with afatinib (an irreversible EGFR inhibitor) causing more skin rash and gefitinib more interstitial lung disease. RTKIs are therefore the standard of care for first-line treatment for advanced non-small cell lung cancer harbouring an EGFR-sensitizing mutation. TKIs have also been studied in patients without a sensitizing mutation ("wild type"). The TAILOR study comparing erlotinib with docetaxel with erlotinib in a second-line setting and showed that wild type patients did better on chemotherapy [56]. As a result of this and other studies, it is generally felt there is little clinical utility in using these agents in wild type EGFR patients.

All patients treated with RTKIs will eventually develop resistance to these agents. In over half of these patients, the mechanism of resistance to current agents is by the T790M secondary mutation. A number of third generation TKIs active in T790M have now been evaluated, and osimertinib has now been approved for use in those with progressive disease who have developed this mutation after a first-line TKI. Rociletinib has also been shown to be active in these patients, but awaits fuller evaluation.

Patients who may have developed resistance to first- or second-line TKIs will require a further biopsy to confirm the presence of a treatable mutation. Obtaining tissue for the second time might not be safe or feasible, but there is now the possibility of identifying circulating tumour DNA (ctDNA) from plasma samples, so-called *liquid biopsy*. The technical aspects of this technique are evolving, but at present the available testing is specific but relatively insensitive.

Humanised Monoclonal Antibodies Against EGFR in NSCLC

An initial study of cetuximab combined with cisplatin/vinorelbine against cisplatin/vinorelbine alone showed superior efficacy for the cetuximab combination, but at the expense of greater toxicity. Subsequently a second trial of chemotherapy with or without cetuximab failed to show any such advantages. A second-generation antibody necitumumab appeared to improve survival in squamous cell cancers, but not adenocarcinomas, and has not been recommended by NICE because of cost and low efficacy.

ALK Inhibitors

The anaplastic lymphoma kinase (ALK) gene on chromosome 2 codes for a receptor tyrosine kinase ALK protein, which is a member of the insulin receptor kinase family. In approximately 5% of non-small cell lung cancer, a rearrangement occurs in chromosome 2 resulting in the EML4 (echinoderm microtubule-associated protein-like 4) gene being transposed next to the ALK gene. This results in a fusion protein where the kinase function is constitutively activated. ALK gene rearrangements occur mainly in ade-

nocarcinoma and never smoker patients, and tend not to occur in patients with EGFR mutations.

Currently there are four methods of detecting ALK rearrangements: immunohistochemistry (IHC), fluorescent in situ hybridisation (FISH), reverse transcription polymerase chain reaction (RT-PCR) and direct sequencing. All of these have different pros and cons, sensitivities and specificities [57].

At this time, there are four small molecule ALK inhibitors in varying stages of clinical development: crizotinib, ceterinib, alectinib, and brigatinib. Crizotinib was the first inhibitor to enter clinical practice. An initial study demonstrated a 57% response rate in ALK-positive NSCLC who had progressed on prior systemic therapy. A subsequent study in ALK-positive NSCLC previously treated with a platinum doublet randomised between crizotinib and docetaxel or pemetrexed demonstrated improved progression free survival, overall response rate, and lung cancer-related symptoms for crizotinib. More recently a randomised study of this agent confirmed the superiority of this agent versus standard chemotherapy, with an improvement in quality of life for crizotinib treated patients. The main toxicities of crizotinib are visual disturbances, nausea, diarrhea, vomiting, oedema, elevated transaminases, constipation, and fatigue. The second-generation ALK inhibitor ceritinib has been shown to be active in ALK-positive patients who have progressed on crizotinib, and has been approved for use in the UK. Side effects include gastrointestinal upset, hyperglycaemia, abnormal liver enzymes, Q Tc prolongation, and pneumonitis. Both alectinib and brigatinib have useful activity in patients who have progressed on crizotinib, and have been approved for use in the United States.

Inhibitors of Tumour Angiogenesis

Tumour angiogenesis is central to the progression, invasion, and metastasis of all solid tumours. Even small tumours have the ability to attract in new blood vessels mediated by the secretion of

Fig. 6.9 VEGF
pathways. Reprinted by
permission from:
Springer Nature, Nature
Biotechnology.
Modeling and predicting
clinical efficacy for
drugs targeting the
tumor milieu. Mallika
Singh, Napoleone
Ferrara. © 2012

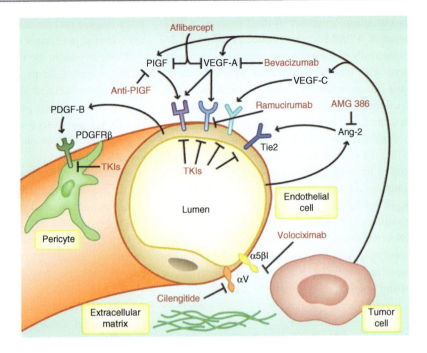

several pro-angiogenic factors (the angiogenic
"switch"). The most notable of these is vascular
endothelial growth factor (VEGF) (Fig. 6.9). As
such, VEGF has been the target of several anti-
angiogenic drugs.

Angiogenesis inhibitors come as either monoclonal antibodies or small-molecule tyrosine
kinase inhibitors. Two monoclonal antibodies,
bevacizumab and ramucirumab, have been used
in non-small cell lung cancer. Bevacizumab works
by inhibiting the binding of VEGF to receptors
VEGFR-1 and VEGFR-2. Ramucirumab works
by targeting the extracellular domain of VEGFR-
2. The benefits of adding these agents to conventional chemotherapy would appear small. Of the
small-molecule anti-angiogenic inhibitors, nintedanib, a triple angiokinase inhibitor, has shown an
improvement in overall survival when combined
with docetaxel versus docetaxel alone, especially
in patients relapsing/progressing within 9 months
of platinum-based chemotherapy.

Immune Checkpoint Inhibitors

It is well known that the immune system is crucial in the development and progression of human

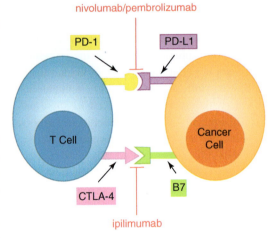

Fig. 6.10 Immune checkpoints in cancer and corresponding inhibitor therapies. T cells express the immune-
checkpoint receptors PD-1 and CTLA-4. Binding and
activation of these immune checkpoint receptors to their
cognate ligands (PD-L1 and B7) expressed on cancer cells
results in T cell inhibition. Monoclonal antibodies inhibit
PD-1 signalling or CTLA-4 activation, resulting in survival and activation of T cells. Figure provided by Bethany
Marshall

cancers. It is also known that tumours can evade
the immune system (Fig. 6.10).

Killer T cells primed by interacting with tumour
antigen-presenting cells will normally destroy

tumour cells. However, tumour cells are able to destroy killer T cells by interaction through the PD-L1/PD1 system. Antibodies to PD1 or PD-L1 can inhibit this process, thus restoring immunocompetence. Currently there are four monoclonal antibodies that inhibit this system in lung cancer: two PD-1 inhibitors (nivolumab and pembrolizumab) and two PD-L1 inhibitors (atezolizumab and tremelimumab). There have been two pivotal studies of nivolumab in non-small cell lung cancer. In the first, Checkmate 017 [58], patients with squamous histology who had failed platinum-based chemotherapy were randomised to nivolumab or docetaxel. Nivolumab improved overall survival by just over 3 months. One-year progression-free survival was 42% with nivolumab versus 24% with docetaxel, and many of these responses seem durable. The overall response rate was 20% for the nivolumab arm as opposed to 9% for docetaxel. Serious toxicity was much lower in the nivolumab arm than in the docetaxel arm. A second and similar study in non-squamous cancers, Checkmate 057 [59], again showed overall survival and response rates favoured nivolumab over docetaxel, and the response rates were better in those whose tumours expressed higher levels of PD-L1. In the Keynote-010 study, patients with both squamous and non-squamous histologies who had relapsed following platinum-based chemotherapy were randomised to docetaxel or one of two differing doses of pembrolizumab [60]. Again, the results favoured the PD-1 inhibitor, but the effect was greater in the non-squamous cell carcinoma patients. Whilst these agents are less toxic than conventional chemotherapy, they do have serious and potentially fatal side effects such as pneumonitis, hepatitis, hypophysititis, and colitis. The two PD-L1 inhibitors are still undergoing clinical trials, but atezolizumab had only a weak survival advantage compared to docetaxel, and is considered too costly.

Lastly, there is considerable confusion and conflicting data about the role of tumour PD1 and/or PD-L1 expression as a predictive biomarker. This is compounded by the fact that the pharmaceutical companies are each using different diagnostic antibodies and different cut-off points for positivity. In Checkmate 017, PD-L1 status did not appear to predict responsiveness to nivolumab, but this was not the case for pembrolizumab, where increased responsiveness was found in patients whose tumours had PD-L1 expression>50%. In the KEYNOTE-024 study, pembrolizumab led to improved response rates and short-term survival compared with chemotherapy in the first-line setting in patients whose tumors expressed $\geq$50% PD-L1 with less toxicity [61]. Nivolumab is now approved for use in advanced or metastatic NSCLC after progressing on chemotherapy, and pembrolizumab for untreated NSCLC if >50% of tumour cells express PD-L1.

Ongoing studies are evaluating combination immunotherapy targeting PD-L1 and CTLA4, and also combined immunotherapy with conventional chemotherapy in advanced lung cancer.

References

1. Royal College of Physicians. National Lung Cancer Audit annual report 2016 (for the audit period 2015). London: Royal College of Physicians; 2017.
2. Walter FM, Rubin G, Bankhead C, Morris HC, Hall N, Mills K, et al. Symptoms and other factors associated with time to diagnosis and stage of lung cancer: a prospective cohort study. Br J Cancer. 2015;112(Suppl 1):S6–13.
3. Lam KY, Lo CY. Metastatic tumours of the adrenal glands: a 30-year experience in a teaching hospital. Clin Endocrinol. 2002;56(1):95–101.
4. NICE. Suspected cancer: recognition and referral. London: National Institute for Health and Care Excellence; 2015.
5. Church TR, Black WC, Aberle DR, Berg CD, Clingan KL, Duan F, et al. Results of initial low-dose computed tomographic screening for lung cancer. N Engl J Med. 2013;368(21):1980–91.
6. NCIN. Routes to diagnosis: exploring emergency presentation. Available at: http://www.ncin.org.uk/publications.
7. Beckett P, Tata LJ, Hubbard RB. Risk factors and survival outcome for non-elective referral in non-small cell lung cancer patients – analysis based on the National Lung Cancer Audit. Lung Cancer. 2013;83(3):396–400.
8. Walters S, Benitez-Majano S, Muller P, Coleman MP, Allemani C, Butler J, et al. Is England closing the international gap in cancer survival? Br J Cancer. 2015;113(5):848–60.
9. Silvestri GA, Gonzalez AV, Jantz MA, Margolis ML, Gould MK, Tanoue LT, et al. Methods for staging non-small cell lung cancer: diagnosis and management of lung cancer, 3rd ed: American College of Chest

Physicians evidence-based clinical practice guidelines. Chest. 2013;143(5 Suppl):e211S–50S.

10. Chopra A, Ford A, De Noronha R, Matthews S. Incidental findings on positron emission tomography/CT scans performed in the investigation of lung cancer. Br J Radiol. 2012;85(1015):e229–37.

11. Evison M, Morris J, Martin J, Shah R, Barber PV, Booton R, et al. Nodal staging in lung cancer: a risk stratification model for lymph nodes classified as negative by EBUS-TBNA. J Thorac Oncol. 2015;10(1):126–33.

12. Kumaran M, Benamore RE, Vaidhyanath R, Muller S, Richards CJ, Peake MD, et al. Ultrasound guided cytological aspiration of supraclavicular lymph nodes in patients with suspected lung cancer. Thorax. 2005;60(3):229–33.

13. Verhagen AF, Bootsma GP, Tjan-Heijnen VC, van der Wilt GJ, Cox AL, Brouwer MH, et al. FDG-PET in staging lung cancer: how does it change the algorithm? Lung Cancer. 2004;44(2):175–81.

14. Pozo-Rodriguez F, Martin de Nicolas JL, Sanchez-Nistal MA, Maldonado A, Garcia de Barajas S, Calero-Garcia R, et al. Accuracy of helical computed tomography and [18F] fluorodeoxyglucose positron emission tomography for identifying lymph node mediastinal metastases in potentially resectable non-small-cell lung cancer. J Clin Oncol. 2005;23(33):8348–56.

15. Detterbeck FC, Boffa DJ, Kim AW, Tanoue LT. The eighth edition lung cancer stage classification. Chest. 2017;151(1):193–203.

16. Goldstraw P, Chansky K, Crowley J, Rami-Porta R, Asamura H, Eberhardt WE, et al. The IASLC lung cancer staging project: proposals for revision of the TNM stage groupings in the forthcoming (eighth) edition of the TNM classification for lung cancer. J Thorac Oncol. 2016;11(1):39–51.

17. Pezzi CM, Mallin K, Mendez AS, Greer Gay E, Putnam JB. Ninety-day mortality after resection for lung cancer is nearly double 30-day mortality. J Thorac Cardiovasc Surg. 2014;148(5):2269–77.

18. Aberle DR, Adams AM, Berg CD, Black WC, Clapp JD, Fagerstrom RM, et al. Reduced lung-cancer mortality with low-dose computed tomographic screening. N Engl J Med. 2011;365(5):395–409.

19. Baldwin DR, Callister ME. The British Thoracic Society guidelines on the investigation and management of pulmonary nodules. Thorax. 2015;70(8):794–8.

20. Field JK, Duffy SW, Baldwin DR, Brain KE, Devaraj A, Eisen T, et al. The UK lung cancer screening trial: a pilot randomised controlled trial of low-dose computed tomography screening for the early detection of lung cancer. Health Technol Assess. 2016;20(40):1–146.

21. Smith-Bindman R, Lipson J, Marcus R, Kim KP, Mahesh M, Gould R, et al. Radiation dose associated with common computed tomography examinations and the associated lifetime attributable risk of cancer. Arch Intern Med. 2009;169(22):2078–86.

22. Spiro SG, Gould MK, Colice GL. Initial evaluation of the patient with lung cancer: symptoms, signs, laboratory tests, and paraneoplastic syndromes: ACCP evidenced-based clinical practice guidelines (2nd edition). Chest. 2007;132(3 Suppl):149S–60S.

23. Inoue M, Sawabata N, Takeda S, Ohno Y, Maeda H. Results of surgical intervention for p-stage IIIA (N2) non-small cell lung cancer: acceptable prognosis predicted by complete resection in patients with single N2 disease with primary tumour in upper lobe. J Thorac Cardiovasc Surg. 2004;127(4):1100–6.

24. Lim E, Baldwin D, Beckles M, Duffy J, Entwisle J, Faivre-Finn C, et al. Guidelines on the radical management of patients with lung cancer. Thorax. 2010;65(Suppl 3):iii1–27.

25. National Institute for Health and Clinical Excellence. Lung cancer: diagnosis and management. Clinical guideline [CG121] Published date: April 2011. Available at: http://guidance.nice.org.uk/CG121.

26. Colice GL, Shafazand S, Griffin JP, Keenan R, Bollinger CT. Physiological evaluation of the patient with lung cancer being considered for resectional surgery: ACCP evidence-based clinical practice guidelines (2nd edition). Chest. 2007;132(3 Suppl):161S–77S.

27. Falcoz PE, Conti M, Brouchet L, Chocron S, Puyraveau M, Mercier M, et al. The thoracic surgery scoring system (Thoracoscore): risk model for in-hospital death in 15,183 patients requiring thoracic surgery. J Thorac Cardiovasc Surg. 2007;133(2):325–32.

28. Bradley A, Marshall A, Abdelaziz M, et al. Thoracoscore fails to predict complications following elective lung resection. Eur Respir J. 2012;40(6):1496–501.

29. Ginsberg RJ, Rubinstein LV. Randomized trial of lobectomy versus limited resection for T1 N0 non-small cell lung cancer. Lung Cancer Study Group. Ann Thorac Surg. 1995;60(3):615–22.

30. Zhang Z, Zhang Y, Feng H, Yao Z, Teng J, Wei D, et al. Is video-assisted thoracic surgery lobectomy better than thoracotomy for early-stage non-small cell lung cancer? A systematic review and meta-analysis. Eur J Cardiothorac Surg. 2013;44(3):407–14.

31. Pezzi CM, Mallin K, Mendez AS, Greer Gay E, Putnam JB. Ninety-day mortality after resection for lung cancer is nearly double 30-day mortality. J Thorac Cardiovasc Surg. 2014;148(5):2269–77.

32. Bezjak A, Rumble RB, Rodrigues G, Hope A, Warde P. Members of the IMRT indications expert panel. Intensity-modulated radiotherapy in the treatment of lung cancer. Clin Oncol (R Coll Radiol). 2012;24(7):508–20.

33. Saunders M, Dische S, Barrett A, Harvey A, Gibson D, Parmar M. Continuous hyperfractionated accelerated radiotherapy (CHART) versus conventional radiotherapy in non-small-cell lung cancer:

a randomised multicentre trial. Lancet. 1997;350: 161–5.

34. Aupérin A, Le Péchoux C, Rolland E, Curran WJ, Furuse K, Fournel P, et al. Meta-analysis of concomitant versus sequential radiochemotherapy in locally advanced non-small-cell lung cancer. J Clin Oncol. 2010;28:2181–90.

35. O'Rourke N, Roqué I, Figuls M, Farré Bernadó N, Macbeth F. Concurrent chemoradiotherapy in non-small cell lung cancer. Cochrane Database Syst Rev. 2010;6:CD002140.

36. Murray L, Ramasamy S, Lilley J, Snee M, Clarke K, Musunuru HB, et al. Stereotactic ablative radiotherapy (SABR) in patients with medically inoperable peripheral early stage lung cancer: outcomes for the first UK SABR cohort. Clin Oncol (R Coll Radiol). 2016;28(1):4–12.

37. PORT Meta-analysis Trialists Group. Postoperative radiotherapy for non-small cell lung cancer. Cochrane Database Syst Rev. 2005;2:CD002142.

38. Robinson CG, Patel AP, Bradley JD, DeWees T, Waqar SN, Morgensztern D, et al. Postoperative radiotherapy for pathologic N2 non–small-cell lung cancer treated with adjuvant chemotherapy: a review of the National Cancer Data Base. J Clin Oncol. 2015;33(8):870–6.

39. Wang EH, Corso CD, Rutter CE, Park HS, Chen AB, Kim AW, et al. Postoperative radiation therapy is associated with improved overall survival in incompletely resected stage II and III non–small-cell lung cancer. J Clin Oncol. 2015;33(25):2727–34.

40. Pignon JP, Arriagada R, Ihde DC, Johnson DH, Perry MC, Souhami RL, et al. A meta-analysis of thoracic radiotherapy for small-cell lung cancer. N Engl J Med. 1992;327(23):1618–24.

41. De Ruysscher D, Pijls-Johannesma M, Vansteenkiste J, Kester A, Rutten I, Lambin P. Systematic review and meta-analysis of randomised, controlled trials of the timing of chest RT in patients with limited-stage, small-cell lung cancer. Ann Oncol. 2006;17:543–52.

42. Takada M, Fukuoka M, Kawahara M, Sugiura T, Yokoyama A, Yokota S, et al. Phase III study of concurrent vs sequential thoracic radiotherapy in combination with cisplatin and etoposide for limited-stage small cell lung cancer: results of the Japan Clinical Oncology Group Study 9104. J Clin Oncol. 2002;20:3054–60.

43. Slotman B, Faivre-Finn C, Kramer G, Rankin E, Snee M, Hatton M, et al. Prophylactic cranial irradiation in extensive small-cell lung cancer. N Engl J Med. 2007;357:664–72.

44. Slotman BJ, van Tinteren H, Praag JO, Knegjens JL, El Sharouni SY, Hatton M, et al. Use of thoracic radiotherapy for extensive stage small-cell lung cancer: a phase 3 randomised controlled trial. Lancet. 2015;385:36–42.

45. Stevens R, Macbeth F, Toy E, Coles B, Lester JF. Palliative radiotherapy regimens for patients with thoracic symptoms from non-small cell lung cancer.

Cochrane Database Syst Rev. 2015;1:CD002143. https://doi.org/10.1002/14651858.CD002143.pub4.

46. Reveiz L, Rueda JR, Cardona AF. Palliative endobronchial brachytherapy for non-small cell lung cancer. Cochrane Database Syst Rev. 2012;12:CD004284. https://doi.org/10.1002/14651858.CD004284.pub3.

47. Sze WM, Shelley M, Held I, Mason M. Palliation of metastatic bone pain: single fraction versus multifraction radiotherapy–a systematic review of the randomised trials. Cochrane Database Syst Rev. 2004;2:CD004721.

48. Hoskin P, Rojas A, Fidarova E, Jalali R, Mena Merino A, Poitevin A, et al. IAEA randomised trial of optimal single dose radiotherapy in the treatment of painful bone metastases. Radiother Oncol. 2015;116: 10–4.

49. Mulvenna P, Nankivell M, Barton R, Faivre-Finn C, Wilson P, McColl E, et al. Dexamethasone and supportive care with or without whole brain radiotherapy in treating patients with non-small cell lung cancer with brain metastases unsuitable for resection or stereotactic radiotherapy (QUARTZ): results from a phase 3, non-inferiority, randomised trial. Lancet. 2016;388(10055):2004–14.

50. Xu YP, Li B, Xu XL, Mao WM. Is there a survival benefit in patients with stage IIIA (N2) non-small cell lung cancer receiving neoadjuvant chemotherapy and/or radiotherapy prior to surgical resection: a systematic review and meta-analysis. Medicine (Baltimore). 2015;94(23):e879.

51. Billingham LJ, Cullen MH. The benefits of chemotherapy in patient subgroups with unresectable non-small-cell lung cancer. Ann Oncol. 2001;12(12):1671–5.

52. Zhong C, Liu H, Jiang L, Zhang W, Yao F. Chemotherapy plus best supportive care versus best supportive care in patients with non-small cell lung cancer: a meta-analysis of randomized controlled trials. PLoS One. 2013;8(3):e58466.

53. Non-small Cell Lung Cancer Collaborative Group. Chemotherapy in non-small cell lung cancer: a meta-analysis using updated data on individual patients from 52 randomised clinical trials. BMJ. 1995;311(7010):899–909.

54. Schiller JH, Harrington D, Belani CP, Langer C, Sandler A, Krook J, et al. Comparison of four chemotherapy regimens for advanced non-small-cell lung cancer. N Engl J Med. 2002;346(2):92–8.

55. Zhou F, Jiang T, Ma W, Gao G, Chen X, Zhou C. The impact of clinical characteristics on outcomes from maintenance therapy in non-small cell lung cancer: a systematic review with meta-analysis. Lung Cancer. 2015;89(2):203–11.

56. Garassino MC, Martelli O, Broggini M, Farina G, Veronese S, Rulli E, et al. Erlotinib versus docetaxel as second-line treatment of patients with advanced non-small-cell lung cancer and wild-type EGFR tumours (TAILOR): a randomised controlled trial. Lancet Oncol. 2013;14(10):981–8.

57. Yatabe Y. ALK FISH and IHC: you cannot have one without the other. J Thorac Oncol. 2015;10(4): 548–50.

58. Brahmer J, Reckamp KL, Baas P, Crino L, Eberhardt WE, Poddubskaya E, et al. Nivolumab versus docetaxel in advanced squamous-cell non-small-cell lung cancer. N Engl J Med. 2015;373(2):123–35.

59. Borghaei H, Paz-Ares L, Horn L, Spigel DR, Steins M, Ready NE, et al. Nivolumab versus docetaxel in advanced nonsquamous non-small-cell lung cancer. N Engl J Med. 2015;373(17):1627–39.

60. Herbst RS, Baas P, Kim DW, Felip E, Perez-Gracia JL, Han JY, et al. Pembrolizumab versus docetaxel for previously treated, PD-L1-positive, advanced non-small-cell lung cancer (KEYNOTE-010): a randomised controlled trial. Lancet. 2016;387(10027): 1540–50.

61. Reck M, Rodríguez-Abreu D, Robinson AG, Hui R, Csőszi T, Fülöp A, et al. Pembrolizumab versus chemotherapy for PD-L1-positive non-small-cell lung cancer. N Engl J Med. 2016;375(19): 1823–33.

Diseases of the Pleura

Jack A. Kastelik, Michael A. Greenstone, and Sega Pathmanathan

Introduction

The visceral and parietal pleural membranes cover the lungs and the inner surface of the chest wall, and are each composed of a single layer of mesothelial cells. The pleural space in health contains a small volume (0.26 ml/kg) of pleural fluid and lubricates the visceral and parietal pleural surfaces. Normal pleural fluid contains approximately 1800 cells/µl which comprise macrophages (75%) and lymphocytes (23%), with small number of mesothelial cells, neutrophils, and eosinophils [1, 2].

Pleural Effusion

Pleural effusion occurs when there is imbalance between pleural fluid formation and reabsorption, and the mechanisms include increased pulmonary capillary pressure (in cases of cardiac failure), decreased oncotic pressure (in hypoalbuminaemia), or increased permeability as seen in pleural infection or malignancy, with the latter having also obstructed lymphatic flow as a contributing factor [3].

J. A. Kastelik (✉) · M. A. Greenstone
S. Pathmanathan
Department of Respiratory Medicine,
Hull and East Yorkshire Hospitals NHS Trust,
Castle Hill Hospital, Cottingham, East Yorkshire, UK
e-mail: Jack.kastelik@hey.nhs.uk;
Sega.pathmanathan@hey.nhs.uk

Imaging and Further Investigation

Pleural effusions can be imaged by chest X-ray, thoracic ultrasound, and computed tomography (CT) (Fig. 7.1a–c). Although rarely the only imaging modality used, the plain chest X-ray is usually the first investigation in the breathless patient, and therefore the one most likely to indicate possible pleural pathology. Between 200 and 500 ml fluid is required before the costophrenic angle is blunted on a plain PA radiograph, but the lateral decubitus view is far more sensitive, although rarely employed. As fluid accumulates, the characteristic "meniscus" may be recognised and is explained by the greater thickness of fluid traversed at the periphery by the X-ray beam. Fluid may accumulate in the fissures and suggest a mass. Subpulmonary effusions are usually transudates and cause elevation of the hemidiaphragm. They are most easily identified on the left because of the separation of the stomach bubble from the apparent left hemidiaphragm. Thoracic ultrasound can provide real-time images of a pleural effusion, allowing assessment of its characteristics and size at the initial visit [2, 4].

Ultrasound scanning is also used to guide pleural needle aspiration (thoracocentesis) for analysis of pleural fluid. It is recommended that thoracocentesis be performed under ultrasound guidance, since concurrent ultrasound imaging is associated with low rates of complications such as pain and pneumothorax [4, 5].

© Springer International Publishing AG, part of Springer Nature 2018
S. Hart, M. Greenstone (eds.), *Foundations of Respiratory Medicine*,
https://doi.org/10.1007/978-3-319-94127-1_7

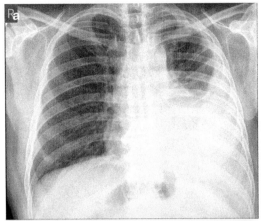

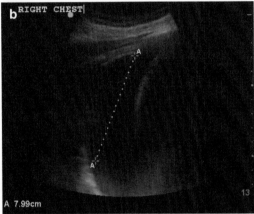

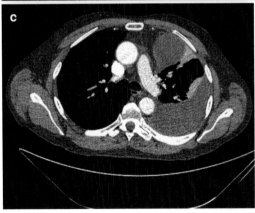

Fig. 7.1 (**a**) Chest X-ray appearance of a patient with a left pleural effusion. (**b**) Thoracic ultrasound image of a simple pleural effusion. (**c**) CT scan of the thorax demonstrating a left pleural effusion. Areas of atelectasis within the underlying lung can also be seen

CT has a complementary role in assessing pleural disorders. CT may provide information on the origin of an effusion (e.g. pulmonary embolism, infection, or malignancy) which cannot be diagnosed by ultrasound alone. Specific findings on CT which support a diagnosis of malignancy include pleural nodules, infiltration of the diaphragm, and circumferential or mediastinal pleural thickening [2, 6]. Moreover, CT-guided biopsy of pleura has been shown to have higher diagnostic yield for malignancy compared to blind Abrams pleural biopsy [7].

Thoracoscopy (insertion of an endoscope into the pleural cavity) allows examination of the pleural cavity, sampling the pleura, drainage of fluid and, if required, pleurodesis by insufflation of talc [8, 9]. Thoracoscopy can be performed with the patient awake under local anaesthesia and sedation (so called local anaesthetic medical thoracoscopy), or in the operating theatre under general anaesthesia using VATS. Local anaesthetic medical thoracoscopy is performed in a lateral position with the unaffected lung in the dependent position [8]. The trocar is introduced under ultrasound guidance, then the fluid is drained and the lung collapsed, allowing for visualisation of the pleural cavity using the optical telescope (single port technique) or using a second smaller trocar to introduce biopsy forceps (double port approach). The most common approach is to use a rigid thoracoscope with a light source size ranging between 5 mm and 7 mm, although smaller (3 mm) thoracoscopes have been used. Semi-rigid thoracoscopes have similar controls to the flexible bronchoscope and are easier to manoeuvre, but the biopsies are smaller and the diagnostic yield lower [8].

Pleural Fluid Analysis

Light's criteria divide pleural effusions into exudates and transudates depending on the pleural fluid and serum levels of protein and lactate dehydrogenase (LDH). Exudates are defined by one or more of the following: a ratio of pleural fluid to serum protein greater than 0.5, a ratio of pleural fluid to serum LDH greater than 0.6, and pleural fluid LDH greater than two-thirds of the upper limit of normal value for serum LDH [2]. The diagnostic accuracy of Light's criteria have been reported at 96% when comparing with other methods, which included measurements of pleural fluid cholesterol or albumin [2]. The cellular composition of exudative pleural effusions may vary. Exudative pleural effusions due to tuberculosis, lymphoma, leukaemia, rheumatoid arthritis, and post cardiac surgery are predominantly (>80%) lymphocytic [2]. Malignant pleural effusions may have lower lymphocyte counts (50–70%). A predominance of eosinophils (>10%) can be seen in haemothorax, pneumothorax, malignancy, infection, drug reactions, pulmonary embolism, or benign asbestos-related pleural effusions [2]. Transudates, which most commonly occur in cardiac failure or liver or renal diseases, are mainly lymphocytic in composition. Rarely chyle (a lymphatic fluid rich in lymphocytes, immunoglobulins, and lipids) may be detected in the pleural space. Chylothorax has been described due to trauma, lymphoma and, less frequently, due to lymphangioleiomyomatosis (LAM) or yellow nail syndrome.

Pleural fluid pH characteristics may be of diagnostic value. Exudates with low pH (defined as <7.2) are reported in pleural infection, tuberculosis, rheumatoid arthritis, and drug reactions. In the context of low pleural fluid pH, an increased neutrophil count would suggest empyema, a raised eosinophil count suggests a drug reaction, and an increased lymphocyte count suggests tuberculosis or cancer.

The most common causes of exudative effusions are malignancy, infection, and pulmonary embolism, [2] but there are numerous other causes (see Table 7.1). Less common causes of exudative pleural effusion include rheumatoid arthritis and connective tissue disorders, coronary artery bypass graft (CABG) surgery, medications, and pleural effusion in the immunocompromised host. Studies on CTPA (computed tomography pulmonary angiography)-diagnosed pulmonary embolism have shown the prevalence of effusion to be almost a half, increasing to 80% when massive pulmonary embolism occurs [10]. Typically, this type of pleural effusion is small, unilateral, and simple in appearance. Pleural effusion on the background of pulmonary embolism is an exudate with neutrophils being the

Table 7.1 Causes of Pleural Effusion

Exudates
Infection
• Parapneumonic
• Empyema
• Tuberculosis
• Viral pleuritis
Malignancy
• Primary: mesothelioma
• Secondary: lung, breast, lymphoma, others
Pulmonary embolism
Connective tissue disease
• Rheumatoid arthritis
• SLE
• Vasculitis
Dressler's syndrome
Post cardiac surgery
Drug hypersensitivity
Benign asbestos pleural effusion
Subphrenic
• Pancreatitis
• Subphrenic abscess
• Liver abscess
Transudates
Heart failure
Nephrotic syndrome
Cirrhosis
Renal failure
Meigs' syndrome
Hypothyroidism
Lymphatic
Chylothorax
Yellow nail syndrome
Lymphangioleiomyomatosis
Others
Haemothorax

main cell type. In most of the cases it is asymptomatic but occasionally may lead to haemothorax or infection.

There are two types of pleural effusion associated with CABG. Firstly, pleural effusion can occur early, within 28 days of surgery, and is eosinophil predominant and thought to be traumatic in origin [11]. Late effusions (more than 30 days after CABG surgery) are mainly lymphocytic in composition and most likely immunological in nature. Rarely, pleural effusion may be seen in pulmonary hypertension (idiopathic or associated with connective tissue disorders).

Pleural effusion may be seen in around 4% of patients with rheumatoid arthritis, may be associated with pleural thickening, and characteristically is an exudate with low pH and glucose levels and cellular composition varying from lymphocyte- to neutrophil-predominant. Rheumatoid arthritis pleural effusions improve spontaneously in 50% of cases, but in a fifth of patients may persist for over a year, and some will develop a cholesterol-rich pleural collection, the so-called pseudochylous effusion. Patients with rheumatoid arthritis have an increased risk of developing empyema. Systemic lupus erythematosus (SLE), systemic sclerosis, or dermatomyositis can be associated with exudative pleural effusions, with the former having characteristically reduced levels of complement and a fluid-to-serum antinuclear antibody ratio of >1. Medications such as methotrexate, amiodarone, phenytoin, or pergolide have been shown to cause pleural diseases, including pleural thickening or pleural effusion [12]. Pleural disorders in an immunocompromised host include pleural infection, tuberculosis, Kaposi's sarcoma, pulmonary lymphoma, and pneumothorax.

Asbestos Pleural Disease

Pleural Plaques

Pleural plaques are discrete areas of fibrosis affecting the parietal pleura of diaphragm, chest wall, and mediastinum, and consist of acellular, avascular, hyalinised collagenous bundles arranged in a "basket weave" pattern. They are caused by occupational or environmental asbestos exposure (and arguably talc, kaolin, and refractory ceramic fibres) and although only small exposures are required, the prevalence is greatest with heavy exposures and with time elapsed from first exposure. They are not normally visible radiographically (Fig. 7.2a, b) until 20 years after first exposure, and calcification only occurs in 10% by 30 years, but more frequently with prolonged follow-up. Plaques are asymptomatic, although occasionally may be associated with a localised grating discomfort in the chest. Uncomplicated plaques do not affect

lung function, and in the breathless patient an alternative explanation must be sought. There are epidemiological associations with minor reductions in vital capacity and small airway obstruction, but these abnormalities are likely to be due to occult fibrosis rather than the plaques per se. Occasionally plaques can become confluent and cause extrapulmonary restriction. The mechanism by which asbestos fibres reach the parietal pleura is unclear, but possibilities include direct penetration from the lung or retrograde flow in the lymphatics.

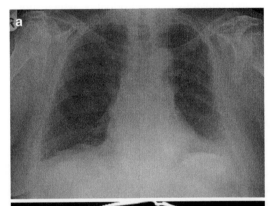

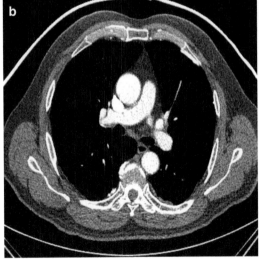

Fig. 7.2 (a) Calcified pleural plaques overlying right third and left first and second ribs anteriorly. Dense calcification of left-sided diaphragmatic plaques can be seen. Both costophrenic angles are blunted, and there is pleural thickening adjacent to the left lateral chest wall. (b) CT of typical pleural plaques. Characteristically positioned: anterior (densely calcified) and bilateral paravertebral posterior lower zones (uncalcified and partially calcified respectively)

Benign Asbestos Pleural Effusion (BAPE)

Unlike malignant mesothelioma, BAPE may be an early complication of previous asbestos exposure. It may be asymptomatic, but is usually misdiagnosed as post-pneumonic, especially as chest pain and systemic upset are often accompanying features. The effusion is frequently bloodstained and is an inflammatory exudate which may contain neutrophils, eosinophils, and mononuclear cells, but not asbestos fibres. Pleural biopsies, when performed, may show non-specific features of an organising effusion: reactive mesothelial cells, proliferating fibroblasts, chronic inflammatory cells and an absence of invasion, bland necrosis, and sarcomatoid areas suggesting mesothelioma, with which it may be confused. Simple aspiration may be sufficient, and spontaneous resolution may also occur, albeit with residual pleural thickening. Recurrence of the effusion, most frequently contralateral, is common (at least 30% of cases) and if this progresses to diffuse pleural thickening, long-term disability may occur.

Diffuse Pleural Thickening (DPT)

This is probably the consequence of a resolved BAPE and involves the visceral pleura fusing with the parietal. There is frequently a history of previous pleurisy or effusion, and the presentation is usually with dyspnoea. Inspiratory and expiratory crackles may be present even if there is no pulmonary fibrosis. Plain chest imaging may show a blunted costophrenic angle, pleural thickening, or fluid. Bands of fibrosis (so-called crow's feet) radiate from the thickened pleura across the lung fields. Computed tomographic imaging shows lower and midzone pleural thickening, with or without calcification (Fig. 7.3). The thickening (which may be 1 cm or more in thickness) circumscribes part (at least a third and maybe more than half) of the hemithorax and may be seen to reduce its circumference. Changes in the lung fields adjacent to the pleural thickening should be distinguished from pulmonary fibrosis. The scan may also show the presence of rounded atelectasis (aka folded lung or Blesovsky's syndrome) which has a characteristic appearance of vessels and bronchi radiating

towards the hilum to form a solid-looking shadow which may be mistaken for tumour (Fig. 7.4).

Lung function testing shows symmetrical reduction in all lung volumes (FEV1, FVC, RV,

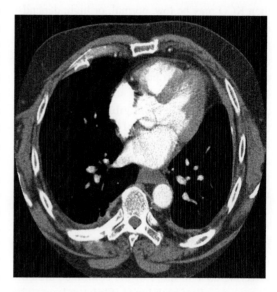

Fig. 7.3 Bilateral diffuse pleural thickening. The thickening is more marked on the left and has caused a reduction in the circumference of the left hemithorax. There is a discrete calcified pleural plaque on the right side anteriorly, which differs from the widespread smooth rind that encircles the entire contralateral hemithorax

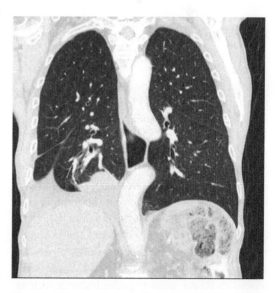

Fig. 7.4 CT coronal views of round atelectasis: whorled infolded thickened pleura leading to distortion of vessels and bronchi, producing the so-called comet's tail. The "mass" may be mistaken for a tumour. There is a small right basal effusion

TLC) and a reduction in gas transfer factor (TLCO). However, if there is no parenchymal lung involvement (i.e. asbestosis is not present) the transfer coefficient (KCO) is normal or supranormal. When both fibrosis and PT are present then KCO may be low, normal, or high, depending on the predominant abnormality.

In a quarter of cases DPT may progress, usually in those with early-onset disease, but the process tends to burn itself out after about 15 years and then there is stability. In the UK patients with DPT are eligible for compensation from the Department of Work and Pensions and whose criteria require unilateral or bilateral diffuse pleural thickening with obliteration of the costophrenic angle and a degree of respiratory disability. Compensation is normally awarded on the basis of a chest X-ray, although CT may be used to substantiate claims. The previous definition required PT (5 mm or more) in a standard chest radiograph covering 25% or more of the combined area of the chest wall of both lungs if bilateral, or 50% or more if unilateral.

Mesothelioma, the commonest primary pleural malignancy, is discussed in the section on malignant effusion below.

Pleural Infection

Approximately, 40% of cases of pneumonia are complicated by pleural effusion [13]. The mortality of pneumonia associated with pleural effusion has been reported at approximately 15% [14]. Empyema due tuberculosis remains an important cause of pleural infection [15]. *Streptococcus milleri, Streptococcus pneumonia, Staphylococcus aureus,* and anaerobes are the most common organisms responsible for community-acquired pleural infection [13]. In contrast, the causative organisms for hospital-acquired pleural infection include Staphyloccci such as Methicillin-resistant *Staphylococcus aureus* (MRSA), gram-negative bacteria such as *Escherichia coli* or Klebsiella species, as well as anaerobes [13]. Pleural effusion due to infection is an exudate with characteristically pH below

7.2 (except for cases of empyema due to Proteus, which may be alkalotic), low glucose, and high protein and LDH.

There are three developmental stages of empyema associated with pneumonia: a simple exudate, fibrinopurulent stage, and organising stage with scar tissue formation [13]. Parapneumonic effusions can be subdivided into simple, complicated (pH < 7.2, LDH > 1000 IU/L and glucose <2.2 mmol/L), and frank pus [13]. The fluid should be sampled under ultrasound guidance and analysed for pH, glucose, LDH, and microbiology. This should include cultures for tuberculosis, with microbiology samples being also inoculated into aerobic and anaerobic blood culture bottles (which may increase the yield by a fifth) [13]. Cases where pleural effusion is 10–20 mm in depth would be expected to settle down without need for drainage. Conversely, in cases of complicated parapneumonic effusion or empyema (Fig. 7.5a, b) pleural fluid drainage should be undertaken under ultrasound or CT guidance. However, when a pleural effusion is loculated and septated, drainage with intercostal chest drains may not be successful. In this situation there may be a role for the use of intra-pleural tissue plasminogen activator (t-PA) and DNase, which in a recent study were shown to improve the drainage of infected fluid, shorten hospital stay, and reduce the requirement for surgical intervention [16]. However, some patients require surgery either in the form of VATS or open thoracotomy and decortication. Recently Rahman et al. proposed a risk stratification score (RAPID) based on the levels of urea, patient's age, pleural fluid purulence, albumin levels, and whether infection is community- or hospital-acquired [17]. The risk stratification (0–2 low; 3 and 4 medium; 5–7 high) with mortality at 3 months for the low-risk group patients being estimated at 1–3% and that for high-risk group between 31% and 51%.

Indications for chest tube drainage include the presence of frank pus, organisms on Gram stain or culture, a loculated effusion, or lack of improvement with antibiotic therapy. A low pleural fluid pH (<7.2) is associated with a greater need for surgical intervention and is often inter-

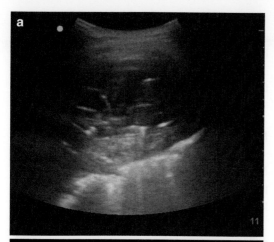

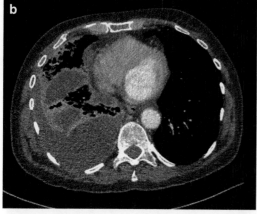

Fig. 7.5 (**a**) thoracic ultrasound images of a complex pleural effusion with septations and loculations. (**b**) A CT image of a patient with a right empyema

infected cavity and removal of the pleural peel to allow the lung to re-expand so obliterating the empyema cavity. Thoracoscopic debridement is effective when the empyema is still in the fibrino-purulent stage, but more established empyemas (usually 4–6 weeks old) with a thickened visceral cortex which prevents apposition of the two pleural surfaces and a trapped lung, requires decortication. Increasingly this is now attempted with thoracoscopy, but conversion to open decortication is still sometimes required. General anaesthesia with single-lung ventilation is usually preferred. In patients unfit for these procedures, rib resection over the most dependent part of the empyema cavity allows drainage, breakdown of loculations, and medium-term intercostal drainage of the residual cavity.

Malignant Pleural Effusion

The pleura are frequently involved in malignant processes, and neoplasia is one of the commonest causes of pleural effusion. The pleura may be invaded directly from adjacent structures such as the lung, chest wall, and mediastinum, but most commonly the invasion occurs because of tumour emboli to the visceral pleura with secondary seeding to the parietal pleura. Fluid accumulation is not invariable with pleural invasion, but when it occurs it is thought that the tumour has effected an inflammatory response with a change in pleural permeability. Normally fluid is removed from the pleural space by lymphatics in the parietal pleura, but when there is direct pleural involvement by tumour or distant lymphatic obstruction in the mediastinum, then pleural fluid is more likely to accumulate. There are significant health care costs associated with malignant pleural effusion, with reportedly over 40,000 cases each year in the United Kingdom [3]. The presence of malignant cells in pleural fluid defines a malignant pleural effusion, with adenocarcinoma being the most common histological type. Lung cancer is the most common primary site, with 30% of cases developing pleural effusion, followed by breast cancer, ovarian cancer, and lymphoma [1, 3].

preted as an indication for early chest tube drainage. Antibiotic therapy should be guided by culture results, or if negative, by the spectrum of possible infecting organisms including anaerobes. Prolonged antibiotic therapy (>3 weeks) may be required, depending on response to treatment as assessed by resolution of fever, improved imaging appearances, and falling blood inflammatory markers.

Failure to improve after 5–7 days with appropriate antibiotic therapy and intercostal drainage of accessible fluid should prompt consideration of surgery. Persistence of fever, rising inflammatory markers, and a persistent collection of loculated pus should prompt consultation with a thoracic surgeon. The surgical approach aims to control sepsis through debridement of the

Management of Malignant Pleural Effusion

The presence of a malignant effusion in patients with lung cancer carries a poor prognosis, with a median survival of only 4 months [3]. The management of patients with malignant pleural effusion depends on patients' symptoms, performance status, and the nature of the primary neoplasm, and requires a multidisciplinary approach. Chemotherapy may be an option, and in many cases can result in reduction or clearance of the pleural effusion [1]. Patients with a life expectancy of less than 1 month may be managed symptomatically by therapeutic drainage of pleural effusion. In patients with a better prognosis, options include surgical video-assisted thoracic surgery (VATS), local anaesthetic medical thoracoscopy, insertion of an indwelling pleural catheter, or chest drain insertion and medical pleurodesis [1, 8]. Pleurodesis is a procedure that aims to produce a symphysis between the visceral and parietal pleura to prevent the re-accumulation of the pleural fluid, and is best achieved with talc [9]. Pleural fluid drainage, pleural biopsy, and pleurodesis can be undertaken using medical thoracoscopy under local anaesthesia, with its diagnostic yield quoted at around 97% [8]. If required, talc poudrage pleurodesis can be performed, with reported success rates at 1 month of 78–84% [8] compared to drain insertion and talc slurry pleurodesis, where success rates at 1 month of 60–71% are reported [8, 9]. Another option is to consider insertion of long-term small-bore indwelling pleural catheters (IPC) and which can be performed in ambulatory settings. The IPC is often used in the context of malignant pleural effusion with a trapped lung, or in patients who had recurrence of pleural effusion following failed pleurodesis. IPCs were shown to improve patients' symptoms of breathlessness and quality of life, as well as a 45% rate of spontaneous pleurodesis and relatively low rates of complications [18]. IPC can be inserted following thoracoscopy with talc pleurodesis, with this strategy resulting in a small reduction in hospital stay and success rates of 92% [18].

The treatment of a chylous effusion may include a low-fat diet containing medium chain triglycerides, which reduces production of chyle, or surgical ligation of the duct, which is successful in up to 90% of patients.

Mesothelioma

Malignant pleural mesothelioma (MPM) usually presents with a unilateral pleural effusion or pleural thickening (Fig. 7.6a, b). Persistent pain

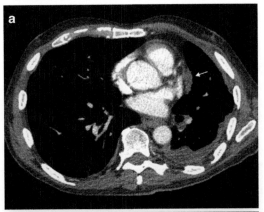

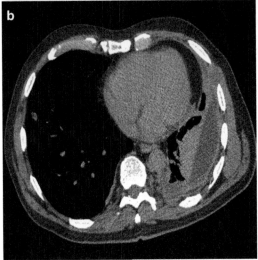

Fig. 7.6 Typical CT appearances of a left-sided mesothelioma. (**a**) the left hemithorax is contracted and there is irregular lumpy pleural thickening, which also involves the mediastinal pleura (arrow). There are non-calcified pleural plaques in the right paravertebral region. There is a faint rim of contrast enhancement posteriorly. (**b**) Loculated pleural fluid, pleural enhancement, and chest wall invasion, with a palpable chest wall mass

is a common feature, and its presence in an asbestos-exposed individual should prompt further investigation, even if the chest X-ray is normal. Presentation with distant metastases is unusual, although these are common at autopsy.

Experienced operators may be able to detect certain characteristics on thoracic ultrasound, such as pleural thickening, pleural nodularity, or diaphragmatic thickening, which may be useful in diagnosing mesothelioma and other pleural malignancies [6]. Compared to CT, ultrasound is less sensitive in the diagnosis of mesothelioma, but has similar specificity [6]. Malignant mesothelioma can be divided according to the World Health Organization (WHO) classification into epithelioid, sarcomatoid, and biphasic (containing elements of both) histological subtypes. Epithelioid histology is the most common (approximately 60% of cases) followed by biphasic, then sarcomatoid subtypes. Desmoplastic mesothelioma is usually regarded as a sarcomatoid mesothelioma with a particularly dense collagenous stroma, and may be misdiagnosed as a benign fibrinous pleuritis. Overall, the epithelioid subtype carries a better prognosis, hence the importance of making a precise diagnosis.

Cytological diagnosis of malignant mesothelioma based on pleural fluid analysis may be difficult, as the malignant cells are difficult to distinguish from reactive mesothelial cells and adenocarcinoma. Cytological examination of pleural fluid is often non-diagnostic and is almost invariably so with sarcomatoid mesothelioma. When performing thoracocentesis in patients with suspected malignant mesothelioma, at least 100 ml of pleural fluid should be collected, allowing for cell block immunohistochemical analysis. However, CT-guided biopsy or VATS biopsy of the abnormal pleura is recommended. This allows for histological analysis as well as immunohistochemical analysis using a panel including mesothelial- and carcinoma-related markers. Epithelioid mesothelioma may have a similar histological appearance to adenocarcinoma of the lung, and sarcomatoid mesothelioma needs to be distinguished from high-grade pleural sarcoma and sarcomatoid carcinomas. Ideally, a firm diagnosis of MPM can be made if the pleural biopsy

Table 7.2 Immunohistochemical markers in malignant mesothelioma

Positive	Negative
Calretinin	BerEp 4
Thrombomodulin	CEA
CK 5/6	TTF-1
CAM 5.2	MOC-31
EMA	Leu-M1
Vimentin	
WT-1	

(or less often, fluid) shows two positive mesothelial markers and two negative adenocarcinoma markers (see Table 7.2 below). Even when a broad immunohistochemistry panel is used, the specific subtyping of mesothelioma may still be difficult. Calretinin, one of the most sensitive and specific markers for epithelioid mesothelioma, is often negative with the sarcomatoid subtype. Generally the diagnosis of MPM should not be made on pleural fluid cytology alone, unless the patient is unfit for a more invasive biopsy procedure.

Biomarkers in MPM

Biomarkers are not yet established in the daily clinical management of patients with mesothelioma, and the limited availability of the assay has restricted its use. The best studied markers are soluble mesothelin-related peptides (SMRP) and osteopontin. A recent meta-analysis of the utility of serum SMRP measurement in the diagnosis of MPM showed sensitivities and specificities of 61% and 80% respectively, increasing to 75% and 76% respectively in pleural fluid. Similar results were found for serum osteopontin measurements. Serum SMRP may reflect tumour bulk and fall with positive response to chemotherapy, but it does not predict stage or survival and has no role in screening. It has recently been suggested that it may have a limited role in patients with suspicious pleural fluid cytology who are not fit for further invasive diagnostic tests.

Staging of mesothelioma requires CT of the thorax and abdomen as well as positron emission tomography (PET-CT), as the latter is more sensitive in detecting lymph node involvement and distant metastases. Various staging systems have been described, but the best established is the TNM system proposed by the International Mesothelioma Interest Group. This system predicts survival in a surgical population, but its role is unclear in the larger group of non-surgical patients. At a time when enthusiasm for radical surgery is waning, it may be still be useful for stratifying patients for clinical trials.

PET-CT may also be helpful in distinguishing between benign pleural disease and malignant mesothelioma, and help identify a suitable site for biopsy. T staging is not well assessed by either modality, and if the precise extent of the tumour is required (for instance the degree of diaphragmatic infiltration), then MRI scanning should be considered. Mesotheliomas are less reliably FDG-avid than lung cancers, and false positive results may occur following pleurodesis. In PET-avid mesotheliomas, disease progression or response to chemotherapy can be assessed.

Treatment of Malignant Mesothelioma

The prognosis of MPM is poor, with a median survival of 9 months from diagnosis, and 1-year survival of only 40%. Treatment options for malignant mesothelioma are limited, with symptom palliation being the main aim. Many patients will undergo surgical or medical thoracoscopy with pleural biopsy to confirm the diagnosis. At the same time, pleural fluid can be drained and pleurodesis performed to prevent recurrence of pleural effusion. Other therapeutic options for the management of the pleural effusion include medical pleurodesis or in cases of recurrent pleural effusion or trapped lung IPC insertion. Pain control will remain the main focus of palliation.

Chemotherapy can be considered in symptomatic patients with good performance status (PS 0–2). The current evidence suggests that doublet chemotherapy with cisplatin and an antifolate (pemetrexed or less commonly raltitrexed) may prolong median survival by 3 months. Prophylactic irradiation of procedure tracts (such as the site of thoracoscopy or intercostal drains) in the hope of preventing tumour seeding is no longer considered necessary. Should a painful tract metastasis develop, then localised irradiation is usually effective. Unfortunately, hemithoracic irradiation for diffuse chest pain is not supported by clinical studies, and in practice is rarely beneficial.

The role of surgery remains controversial. Case series from North America suggested a possible role for trimodality treatment in highly selected groups of early-stage good PS patients. This consists of extrapleural pneumonectomy (EPP, an en-bloc resection of parietal pleura, lung, diaphragm, pericardium) preceded by preoperative chemotherapy and hemithoracic radiation given post-operatively. The MARS (Mesothelioma and Radical Surgery) trial examined the feasibility of conducting a randomised trial of trimodality treatment versus chemotherapy. Of the 50 randomised patients, survival was worse in the trimodality group (14.4 versus 19 months) and there was a 10% perioperative mortality. EPP is no longer considered an acceptable treatment option in the UK and should not be offered. There may, however, be a role for more limited surgery although that, too, is unproven. MesoVATS compared talc pleurodesis versus thoracoscopic partial pleurectomy and talc and found no effect on lung function or survival, but better early fluid control and slight improvement in quality of life in the longer survivors treated with surgery. Whether more extensive decortication combined with chemotherapy can extend survival is currently being tested in MARS2.

Other Pleural Neoplasms

Pleural metastases followed by solitary fibrous tumour, primary pleural lymphoma, pleural sarcoma, or pleural haemangioendothelioma are examples of other pleural neoplasms. Well differentiated papillary mesothelioma is rare, occurs almost exclusively in women, and is usually peritoneal. It appears to be unrelated to asbestos exposure and behaves as an indolent tumour with a good prognosis. Very occasionally it involves

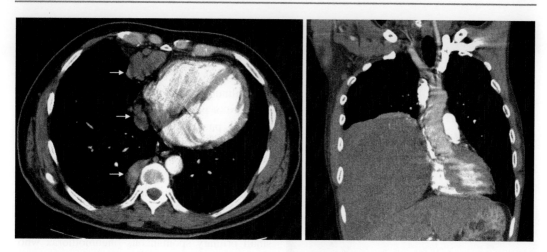

Fig. 7.7 CT scans of two patients with benign pleural fibromas. Pleural fibromas can be multiple (arrowed, left panel) or massive (right panel)

the pleura, in which case men and women are equally affected.

Solitary fibrous tumour of the pleura (pleural fibroma) is a mesenchymal spindle-type neoplasm usually presenting as a soft tissue mass varying in size and most commonly arising from the visceral pleura (Fig. 7.7). This type of neoplasm may present with hypoglycaemia, due to production of insulin-like growth factor II (IGF-II)—so called Doege-Potter syndrome. Occasionally, solitary fibrous tumour can be associated with finger clubbing (Pierre-Marie-Bamberg syndrome). Solitary fibrous tumours are potentially treated with surgical resection but can recur locally. Primary effusion lymphoma is a neoplasm of large B-cell type, presents as pleural effusion in the context of immunodeficiency caused by human immunodeficiency virus (HIV), and in association with human herpes virus 8. This type of neoplasm is very aggressive. Pyothorax associated lymphoma is a neoplasm of large B cells associated with Epstein-Barr virus, usually occurring in patients from the Far East with a history of pyothorax due to old tuberculosis. This type of neoplasm usually presents as a pleurally based mass which frequently invades adjacent structures and generally has a very poor prognosis, but may benefit from chemotherapy and radiotherapy. Synovial sarcoma is a mesenchymal neoplasm composed of epithelial and spindle cells and is an aggressive form of pleural

neoplasm occurring in young people, which may present as a localised neoplasm or diffuse pleural thickening. Pleural haemangioendothelioma is a vascular neoplasm presenting as diffuse pleural thickening, and behaves aggressively with poor response to treatment. Biopsy is required to distinguish it from malignant mesothelioma.

Pneumothorax

Pneumothorax is defined as the presence of air in the pleural cavity (Fig. 7.8a, b). The incidence of pneumothorax is not precisely known, with reports suggesting 18–28/100,000 cases per annum for men and 1.2/100,000 for women [19]. Pneumothoraces can be broadly divided into spontaneous, traumatic, or iatrogenic. Spontaneous pneumothoraces can be further subdivided into primary and secondary, depending on whether or not there is pre-existing pulmonary disease. Pneumothorax requires to be distinguished from pneumomediastinum, which is defined as free air within the mediastinum. Older epidemiological studies suggested that up to 50% of spontaneous pneumothoraces are secondary spontaneous pneumothoraces, but a recent report suggested a much lower figure (14%) [20]. The underlying aetiology of pneumothorax is not fully understood, with suggested mechanisms including rupture of pleural blebs, emphysema-

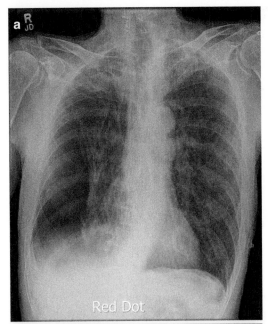

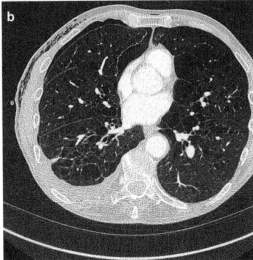

Fig. 7.8 (**a**) Chest X-ray of a patient with a right pneumothorax. (**b**) CT scan following chest tube drainage (not seen) reveals a small residual right pneumothorax and extensive pulmonary emphysema. Subcutaneous emphysema can also be seen in the chest wall

like changes, pleural inflammation, or porosity due to replacement of mesothelial cells by inflammatory cells [19]. Studies have shown that the presence of pleural blebs on CT imaging increases the risk of recurrence of ipsilateral as well as contralateral pneumothoraces.

Iatrogenic pneumothorax is a recognised complication of any procedures involving close proximity to the lungs, including central venous line placement, thoracocentesis, CT-guided biopsy of intrapulmonary lesions, or occasionally, acupuncture or pain-management interventions. For example, pneumothorax following thoracocentesis has been reported in meta-analysis at a rate of 6%, with a third of cases requiring intercostal chest drain insertion [21]. An experienced operator and ultrasound guidance reduce this risk considerably.

It is generally accepted that patients with a small primary spontaneous pneumothorax who are not symptomatic could be managed conservatively. The rate of resolution of spontaneous pneumothorax has been suggested at between 1.25% and 2.2% of volume of hemithorax per 24 h [19, 22]. Conversely, patients with a large pneumothorax or those with small pneumothorax who are symptomatic require intervention. The BTS guidelines suggest that for a large pneumothorax, defined as greater than 2 cm inter-pleural distance at the level of hilum, aspiration using a 16–18G cannula should be considered, and if not successful, then insertion of a chest drain should be undertaken [19]. The success rate of needle aspiration have been reported as between 30% and 80% [19]. However, if needle aspiration fails, there is good evidence that small-bore (<14 Fr) drains have a similar success rate in treatment of pneumothorax compared to larger drains, and result in less discomfort to the patients. The American College of Chest Physicians (ACCP) guidelines differ, as they define a large pneumothorax as ≥3 cm apex-to-cupola distance and favour chest drain insertion over simple aspiration [22]. The reason for the differences is the different weight given to the absence of randomised controlled studies.

The insertion of a small drain [18] with or without minocycline pleurodesis [19] may be associated with a lower risk of recurrence and raises the possibility that intervention (intercostal drainage and pleurodesis) might be considered when patients first present with their primary spontaneous pneumothorax (PSP). The recurrence rate for PSP is about 30%, increasing to at least 60% after a second episode [14]. Current guidelines recommend consideration of surgical treatment for patients with their first episode of primary pneumothorax, with persistent air leak lasting for more than 5–7 days, in professions at risk such as pilots and divers, or those occurring during pregnancy [19]. Moreover, surgery is recommended for recurrent ipsilateral pneumothorax, contralateral pneumothorax, or bilateral simultaneous pneumothoraces [19]. Surgery, which usually involves resection of a bullous lesion, emphysematous pleural blebs, and emphysema-like changes, together with pleurodesis, is relatively safe and carries high success rates with low (3%) recurrence rates and may be cost-effective [19].

References

1. Roberts ME, Neville E, Berrisford RG, Antunes G, Ali NJ. Management of a malignant pleural effusion: British Thoracic Society pleural disease guideline 2010. Thorax. 2010;65(Suppl 2):ii32–40.
2. Hooper C, Lee YC, Maskell N. Investigation of a unilateral pleural effusion in adults: British Thoracic Society pleural disease guideline 2010. Thorax. 2010;65(Suppl 2):ii4–17.
3. Kastelik JA. Management of malignant pleural effusion. Lung. 2013;191:165–75.
4. Rahman NM, Singanayagam A, Davies HE, Wrightson JM, Mishra EK, Lee YC, et al. Diagnostic accuracy, safety and utilisation of respiratory physician-delivered thoracic ultrasound. Thorax. 2010;65:449–53.
5. Havelock T, Teoh R, Laws D, Gleeson F. Pleural procedures and thoracic ultrasound: British Thoracic Society pleural disease guideline 2010. Thorax. 2010;65(Suppl 2):ii61–76.
6. Qureshi NR, Rahman NM, Gleeson FV. Thoracic ultrasound in the diagnosis of malignant pleural effusion. Thorax. 2009;64:139–43.
7. Maskell NA, Gleeson FV, Davies RJ. Standard pleural biopsy versus CT-guided cutting-needle biopsy for diagnosis of malignant disease in pleural effusions: a randomised controlled trial. Lancet. 2003;361:1326–30.
8. Rahman NM, Ali NJ, Brown G, Chapman SJ, Davies RJ, Downer NJ, et al. Local anaesthetic thoracoscopy: British Thoracic Society pleural disease guideline 2010. Thorax. 2010;65(Suppl 2):ii54–60.
9. Dresler CM, Olak J, Herndon JE 2nd, Richards WG, Scalzetti E, Fleishman SB, et al. Phase III intergroup study of talc poudrage vs talc slurry sclerosis for malignant pleural effusion. Chest. 2005; 127:909–15.
10. Porcel JM, Madronero AB, Pardina M, Vives M, Esquerda A, Light RW. Analysis of pleural effusions in acute pulmonary embolism: radiological and pleural fluid data from 230 patients. Respirology. 2007;12:234–9.
11. Light RW, Rogers JT, Cheng D, Rodriguez RM. Large pleural effusions occurring after coronary artery bypass grafting. Ann Intern Med. 1999;130:891–6.
12. Kastelik JA, Aziz I, Greenstone MA, Thompson R, Morice AH. Pergolide-induced lung disease in patients with Parkinson's disease. Respir Med. 2002;96:548–50.
13. Davies HE, Davies RJ, Davies CW. Management of pleural infection in adults: British Thoracic Society pleural disease guideline 2010. Thorax. 2010;65(Suppl 2):ii41–53.
14. Sahn SA. Diagnosis and management of parapneumonic effusions and empyema. Clin Infect Dis. 2007;45(11):1480–6.
15. Sahn SA, Iseman MD. Tuberculous empyema. Semin Respir Infect. 1999;14:82–7.
16. Rahman NM, Maskell NA, West A, Teoh R, Arnold A, Mackinlay C, et al. Intrapleural use of tissue plasminogen activator and DNase in pleural infection. N Engl J Med. 2011;365:518–26.
17. Rahman NM, Kahan BC, Miller RF, Gleeson FV, Nunn AJ, Maskell NA. A clinical score (RAPID) to identify those at risk for poor outcome at presentation in patients with pleural infection. Chest. 2014;145:848–55.
18. Van Meter ME, McKee KY, Kohlwes RJ. Efficacy and safety of tunneled pleural catheters in adults with malignant pleural effusions: a systematic review. J Gen Intern Med. 2011;26:70–6.
19. MacDuff A, Arnold A, Harvey J. Management of spontaneous pneumothorax: British Thoracic Society pleural disease guideline 2010. Thorax. 2010;65(Suppl 2):ii18–31.
20. Bobbio A, Dechartres A, Bouam S, Damotte D, Rabbat A, Regnard JF, et al. Epidemiology of spontaneous pneumothorax: gender-related differences. Thorax. 2015;70:653–8.
21. Gordon CE, Feller-Kopman D, Balk EM, Smetana GW. Pneumothorax following thoracentesis: a systematic review and meta-analysis. Arch Intern Med. 2010;170:332–9.
22. Baumann MH, Strange C, Heffner JE, Light R, Kirby TJ, Klein J, et al. Management of spontaneous pneumothorax: an American College of Chest Physicians Delphi consensus statement. Chest. 2001;119:590–602.

Sleep

8

Michael A. Greenstone

Sleep Physiology

The function of sleep is still largely unknown, but it should be considered a homeostatic drive just like thirst and hunger, and can be divided into phases defined by muscle activity and eye movement. Sleep usually consists of four or five cycles of quiet non-rapid eye movement (NREM) sleep, alternating with periods of rapid eye movement (REM), the latter usually beginning after about 90 min and increasing in length throughout the night. Stage 1 is brief and transitional, then briskly followed by stage 2 sleep when electroencephalography (EEG) shows evidence of sleep spindles, the appearance of delta and theta rhythms, and reduced muscular activity, with a slight decrease in heart rate and respiratory frequency. Stage 2 sleep occupies approximately half of total sleep time, and increases in old age. Stages 3 and 4 are known as slow-wave sleep (SWS) because of the increasing predominance of high-amplitude slow delta waves, and it is during this phase that body restoration occurs. SWS is most prevalent in the early part of the night, but with age, the amount of SWS progressively diminishes as stage 2 sleep lengthens. Eye move-

ment is absent and muscle tone reduced in stages 2–4 sleep. REM occupies about 20% of adult sleep (although it predominates in neonates) and is associated with EEG evidence of cortical activity, but accompanied by muscular paralysis apart from the extraocular muscles, the diaphragm, and the posterior crico-arytenoid muscles which abduct the vocal cords. REM is when most dreaming takes place, and this loss of muscle activity is an important mechanism which prevents individuals from acting out dreams. Following sleep deprivation there is a rebound catch-up of SWS and then REM.

Sleep and Respiration

During wakefulness, activation of the upper airway and intercostal muscles ensure that the subatmospheric intrapleural pressure of inspiration does not narrow the upper airway or reduce the outward motion of the ribcage when the diaphragm descends. NREM sleep inhibits neural activity in the medulla, with a resultant reduction in output to the hypoglossal and phrenic nerves. Minute ventilation decreases by 10–15% during both NREM and REM sleep, and there are small decreases in arterial oxygen saturation and increases in alveolar and arterial CO_2 [1]. This is partly due to a blunted ventilatory response of the peripheral and central chemoreceptors, but also there is reduced upper airway calibre and an

M. A. Greenstone
Department of Respiratory Medicine, Hull and East Yorkshire Hospitals NHS Trust, Castle Hill Hospital, Cottingham, East Yorkshire, UK
e-mail: mike.greenstone@hey.nhs.uk

© Springer International Publishing AG, part of Springer Nature 2018
S. Hart, M. Greenstone (eds.), *Foundations of Respiratory Medicine*,
https://doi.org/10.1007/978-3-319-94127-1_8

increase in upper airway resistance (UAR). Imaging confirms that the airway lumen is narrowed, opens at transition to expiration, and then narrows again during mid and late expiration. The increase in resistance may be minor in the young and thin but sizeable in obese snorers. With the rise in UAR there is increased EMG input to the diaphragm and accessory muscles, which persists until the airway narrowing resolves. In REM sleep diaphragmatic activity predominates over intercostal activity and inhibition of the upper airway dilator muscles predisposes to airway closure.

Obstructive Sleep Apnoea

The human upper airway is crucial for respiration, swallowing, and speech, and the latter requires pharyngeal mobility so that the hyoid bone, an important anchoring site for pharyngeal muscles, is not firmly attached to the skeleton, as it is in other species. The nasal and laryngeal segments of the upper airway are rigid, but the pharynx is a collapsible tube subject to surrounding pressure and muscular activation. A key physiological abnormality in the airway of obstructive sleep apnoea (OSA) patients is the presence of a higher critical closing pressure (Pcrit), so when muscular activation is negated (for instance by general anaesthesia) the upper airway may collapse at atmospheric pressure, whereas normal individuals require a negative pressure. This increased tendency of the airway to collapse is due to a combination of anatomical crowding and abnormalities of neuromuscular control, although in an individual patient one or other may predominate.

Numerous imaging studies in OSA patients confirm lumen size is compromised compared to non-apnoeic subjects. Luminal anatomy may be influenced by a number of factors including obesity, jaw position, tongue size, and craniofacial anatomy. Mandibular and hyoid position and maxillary height are factors which can increase the risk of OSA, and are a plausible explanation for familial aggregation. During wakefulness, OSA patients show increased pharyngeal dilator muscle activity compared to non-apnoeic controls, that is they offset their airway's tendency to collapse. However, they have less activation when asleep, and this has been attributed to subtle muscle denervation and neuropathy in the upper airway.

The strong association between OSA and obesity is multifactorial: firstly the tongue may contain relatively more fat, and secondly, increased thickness of the lateral pharyngeal wall may explain the reduced lateral diameter of the airway over and beyond fat pad thickness. In health, negative intrathoracic pressure and diaphragm descent on inspiration increases traction on the trachea and reduces upper airway resistance. However, if end-expiratory lung volume is reduced by recumbency and obesity, then upper airway calibre is also likely to be reduced, making it more prone to collapse. The reestablishment of tone in the upper airway musculature which leads to the termination of the apnoea is often associated with EEG evidence of electrophysiological arousal (defined as an abrupt shift in EEG frequency of 3s preceded by a minimum of 10s sleep). At sleep onset and during REM, reflex upper airway muscle activation is reduced, as is the response to arousal. This explains the observation that apnoeas are more common in light sleep (stages 1 and 2) and REM, but relatively uncommon in SWS. Blunted responsiveness in a compromised airway may be sufficient to result in an apnoea or hypopnoea, following which hypoxia and minor hypercapnia develops, respiration is stimulated, and arousal occurs, with activation of the upper airway dilators to restore airway patency. These muscles can respond to resistive loading and rising CO_2 without necessarily eliciting an arousal, which explains why despite their compromised anatomy, most OSA patients maintain normal ventilation for at least part of the night, and why not all sleep-disordered breathing is accompanied by sleep fragmentation. Hypoxia, hypercapnia, and increased airflow resistance *per se* do not seem to be the cause of the arousal, and the signal to the brain may be the increasingly negative pleural pressure, although whether the sensor is in the lungs or the chest wall is still unclear.

The Epidemiology of OSA

The obstructive sleep apnoea syndrome (OSAS) is defined as an abnormal number of events in sleep caused by repetitive upper airway obstruction, and associated with symptoms of sleep fragmentation. A landmark epidemiological study in North America [2] showed that sleep-disordered breathing (defined here as an apnoeic-hypopnoeic index (AHI) >5 events per hour) was present in 24% of middle-aged men and 9% of women, but when combined with symptoms of excessive daytime somnolence (EDS) the prevalence was 4% and 2% respectively. Similar figures have been obtained in Hong Kong, Korea, and India [3]. Most studies show a male: female ratio of 2:1, and follow-up studies show a tendency of the condition to deteriorate with time. Even moderately severe OSAS (AHI >15 plus frequent sleepiness) is underdiagnosed, with only 18% of men and 7% of women in the Wisconsin Sleep Cohort Study known to have the condition. Snoring, a strong predictor of OSA, is less likely to be reported by women, but does not fully explain the gender bias. A variant of OSA is the upper airway resistance syndrome (UARS), although its existence has been disputed. Patients present with snoring and EDS, but tend to be female, not overtly overweight, and may have a high, narrow hard palate with an abnormal overjet. They do not fulfil the usual AHI criteria for OSA, but sleep studies show multiple respiratory effort-related arousals (RERAs) which cause sleep fragmentation. Identification of RERAs requires measurement of oesophageal pressure or pulse transit time to demonstrate increasing respiratory effort with evidence of inspiratory flow limitation [4].

The Physiology of an Apnoea

Intermittent obstruction of the upper airway has profound effects on a number of organs, but particularly the cardiovascular system. Increasing respiratory effort against an obstructed airway produces abnormally large swings in pleural pressure, and affects the heart. Feedback from respiratory muscles, reduced lung inflation, and chemoreceptor stimulation due to blood gas derangement lead to an increase in respiratory effort. The fall in intra-thoracic pressure lowers intracardiac pressure in relation to extrathoracic structures with reduced perfusion pressure, reduced stroke volume, and a fall in cardiac output. Sympathetic tone increases and muscle bed vasoconstriction occurs. Blood pressure (BP) and heart rate fall, but when the apnoea terminates, blood pressure, heart rate, and cardiac output all rise. The rise in BP, which may be of the order of 15–50 mmHg, is due to arousal and increased sympathetic tone rather than hypoxia *per se*.

It is assumed that excessive daytime somnolence (EDS) in OSAS is due to sleep fragmentation as a result of multiple arousals. This results in a greater time spent in light sleep, reduced SWS, hypoxaemia, and autonomic activation, all of which *might* contribute to EDS. However, many individuals have markedly abnormal sleep studies without EDS, whereas others remain somnolent despite treatment effecting a dramatic reduction in the number of apnoeas. There is surprisingly little correlation between the severity of OSA (as judged by either AHI or the number of arousals) and more objective tests of daytime sleepiness such as MSLT (multiple sleep latency test).

Symptoms of OSA
- Excessive daytime somnolence or unrefreshing sleep
- Snoring
- Witnessed apnoeas, choking, waking with gasping
- Nocturia
- Erectile dysfunction, low libido
- Irritability, impaired concentration, depression, cognitive blunting

EDS has a number of different causes, of which inadequate sleep time is probably the commonest:

Differential diagnosis of excessive daytime somnolence

- Inadequate sleep time
- Sleep apnoea
- Chronic ventilatory failure caused by restrictive or obstructive lung disease
- Circadian rhythm disorder including shift work
- Medical condition (diabetes, pituitary or thyroid disease, renal failure)
- Chronic fatigue syndrome and fibromyalgia
- Drugs (prescribed or recreational)
- Alcohol
- Depression
- Chronic pain syndromes
- Neurological (narcolepsy, idiopathic hypersomnia, Parkinson's Disease, tumour, post stroke, epilepsy)
- Chronic insomnia

Chronic fatigue ("tired all the time") is a common presentation in both primary and secondary care, but if it occurs without daytime naps is unlikely to be due to OSAS. Somewhat counterintuitively, insomnia (often of the sleep maintenance type) may co-exist with OSAS, and complicates both diagnosis and management. It is more common in women, and may be indicative of recurrent arousals with brief awakenings secondary to obstructive events. The Epworth Sleepiness Score (ESS) is a subjective quantification of an individual's propensity to fall asleep in eight different situations (Fig. 8.1) and has a maximum possible score of 24. The ESS has high test-retest reliability, but the cut-off is poorly defined. Although a score of 10 or less is considered normal, scores of 11 are seen in 10% of the population, and scores of 12 or greater are probably abnormal.

The STOP-Bang questionnaire (Fig. 8.2) concentrates less on EDS, but identifies associated features of OSAS such as snoring, witnessed apnoeas, hypertension, and obesity. The probability of OSA is low with scores of 2 or less, whereas scores of 6 or more have high sensitivity and specificity. It has been validated in the preoperative setting as a useful screening tool (albeit with high sensitivity and low specificity) for those who may require further investigation. Local factors may determine the threshold for performing respiratory polysomnography, and common indications are listed in the Table 8.1 below. Isolated snoring or occasional witnessed apnoeas do not require investigation with a sleep study unless upper airway surgery is being considered, there are other features to suggest sleep fragmentation, or reassurance is needed.

Sleep Studies

Overnight oximetry is widely available, but not sufficiently sensitive for the diagnosis of all cases of OSA [5]. The ODI (oxygen desaturation index) measures the number of episodes per hour where saturation falls by 4%, with diagnostic cut-offs of greater than 10 or 15 per hour being suggestive of OSA. Some services use oximetry as a screening test, referring on for more detailed studies if the clinical picture requires it, or directly for treatment if repetitive desaturation is shown. Arrhythmias can lead to imprecise estimation of oxygen saturation, and comorbidities such as COPD with low baseline saturations confound the interpretation of desaturation events. Conversely, individuals with a large lung capacity can have prolonged apnoeas but with little desaturation, as they are on the upper flat portion of the oxygen dissociation curve.

More accurate systems are now widely available and monitor saturation, heart rate, airflow, and respiratory effort (Fig. 8.3). Airflow is measured at the nose with a thermistor or nasal pressure transducer and can detect apnoeas and flow limitation. The reliability of the signal is compromised by mouth breathing and nasal obstruction. Movement sensors detect changes in the volume of chest and abdomen by inductance plethysmography and can distinguish between obstructive and central events by recording either paradoxical or absent movement of chest

Fig. 8.1 The Epworth Sleepiness Scale. The patient is asked to rate their likelihood of falling asleep in eight different situations. The maximum possible score is 24. From ESS © MW Johns 1990-1997. Used under License. Johns MW. A new method for measuring daytime sleepiness: the Epworth Sleepiness Scale. Sleep 1991;14(6):540–5.Mapi Research Trust, Lyon, France https://eprovide. mapi-trust.org. Reproduced with permission

Epworth Sleepiness Scale

Name: _____ Today's date: _____

Your age (Yrs): _____ Your sex (Male = M, Female = F): _____

How likely are you to doze off or fall asleep in the following situations, in contrast to feeling just tired?

This refers to your usual way of life in recent times.

Even if you haven't done some of these things recently try to work out how they would have affected you.

Use the following scale to choose the **most appropriate number** for each situation:

0 = would **never** doze
1 = **slight chance** of dozing
2 = **moderate chance** of dozing
3 = **high chance** of dozing

It is important that you answer each question as best you can.

Situation	Chance of Dozing (0-3)
Sitting and reading _____	—
Watching TV _____	—
Sitting, inactive in a public place (e.g. a theatre or a meeting) _____	—
As a passenger in a car for an hour without a break _____	—
Lying down to rest in the afternoon when circumstances permit _____	—
Sitting and talking to someone _____	—
Sitting quietly after a lunch without alcohol _____	—
In a car, while stopped for a few minutes in the traffic _____	—

THANK YOU FOR YOUR COOPERATION

© M.W. Johns 1990-97

Fig. 8.2 The STOP-Bang Questionnaire: a pre-operative screening tool for identifying individuals requiring a sleep study for exclusion or confirmation of OSA. Reproduced with permission

STOP-BANG Questionnaire

S – Snoring: Do you snore loudly?

T – Tired: Do you feel tired, sleepy during daytime?

O – Observed: Has anyone observed you stop breathing during sleep?

P – Blood Pressure: Are you being treated or have you been treated for hypertension?

B – BMI: Body mass index > 35

A – Age: Age over 50 years

N – Neck: Neck circumference greater than 40 cm

G – Gender: Male gender

Table 8.1 Possible indications for respiratory sleep study

- Excessive daytime somnolence
- Recurrent witnessed apnoeas
- Nocturnal choking, gasping or "dyspnoea"
- Restless sleep, excessive limb movements, parasomnia
- Drug resistant hypertension or refractory atrial fibrillation
- Unrefreshing sleep despite adequate sleep time and continuity
- Near-miss events or accidents caused by reduced vigilance
- Screening prior to bariatric surgery or upper airway surgery for snoring
- Otherwise unexplained polycythaemia, pulmonary hypertension or ventilatory failure

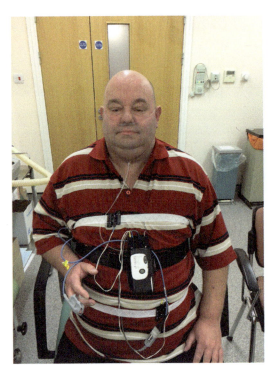

Fig. 8.3 Patient set up for outpatient multichannel respiratory polysomnography. The nasal cannulae are connected to a pressure transducer to measure changes in nasal airflow and snoring, while the two belts measure thoracic and abdominal movement respectively and detect body position. Pulse oximetry provides continuous monitoring of oxygen saturation and pulse rate

and abdomen respectively (Figs. 8.4 and 8.5). Changes in tidal volume are used to detect hypopnoeas, although there is controversy about the optimal definition and whether or not such

an event requires an element of desaturation. These studies can be performed in patients' homes and are widely used. More sophisticated polysomnography—so-called level 1 or, if performed unsupervised, level 2 studies—are expensive, technically demanding, and rarely used in the UK except in equivocal cases or where parasomnias are suspected. In addition to respiratory monitoring, recording of EEG (for sleep staging), chin EMG (for REM detection), limb movements, and perhaps oesophageal manometry (for detection of RERAs) are recorded. Level 3 studies monitor at least three different parameters (e.g. oximetry, snoring, airflow, respiratory effort, position) using portable monitors in the patient's home and are more than adequate for patients with a moderate probability of OSA. Position-dependent OSA (Fig. 8.6), defined as a difference of 50% or more in apnoea index between supine and non-supine positions, is surprisingly common, with a prevalence of >50% reported in several studies.

NICE stratifies OSAS by AHI as follows: mild (5–14 events/h), moderate (15–30), severe (greater than 30), but this classification makes no allowance for the severity of symptoms, which may be severe in patients with "mild" disease.

Sleep Apnoea and Vascular Risk

OSA has been associated with a number of adverse cardiovascular consequences, including hypertension, stroke, coronary artery disease, heart failure, and arrhythmias, but causality has been hard to prove, except for systemic hypertension.

Most, but not all, studies confirm the association of hypertension with OSA. The Wisconsin Sleep Cohort Study prospectively demonstrated a dose-response relationship between the severity of sleep apnoea and the development of hypertension over a 4-year follow-up period [6]. During a longer period of follow-up, a Spanish cohort also found the incidence of hypertension increased with disease severity, and that those adherent to CPAP treatment had the lowest risk of developing hypertension [7]. Patients with resistant hypertension seem more likely to have

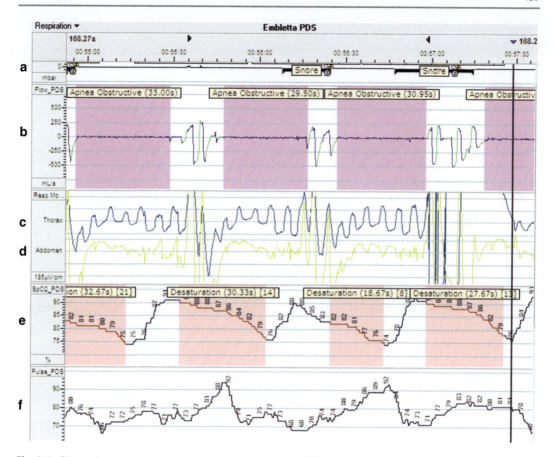

Fig. 8.4 Obstructive sleep apnoea. Apnoeas are registered as periods of absent air flow detected by nasal cannulae (channel B) and are followed by normal breaths as the apnoea is terminated. Channels C and D allow categorisation of these apnoeas as obstructive events. During normal breaths there is synchronisation of thoracic (C) and abdominal (D) movements, which are of similar amplitude and direction. During the obstructive apnoea there is uncoupling of the movements which are out of phase and in different directions. This multichannel recording also shows that the apnoea is associated with snoring (channel A), desaturation (channel E), and pulse rate change (F)

OSA than their well-controlled counterparts, and screening for OSA is often recommended. The mechanism of the association between OSA and hypertension is complex and incompletely understood. Intermittent hypoxia leads to increased oxidative stress, systemic inflammation, and sympathetic activity. Changes in intrathoracic pressure lead to mechanical pressures on the heart, and arousals cause sympathetic activation. Chemoreflex activation with increased sympathetic neural outflow in response to hypoxia seems to be exaggerated during wakefulness in subjects with OSA [8], but resetting of baroreflexes and endothelial activation are also likely to be important. Meta-analysis suggests the overall hypotensive effect of treating OSA is modest, perhaps in the order of 2 mm Hg, but there may

be greater benefits to be had in patients with difficult hypertension or more severe OSA [9]. In patients with minimal symptoms of sleep fragmentation, the effects on BP are trivial, and only present if treatment is used >4 h/night. Pulmonary hypertension is present in about 20% of patients with OSA, but is usually mild and improves with treatment. The mechanism is unclear, but the contribution of recurrent nocturnal hypoxia and left ventricular dysfunction will vary from patient to patient.

Sleep-disordered breathing is common in heart failure patients, and both heart failure and incident coronary disease were increased in populations with severe sleep apnoea [10, 11]. Severe OSA appears to be an independent risk factor for stroke, [12] even allowing for confounders such as hyper-

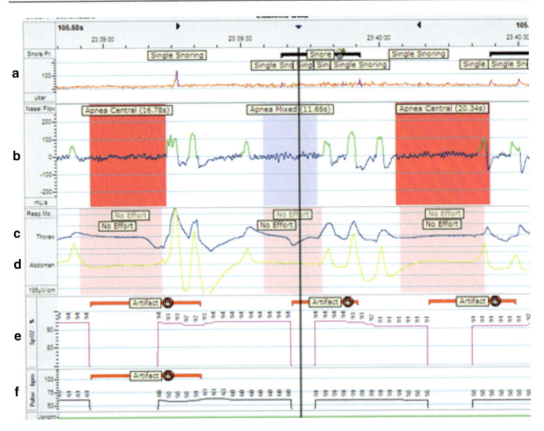

Fig. 8.5 Central sleep apnoea. Multichannel recording shows absence of nasal flow (channel B) accompanied by no movement recorded by either the thoracic (C) or abdominal (D) sensors. The termination of the apnoea is indicated by resumption of nasal flow as synchronised chest and abdominal movements return

tension, atrial fibrillation, and obesity. The risk of atrial fibrillation is much increased in OSA patients, and emerging data suggests that treatment of the latter may be associated with more successful treatment of the arrhythmia. Following stroke, obstructive sleep apnoea is common, but it is unclear if treatment improves outcomes from the acute event. The association of heart disease with OSA is complex, and it is likely that there are common mechanisms which also lead to the development of hypertension. The hypoxia-reoxygenation cycle which accompanies obstructive apnoeas generates reactive oxygen species, and this oxidative stress is thought to result in endothelial dysfunction and atherosclerosis mediated through nuclear transcription factor-kappa B and the expression of pro-inflammatory cytokines such as tumour necrosis factor-alpha (TNF-α) and interleukin-8 (IL-8).

The prevalence of OSA (ODI >10/h) in type 2 diabetics was high (23%) in a community-based UK study, [13] and was even higher (86%) in a more obese North American population using a cut-off AHI of >5/h [14]. Such is the strength of the association that it has recently been suggested that OSA should be regarded as part of the metabolic syndrome, and it is recognised that OSA has an adverse impact on glucose homeostasis and lipid metabolism, perhaps mediated through oxidative stress, inflammation, and intermittent hypoxia. Animal models challenged with the latter develop decreased insulin sensitivity, increased sympathetic activation, and hypertension. Poor diabetic control is associated with more severe OSA, and it was hoped that treatment of the latter might improve insulin sensitivity and glycaemic control. Most studies are short-term, with highly variable adherence, and while some show

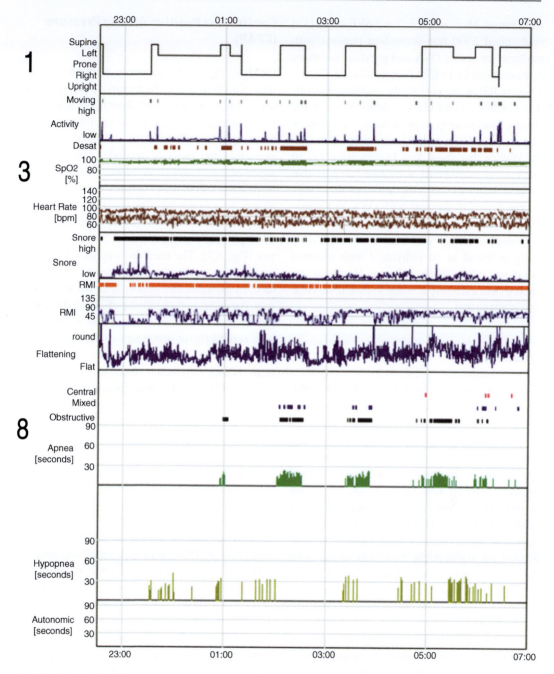

Fig. 8.6 Positional sleep apnoea. Desaturation (channel 3) and clusters of apnoeas (channel 8) occur when subject is in supine position (topmost horizontal "supine" signal in channel 1)

improvement in insulin sensitivity, there is an inconsistent effect on HbA1c, so CPAP remains unproven as adjunctive therapy [15].

A non-randomised observational study [16] indicated that the risk of fatal and non-fatal cardiovascular events was three times higher in patients with untreated severe OSA, and that this risk was attenuated in a control group of severe patients who were compliant with treatment and whose risk was similar to healthy individuals and snorers. More recently, the SAVE study [17] randomised 2700 non-somnolent patients with moderate or severe OSA and previous coronary disease or stroke to CPAP or usual care. Over a 3.7-year follow-up period, the incidence of further vascular events did not differ between the groups. Thus there is no prospective data to show that treating OSA reduces mortality, although the studies that show less hypertension [7] or markers of endothelial activation suggest that some of the underlying risk factors might change for the better. In patients with OSA and symptoms of sleep fragmentation, the decision to treat is uncontroversial; when an abnormal sleep study is found in an individual with minimal symptoms, then the benefits of treatment are unclear, and currently it is not known if vascular risk is attenuated.

Treatment

General measures include advice about weight, alcohol, and sleep position. Obesity is prevalent in the OSA population but, realistically, sustained weight loss sufficient to cure the condition is rarely achieved. Bariatric surgery is remarkably effective in this respect, but invasive and resource-intensive. Weight loss might be an option for patients who are not very symptomatic and only mildly overweight. However, for patients with significant sleep fragmentation, there is no justification for withholding treatment in the hope that they might eventually lose sufficient weight to cure their condition. Alcohol undoubtedly worsens OSA, but there are no long-term studies of the effects of abstention or moderation. Given the prevalence of positional sleep apnoea, treatments to encourage avoidance of the supine position therapy have received surprisingly little attention. Positional therapy usually consists of a device such as a modified vest or backpack which makes the supine position uncomfortable, and appears moderately effective in short-term case series. Recent developments include signal-emitting position sensors that provide feedback for the sleeping patient, but long-term compliance is untested.

Continuous Positive Airway Pressure (CPAP)

CPAP is the most commonly prescribed treatment for OSA, and is the treatment of choice for severe OSA. As discussed, flow in the upper airway depends on minimal upstream intraluminal airway pressure (Pcrit) of the collapsible segment exceeding the pressure around it—namely the negative intraluminal pressure resulting from inspiration. CPAP pneumatically opens the upper airway by constant pressure throughout the respiratory cycle. CPAP machines generate large flows passing via tube and mask into the oropharynx (Fig. 8.7). The mask incorporates a leakage that induces resistance, and thus positive pressure, in the mask that splints open the upper airway. An additional stabilising effect on the upper airway by a CPAP-induced increase in lung volume is unlikely, as upper airway muscular activity has been shown to be reduced by CPAP. In the heart failure population, there are likely to be additional benefits because positive intrathoracic pressure reduces venous return (preload) and left ventricular transmural pressure (afterload). CPAP should be distinguished from non-invasive ventilation (NIV), where cyclical positive pressure applied to the airway increases tidal volume, thereby augmenting lung inflation and improving gas exchange in patients with ventilatory failure.

Treatment usually results in a dramatic improvement in symptoms of sleep fragmentation (namely EDS, poor concentration, loss of energy), snoring, and sometimes nocturia. A Cochrane review comparing CPAP with placebo or an oral appliance showed large improvements in Epworth sleepiness score (mean 3.8) and various quality-of-life indicators [18]. Individuals with very abnormal sleep studies who agree to a trial of CPAP may volunteer improvement in hitherto underappreciated symptoms. Early problems are common, and a good sleep service should be responsive to patients struggling to acclimatise themselves to treatment, with often minor modifications (mask fit, humidification) making an important contribution to long-term adherence (Table 8.2). The minimum effective usage time is unknown, but 4 h use per night is

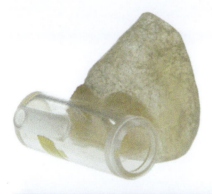

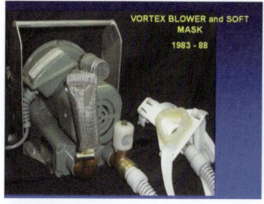

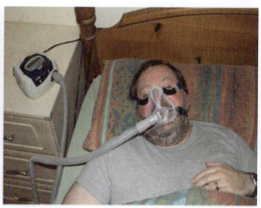

Fig. 8.7 CPAP treatment. On the left is an early individually moulded nasal mask and, below, the bulky flow generator. On the right is a modern CPAP machine with a full face mask

Table 8.2 Troubleshooting CPAP

Symptom	Possible solution
Rhinitis	Humidification; topical steroids
Dry nose or mouth	Humidification; if leak, full face mask
Mask removal in sleep	Review mask fitting; pressure adjustment
Intolerant to pressure	Gradual pressure increment during sleep onset (ramp function); consider auto-adjusting CPAP or bilevel ventilation
Difficulty initiating sleep	Ramp function; sleep hygiene; short course of non-benzodiazepine hypnotic
Swallowing air (aerophagy)	Reduce pressure transiently; sleep propped up
Skin irritation	Mask hygiene; liners; change interface
Claustrophobia	Nasal cushions; acclimatisation; address anxiety

generally considered a minimum for symptom control, and may be higher to achieve any putative cardiovascular benefit. At least 20% of patients are unable to tolerate treatment, and if adherence is defined as >4 h use per night, then 46–83% of patients fail to achieve this.

All modern CPAP machines can measure hours of usage, and diagnostic devices can detect persistent apnoeic events, the CPAP pressure required to abolish them, and quantify the presence of mask leak. Most patients will be treated in the first instance with a fixed-pressure CPAP machine set at about 10 cm H_2O, perhaps determined by an auto-titrating CPAP study which can determine the pressure required to abolish the majority of apnoeic events. Auto-CPAP machines can respond flexibly to the state of the upper airway, where the pressure required to eliminate the apnoeas may vary with position, sleep stage, or alcohol consumption. Direct comparison of auto-CPAP and fixed-pressure CPAP suggests that while the former allows a reduction in mean pressure, there is only a trivial improvement in compliance, and no major difference in AHI or

Table 8.3 Persisting EDS in CPAP patient

Cause	Possible solution
Inadequate use	Aim for >4 h/night; small increase may be worthwhile
Failure to control apnoeas	Identify mask leak, pressure titration; consider missed central apnoeas
Wrong or additional sleep diagnosis	Repeat equivocal sleep study, other sleep investigation (MSLT, full polysomnography, sleep diary)
Inadequate sleep time	Education
Medication	Alternative drug where possible
Comorbidities	Address, but often chronic and intractable
Depression	Treat, if indicated
Unrealistic expectation	Education

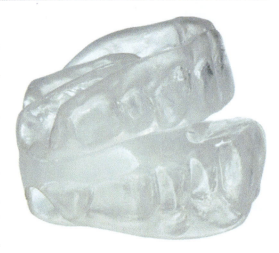

Fig. 8.8 A semi-bespoke commercially available mandibular advancement device. Courtesy of Meditas/SleepPro Ltd.

sleepiness scores [19]. Autotitrating CPAP is more expensive, but is often preferred by patients, and should be considered when patient intolerance is preventing effective treatment. Failure to improve should prompt consideration of an alternative explanation (Table 8.3). Drug therapy is generally ineffective in OSAS, but wake-promoting agents such as modafanil have been used as adjunctive off-license treatment in CPAP patients complaining of residual EDS.

Oral Appliances (OAs)

These work by enlarging the upper airway, either by protruding the mandible (mandibular advancement devices or MADs, Fig. 8.8) or advancing the position of the tongue (tongue retaining devices, Fig. 8.9). Mandibular advancement devices move the tongue anteriorly as well as enlarging the lateral dimensions of the velopharynx, the area between the margin of the hard palate and the soft palate. The further the mandible can be advanced, the greater the efficacy. Customised devices made with dental casts and supervised by dental practitioners are probably the ideal, but semi-personalised devices are cheaper (yet broadly as efficacious) and tend to be preferred to thermoplastic ("boil and bite") appliances. The development of materials that improve intraoral retention,

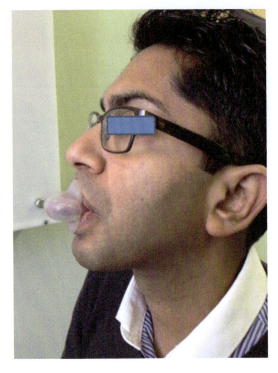

Fig. 8.9 A commercially available tongue-retaining device

and adjustable appliances that allow progressive advancement of the mandible, have made devices more acceptable and effective. Unfortunately, the acclimatisation and advancement process takes many months. Common side effects include excess salivation, xerostomia, dental and temporomandibular joint pain, and gum irritation. Partially or totally edentulous patients are unsuitable for MADs. Compared to CPAP, OAs are not as effective at reducing AHI, but are probably as effective in improving daytime somnolence and health status [20]. A complete response is achieved in approximately half the population of users. Perhaps surprisingly, patient preference outcomes tend to favour OAs over CPAP, and this may be the result in greater hours of use per night, but most commercially available devices do not have any way of measuring compliance. Currently the provision of these devices in the UK is patchy, whereas they have become part of the standard treatment armamentarium in Europe and North America. In patients with severe OSA, CPAP remains first-line treatment, but in mild and moderate disease, OAs can be considered as a potentially effective treatment that may be preferred by the patient, or as second-line if CPAP is not tolerated. Uncomplicated non-apnoeic snoring can also be treated with OAs if nasal obstruction is not the cause.

Hypoglossal Stimulation

Recently it has been shown that implantable hypoglossal nerve stimulators can dramatically improve OSA by dilating the muscles of the upper airway [21]. No randomised data is available, but trials suggest at least a 50% fall in AHI, with greater likelihood of success if patients with concentric upper airway collapse are excluded by nasendoscopy. The equipment is expensive, but might be an option in the future for patients who are CPAP intolerant.

Surgery for OSA

Although superficially an attractive option for what might be seen as an anatomical problem, the results of surgery have been disappointing, perhaps because obstruction often occurs at multiple levels. There is a dearth of rigorously controlled trials, and the reported outcomes often lack detail on sleep parameters or measures of daytime somnolence.

Palatoplasty may help non-apnoeic snoring, but produces inconsistent and rather small improvements in OSA. The previously popular radical uvulopalatopharyngoplasty (UVPPP) is painful, and may cause palatal incompetence and stenosis. The benefit on OSA is unclear, but may make subsequent CPAP harder to tolerate because of problems creating an effective palatal seal. In adults with a particular palatal phenotype and without severe obesity, UVPPP can be effective [22]. Laser-assisted palatoplasty is less invasive, but has not been rigorously evaluated, and reported benefits deteriorate with time. Radiofrequency thermoplasty aims to produce scarring and stiffening of the soft palate and tongue base, but the improvements in sleep parameters are disappointing, long term data are lacking, and multiple treatments may be required. Hyoid suspension aims to prevent hypopharyngeal tongue base collapse and is ineffective in isolation, although it may have a role when it is a component of multilevel surgery [23].

Maxillo-mandibular advancement (MMA) enlarges the velo-orohypopharynx by advancing the structures (soft palate, tongue base, and suprahyoid musculature) attached to the maxilla, mandible, and hyoid bone and, apart from tracheostomy, is probably the most successful surgical option in adults. It is achieved by bilateral osteotomies that are stabilised with plates or bone grafts. Meta-analysis showed mean reductions in AHI from 64 to10 events/h and a cure rate of 67% in those with AHI < 30/h [24]. These results are impressive, but the surgery is invasive, technically challenging, and carries an attendant risk. It seems to be particularly suited to individuals with hypopharyngeal narrowing, which is often found with co-existent skeletal hypoplasia such as retrognathia.

Surgical correction of an obstructed nasal airway hardly ever cures sleep apnoea, but the identification and correction of obstructive pathology may improve CPAP compliance by reducing nasal symptoms and allowing lower treatment pressures.

OSA in Childhood

Childhood OSA is said to have a prevalence of 1–5%, and is associated with tonsillar hypertrophy, obesity, and various craniofacial syndromes. Snoring, restless sleep, sweating, and enuresis are common features, but EDS is rarer than hyperactivity. Adenoidal enlargement is not visible in clinic, but can be inferred by the presence of tonsillar hypertrophy. In the UK, ENT surgeons rarely carry out sleep studies in children because adenotonsillectomy is almost invariably effective treatment in the non-obese child. In less clear-cut cases there may be spontaneous improvement if surgery is deferred. If mild disease is present, weight loss (where appropriate) and topical steroids and/or oral montelukast may reduce adenoidal size sufficiently to effect an improvement, but this is not widely practised. CPAP may be indicated for children with persistent OSA post-surgery, obesity, craniofacial abnormalities, or neuromuscular disorders.

OSA and the Surgical Patient

The risks of desaturation, respiratory failure, reintubation, ICU transfer, and cardiac events are doubled in the OSA population undergoing surgery [25]. General anaesthesia and post-operative analgesia pose a particular risk for the patient with OSA. Anaesthetic agents reduce ventilatory drive, increase the tendency to upper airway collapse, and impair normal arousal mechanisms, all of which will increase the pre-existing tendency to obstructive apnoeas. Not only may the upper airway anatomy of the OSA patient contribute to a difficult intubation, but the timing and monitoring of extubation is critical. If the patient is known to have treated OSA, they should bring their CPAP machine with them to hospital, and post-extubation CPAP is tolerated and safe. If the OSA only becomes apparent post-extubation, then urgent management with an oropharyngeal or nasal airway can be followed by CPAP, although if the patient is not familiar with this treatment it may be poorly tolerated. The risk of adverse outcomes is highest in the first 24 h, and

reversal of anaesthesia and narcotics may be necessary. Increasingly, patients scheduled for elective surgery undergo questionnaire screening for OSA and are referred for diagnostic studies. Surgery may then be delayed until patients with abnormal studies are established on CPAP regardless of symptoms, yet the evidence for the necessity of this strategy is far from convincing [26]. In the bariatric population (where there is a particularly high prevalence of OSA), acclimatising affected patients to treatment means that perioperative CPAP is less likely to cause aerophagy and threaten the integrity of the surgical anastomosis.

Central Sleep Apnoea (CSA)

Central apnoeas and hypopnoeas arise from complete or partial cessation of neural output to the respiratory muscles, and are much rarer then obstructive apnoeas. In the latter there are continuing efforts to overcome an obstructed airway, and this is detected by out-of-phase thoracic–abdominal movement detected by respiratory impedance plethysmography or flow limitation on a nasal pressure signal. Distinguishing central from obstructive hypopnoeas is more difficult, as in both cases diminished respiratory efforts continue. There are no consistent diagnostic criteria to define a clinically significant degree of CSA, but arbitrarily CSA is considered the primary diagnosis if >50% apnoeas are central. Obstructive and central events frequently co-exist in the same patient, and central apnoeas can lead to obstructive events and vice versa.

Central sleep apnoea is less well understood than OSA, and has varying aetiologies. One classification of CSA is based on the presence or absence of hypercapnia.

Hypercapnia CSA

Neurological Disease

Any brainstem pathology (trauma, infarcts, tumours) can adversely affect ventilatory output. The cause is usually obvious, and the other neurological consequences of the brainstem injury tend to dominate the clinical picture. Congenital central hypoventilation syndrome (previously known as Ondine's curse) usually presents in infancy or childhood, and is due to inherited mutation in the PHOX2B gene. There are impaired responses to hypoxia and hypercapnia and daytime ventilatory failure due to low tidal volume and marked alveolar hypoventilation, which is worse in NREM sleep.

Opiate-Induced CSA

Opioids are potent respiratory depressants, particularly in overdose, but it is increasingly recognised that chronic opiate use is associated with CSA, with a quoted prevalence of 24%. This ill-understood phenomena is dose-related and is particularly likely with a morphine equivalent daily dose >200 mg. The central depressant effect is probably due to their effect on brainstem and carotid bodies. Mild hypoxia is common in chronic opiate use, and if further central respiratory depression occurs, worsening hypoxaemia will result. The peripheral chemoreceptor response corrects hypoxaemia and blows off CO_2, but blunting of central chemoreceptors prevents a brisk response to CO_2 tension changes, and continuing exposure to the opiate propagates the cycle.

Obesity Hypoventilation Syndrome (OHS)

This is the combination of obesity (BMI > 30 kg/m^2) and hypercapnia during wakefulness that is unexplained by neuromuscular, metabolic, or ventilatory defects (FEV1/FVC ratio >60%) and is an increasingly prevalent condition, albeit prone to diagnostic delay. Patients normally present with oedema, and this is often misdiagnosed as cardiac failure. Morning headache, somnolence, and neurocognitive impairment are usually present. Obesity impairs respiratory mechanics and there may be an element of respiratory muscle weakness. Obstructive sleep apnoea is present in up to 90% of individuals,

and the condition is present in 10% of OSA patients. Why some individuals develop OHS is incompletely understood, but differences in fat distribution and blunted chemosensitivity have been invoked, and perhaps permit tolerance to the hypercapnia that develops during sleep. Leptin is an adipose tissue-derived protein that controls appetite and acts on central respiratory pathways to increase respiration. In OHS patients leptin levels are higher than weight-matched controls, and this has led to the theory that OHS represents a state of reduced drive and hypercapnic response caused by leptin resistance. OHS patients frequently present in extremis with acidotic exacerbations of chronic ventilatory failure and temporary mild left ventricular impairment. Treatment usually involves long-term, non-invasive bilevel ventilation with high expiratory pressures to treat the associated OSA.

Mixed CSA and OSA

This is encountered in the early stages of CPAP treatment of patients with OSA, and is known variously as "complex sleep apnoea" or "treatment-emergent central apnoeas." It may become apparent during the initial CPAP titration if the pressure is increased too rapidly. Why this develops is unclear: pressure-activated lung stretch receptors may inhibit central motor output via the Hering-Breuer reflex, or mask leak might increase CO_2 excretion and lead to readier crossing of the apnoeic threshold. These central events almost invariably resolve with continued CPAP over the ensuing month, and although quite common, are of uncertain significance.

Non-hypercapnic CSA

Cardiac Failure

Approximately 50% of all patients with cardiac failure have some form of sleep apnoea, either central, obstructive, or both. Although initially thought to be a marker of severe cardiac dysfunction, it is now clear that central apnoeas may be present with mild disease. Some, but not all, studies have associated CSA with increased mortality, but when adequately controlled for heart failure severity, the association is not strong. Cheyne-Stokes (CS) breathing is the waking manifestation of the central apnoeas, and both are characterised by 20–30 s of hyperventilation followed by 10–40 s of hypopnoeas or apnoeas. The waxing and waning in tidal volume distinguishes CSA-CS from other causes of CSA. Unlike OSA, these events occur in wakefulness or stages 1 and 2 non-REM rather than REM sleep.

Pathophysiology of CSA-CS

Raised left atrial pressure and pulmonary venous congestion are consequences of heart failure and stimulate pulmonary receptors, causing hyperventilation and lowering the $PaCO_2$ nearer to the apnoeic threshold. With sleep onset, the waking drive to breath is removed and as the $PaCO_2$ falls below this threshold, the patient remains apnoeic until the CO_2 rises again and ventilation is re-established. Shortly after the arousal occurs, sleep is resumed and the cycle begins again. This oscillation of the feedback loop around the apnoeic threshold is critical to the perpetuation of CSA, but there is no single unifying explanation as to why the system is inherently more unstable than in health, and with a tendency to both overshoot and undershoot. The length of the ventilatory phase is proportional to cardiac output, suggesting (oversimplistically) that the low cardiac output results in a prolonged transit time between lungs and chemoreceptors, and that there is a delay before the $PaCO_2$ in the lungs is sensed in the brainstem and carotid bodies. Supine low-volume lungs, fluctuations in alveolar ventilation, and changes in sleep stage destabilise ventilatory control and predispose to CSA.

Increased central and peripheral chemoreceptor responses to CO_2 have been described in heart failure patients with CSA, and may predispose to instability, indeed central apnoeas can be abolished by small increments in inspired CO_2. While cardiac-induced central apnoeas can cause sleep fragmentation and swings in intrathoracic pressure, the effects on daytime sleepiness and left ventricular afterload appear less than in the OSA population. Bronchoscopic measurements show that during a central apnoea, upper airway closure on expiration may occur, blurring the distinction between the two forms of apnoea.

Patients with CSA may complain of EDS and choking, but are more likely than OSA patients to be elderly and complain of difficulty initiating and maintaining sleep. Treatment for heart failure, including cardiac resynchronisation therapy, improves CSA, but if it persists and is accompanied by symptoms of sleep fragment, targeted treatment should be considered. The CANPAP study [27] randomised patients with heart failure and predominant CSA (mean AHI 40 events/h) to medical treatment or non-titrated CPAP. Although the primary endpoint of transplant-free survival was no different between the groups, the CPAP group had significant falls in AHI, nocturnal desaturation, and noradrenaline levels. A post-hoc analysis suggested that in those patients where CPAP suppressed AHI <15 events/h, survival was improved [28]. Adaptive Servo-Ventilation (ASV) is a pressure preset form of non-invasive ventilation which can be volume- or flow-cycled, and can have variable inspiratory and expiratory pressure to ensure upper airway patency. ASV attenuates hyperventilation and hypocapnoea by delivering preset minute ventilation and providing CPAP to reverse any upper airway obstruction. Early studies suggested ASV was very effective at reducing AHI and improving left ventricular ejection fraction, and it was widely anticipated that in patients with heart failure and CSA this form of ventilatory support would improve sleep quality, left ventricular function, and survival. SERVE-HF was a large multicentre trial examining use of ASV in patients with systolic heart failure and predominant CSA [29]. Although ASV was effective in reducing AHI (from a mean of 25 to 3 central events/h) and improving Epworth scores, there were no improvements in functional outcomes or quality-of-life measurements, and an unexpected increase in all cause and cardiovascular mortality (28% and 34% respectively), with the risk of death greatest in the patients with more severe heart failure. ASV is now contraindicated in patients with chronic heart failure (NYHA 2–4) and left ventricular ejection fraction (LVEF) <45%, but may still be useful in patients with CSA and other forms of heart failure, including those with a preserved ejection fraction. Oxygen treatment suppresses chemoreceptor drive and dampens the oscillations of the respiratory control system. Meta-analyses from a limited number of trials confirm considerable improvement in AHI, arterial desaturation and, to a lesser extent, left ventricular ejection fraction.

Idiopathic CSA

Idiopathic CSA is rare and poorly understood. The key seems to be an unexplained tendency to hyperventilate during wakefulness and sleep, and increased peripheral and central responsiveness to CO_2. When the waking drive to breathe is withdrawn at sleep onset, the low CO_2 from previous hyperventilation is below the apnoeic threshold, which results in an apnoea, then an arousal. Once sleep is firmly established, the apnoeas become less frequent. Only small changes in CO_2 seem to be necessary to perpetuate the cycle of apnoea and hyperventilation, and the degree of oxygen desaturation is typically small. Generally this seems to be a benign condition, but can be symptomatic with either insomnia or excessive daytime somnolence Because of the rarity of the condition, treatment is not clearly established. Acetazolamide and sedatives such as zolpidem and triazolam appear to have some efficacy, [30] by either providing a constant non-fluctuating respiratory stimulus or deliberately blunting the arousal threshold. CPAP seems to be effective, but there is no long-term data, and the mechanism of action is probably different from in OSA.

Non-apnoeic Sleep Disorders

A number of non-apnoeic sleep disorders may present to respiratory physicians because of their expertise in the diagnosis of somnolent patients with sleep-disordered breathing. Although traditionally these patients may be regarded as having a neurological disorder, familiarity with these conditions is useful.

Myotonic Dystrophy

This autosomal dominant disorder is not uncommon, but sporadic cases occur or the classical facial features or muscle weakness may be absent. Obstructive sleep apnoea is common, but if respiratory muscle weakness is present, then nocturnal hypoventilation and diurnal ventilatory failure may develop. Adherence to the recommended form of respiratory support (be it CPAP or bilevel ventilation) may be patchy, as a degree of apathy is often part of the condition. Somnolence may be present without any evidence of sleep-disordered breathing, and REM sleep dysregulation has been identified. Trials of stimulants such as modafanil are sometimes helpful.

Narcolepsy

This condition is now known to be caused by a deficiency of the neurotransmitter hypocretin in the lateral hypothalamus. It can be regarded as a disorder where the demarcation between wakefulness, NREM, and REM sleep is disorganised. It has a bimodal age of onset, with peaks at 16 and 36, and diagnostic delay is usual. Sleep may be irresistible, with a need to take frequent short naps (which are characteristically refreshing), but often occurring in highly inappropriate circumstances. Microsleeps and semi-automatic behaviours are common, but nighttime sleep is often fragmented, and other parasomnias can occur. Cataplexy develops in 60–70% of cases and, if recognised, confirms the diagnosis. Attacks of transient muscular weakness of neck (head nod), leg, arm or facial sagging, or slurred speech with preserved consciousness, usually precipitated by laughter or anger, should be specifically enquired about. Vivid dreams at sleep onset or termination which are hard to distinguish from wakefulness, and routinely dreaming during short naps, is suggestive. Sleep paralysis completes the tetrad, but is sometimes seen in normal individuals as an isolated phenomenon. Although essentially a clinical diagnosis, investigation may be helpful. The Multiple Sleep Latency Test (MSLT) offers up to five nap opportunities at two hourly intervals with EEG monitoring, and can provide useful confirmation if rigorously performed. Narcoleptics have a short sleep latency and may show episodes of REM within 15 min of falling asleep (so-called sleep onset REM). The DQB1*0602 haplotype is found in over 95% of patients with narcolepsy and cataplexy, but is also found in about 30% of the normal population, so has little diagnostic utility. Recently, cases of narcolepsy were associated with vaccination with H1N1 influenza vaccine and the development of antibodies to the hypocretin receptor, suggesting an autoimmune basis to the condition. Management of the EDS requires stimulant medication (modafinil, dexamphetamine) and cataplexy may respond to tricyclics or SSRIs, which suppress REM sleep. Sodium oxybate improves both symptoms, but has an inconvenient dosing schedule and is very expensive.

Another primary sleep disorder that is sometimes hard to distinguish from narcolepsy is idiopathic hypersomnolence. The aetiology is unknown, but subjects need more sleep than normal people and have prolonged nighttime sleep, difficulty waking, unrefreshing daytime naps, and confusional arousals (sleep drunkenness) on waking. There are no other features of the narcolepsy tetrad, and the response to modafinil is often disappointing.

Parkinson's Disease (PD) and Other Neurodegenerative Disorders

Sleep disturbance is common, particularly daytime sleepiness, which may occur with little warning and which may be due to initiation of treatment with dopamine agonists. A surprisingly common parasomnia in this group of patients is REM sleep behaviour disorder (REMBD), where there is a failure of the normal muscle atonia during REM sleep. Subjects act out dreams with often violent limb movements and injuries to themselves or bed partner. If woken, confusion is unusual, and dreams may be recalled. Polysomnography, if performed, shows muscle tone to be preserved during REM sleep. REMBD may develop in otherwise healthy individuals, but at least half of these patients will eventually develop PD or some other neurodegenerative disease. Treatment with clonazepam is usually effective, and failing that, melatonin. The syndrome may be caused by antidepressants, which should be stopped on a trial basis.

Restless Legs Syndrome

This is a common movement disorder that often presents with daytime somnolence due to sleep initiation insomnia or more subtle sleep fragmentation. Uncomfortable legs, worse in the evening and at rest and relieved by movement, are essential to diagnosis. A useful screening question is: "When you try and relax in the evening or sleep at night, do you ever have unpleasant restless feelings in your legs that can be relieved by walking or movement?". The diagnosis is a clinical one and sleep studies are rarely required, although repetitive clusters of periodic limb movements (PLM) may be detected with actigraphy, and are a frequent association. Milder cases may respond to non-pharmacological interventions such as warm baths or avoidance of caffeine and alcohol. Drugs prescribed for comorbid conditions, particularly dopamine antagonists and antidepressants, may exacerbate RLS and can be temporarily withdrawn. Drug therapy is often considered necessary for moderate/severe disease, and transdermal (rotigotine) and oral dopamine agonists (ropinirole and pramipexole) are usually effective. However, there is growing concern about their role in the eventual development of augmentation (earlier timing of symptom onset, reduced response to medication, extension to other body parts) and gabapentin or low-dose opiates may be preferred as initial treatment. Iron deficiency if present, requires replacement therapy.

Circadian Rhythm Disorders

Identification of these conditions is usually clear from the history. Jet lag is transient, but shift work disorder is commoner with age, and a cause of daytime somnolence which is rarely amenable to treatment other than job change. Delayed sleep phase syndrome is common in adolescents and young adults, and is an inability to initiate sleep until the early hours of the morning, and a need to wake later than traditional employment usually demands. Increasingly, abnormalities of the intrinsic clock mechanism are recognised.

References

1. Stradling JR. Handbook of sleep-related breathing disorders. 1st ed. Oxford: Oxford University Press; 1993.
2. Young T, Patta M, Dempsey J, Skatrud J, Weber S, Badr S. The occurrence of sleep-disordered breathing among middle-aged adults. N Engl J Med. 1993;388:1230–5.
3. Lindberg E. Epidemiology of OSA. In: McNicholas WT, Bonsignore MR, editors. Sleep apnoea. European Respiratory Society monograph. Plymouth: European Respiratory Society; 2010. p. 51–68.
4. Pepin JL, Guillot M, Tanisier R, Levy P. The upper airway resistance syndrome. Respiration. 2012;83:559–66.
5. Netzer N, Eliasson AH, Netzer C, Kristo DA. Overnight pulse oximetry for sleep-disordered breathing in adults: a review. Chest. 2001;120:625–33.
6. Peppard PE, Young T, Palta M, Skatrud J. Prospective study of the association between sleep-disordered breathing and hypertension. N Engl J Med. 2000;342:1378–84.
7. Marin JM, Agusti A, Villar I, Forner M, Nieto D, Carrizo SJ, et al. Association between treated and untreated obstructive sleep apnoea and risk of hypertension. JAMA. 2012;307:2169–76.
8. Mansukhani MP, Kara T, Caples S, Somers VK. Chemoreflexes, sleep apnea and sympathetic dysregulation. Curr Hypertens Rep. 2014;16:476. https://doi.org/10.10007/s11906-014-0476-2.
9. Parati G, Lombardi C, Hedner J, Bonsignore MR, Grote L, Tkavoca R, et al. Recommendations for the management of patients with obstructive sleep apnoea and hypertension. Eur Resp J. 2013;41:523–38.
10. Hla KM, Young T, Hagen EW, Stein JH, Finn LA, Nieto FJ, et al. Coronary heart disease incidence in sleep disordered breathing: the Wisconsin Sleep Cohort Study. Sleep. 2015;38:677–84.
11. Shakhar E, Whitney CW, Redline S, Lee ET, Newman AB, Nieto FJ, et al. Sleep-disordered breathing and cardiovascular disease: cross sectional results of the Sleep Heart Health Study. Am J Respir Crit Care Med. 2001;163:19–25.
12. Yaggi HK, Concato J, Kernan WN, Lichtman JH, Brass LM, Mohsenin V. Obstructive sleep apnea as a risk factor for stroke and death. N Engl J Med. 2005;353:2034–41.
13. West SD, Nicoll DJ, Stradling JR. Prevalence of obstructive sleep apnoea in men with type 2 diabetes. Thorax. 2006;61:945–50.
14. Foster GD, Sanders MH, Millman R, Zammit G, Borradaile KE, Newman AB, et al. Obstructive sleep apnea among obese patients with type 2 diabetes. Diabetes Care. 2009;32:1017–9.
15. Kent BD, McNicholas WT, Ryan S. Insulin resistance, glucose intolerance and diabetes mellitus in obstructive sleep apnoea. J Thorac Dis. 2015;7:1343–57.
16. Marin JM, Carizzo SJ, Vicente E, Agusti AG. Long-term cardiovascular outcomes in men with obstructive sleep apnoea-hypopnoea with or without treatment with continuous positive pressure: an observational study. Lancet. 2005;365:1046–53.
17. McEvoy RD, Antic NA, Heeley E, Luo Y, Ou Q, Zhang X, et al. CPAP for prevention of cardiovascular events in obstructive sleep apnea. N Engl J Med. 2016;375:919–31.
18. Giles TL, Lasserson TJ, Smith B, White J, Wright JJ, Cates CJ. Continuous positive airway pressure for obstructive sleep apnoea in adults. Cochrane Database Syst Rev. 2006;1:CD001106.
19. Weaver TE, Grunstein RR. Adherence to continuous positive airway pressure therapy. Proc Am Thorac Soc. 2008;5:173–8.
20. Health Quality Ontario. Oral appliances for obstructive sleep apnea: an evidence-based analysis. Ont Health Technol Assess Ser. 2009;9:1–51.
21. Strollo PJ, Soose RJ, Maurer JT, de Vries N, Cornelius J, Froymovich O, et al. Upper airway stimulation for obstructive sleep apnea. N Engl J Med. 2014;370:139–49.
22. Browaldh N, Nerfeldt P, Lysadahl M, Bring J, Friberg D. SKUP3 randomised controlled trial: polysomnographic results after uvulopalatopharyngoplasty in selected patients with obstructive sleep apnoea. Thorax. 2013;68:846–53.
23. Kotecha BT, Hall AC. Role of surgery in adult obstructive sleep apnoea. Sleep Med Rev. 2014;18:405–13.
24. Holty JE, Guilleminault C. Maxillomandibular advancement for the treatment of obstructive sleep apnea: a systematic review and meta-analysis. Sleep Med Rev. 2010;14:287–97.
25. Kaw R, Chung F, Pasupuleti V, Mehta J, Gay PC, Hernandez AV. Meta-analysis of the association between obstructive sleep apnoea and postoperative outcome. Br J Anaesth. 2012;109:897–906.
26. Nagappa M, Mokhlesi B, Wong J, Kaw R, Chung F. The effects of continuous positive airway pressure on postoperative outcome in obstructive sleep apnea patients undergoing surgery: a systematic review and meta-analysis. Anesth Analg. 2015;120:1013–23.

27. Bradley TD, Logan AG, Kimoff RJ, Series F, Morrison D, Ferguson K, et al. Continuous positive airway pressure for central sleep apnea and heart failure. N Engl J Med. 2005;353:2025–33.

28. Arzt M, Floras JS, Logan AJ, Kinoff RJ, Series F, Morrison D, et al. Suppression of central apnea by continuous positive airway pressure and transplant-free survival in heart failure: a post hoc analysis of the Canadian continuous positive pressure for patients with Central Sleep Apnea and Heart Failure Trial (CANPAP). Circulation. 2007;115:3173–80.

29. Cowie MR, Woehrle H, Wegscheider K, Angermann C, d'Ortho MP, Erdmann E, et al. Adaptive servo-ventilation in central sleep apnea in systolic heart failure. N Engl J Med. 2015;373:1095–105.

30. Aurora RN, Chowdhuri S, Ramar K, Bista SR, Casey KR, Lamm CI, Kristo DA, et al. The treatment of central sleep apnea syndromes in adults: practice parameters with an evidence-based literature review and meta-analyses. Sleep. 2012;35:17–40.

Respiratory Failure and Non-invasive Ventilation

9

Mark Elliott and Dipansu Ghosh

Pathophysiology

Respiratory failure implies an inability of the respiratory system to carry out gas exchange. It can be broadly classified as hypoxaemic, Type I, and hypercapnic, Type II.

Type I respiratory failure is defined by a PaO_2 of less the 8 KPa with a normal or low arterial carbon dioxide tension ($PaCO_2$). This is commonly seen in acute respiratory conditions where there is impaired gas transfer, including acute pulmonary oedema, pneumonia, interstitial lung disease, or collapse of a pulmonary segment. It may also be present when there is lack of oxygen delivery to the alveoli, e.g. due to broncho-constriction, asthma, or COPD.

Type II respiratory failure is characterized by a raised $PaCO_2$ of more than 6.0 KPa with or without hypoxaemia, and occurs when there is a failure to clear carbon dioxide from blood into the alveoli and, subsequently, into the air.

Respiratory failure can occur due to a malfunction of any aspect of the respiratory system, starting from reduced respiratory drive in the brain, upper airways, bronchial tree, alveoli, chest wall, or respiratory muscles. It can also happen in systemic abnormalities like shock, where there is lack of oxygen delivery to the lungs.

Fundamentally there are five processes involved in respiration: (1) delivery of oxygen to alveoli; (2) delivery of oxygen to blood from alveoli; (3) utilization of oxygen by tissues; (4) removal of CO_2 from blood into alveoli; and (5) removal of CO_2 from alveoli into the environment.

Gas Exchange

Gas exchange occurs in the alveolar-capillary units where oxygen diffuses though the membranes and binds with haemoglobin. The amount of oxygen binding with haemoglobin depends on the blood PaO_2 (arterial oxygen). This relationship, expressed as the oxygen haemoglobin dissociation curve, is not linear but has a sigmoid-shaped curve. It has a steep slope between a PaO_2 of 1.3 and 6.6 kPa and a flat portion above a PaO_2 of 9.3 kPa.

Approximately 5% of the total body CO_2 dissolves in the plasma, 5% is carried as carboxy-haemoglobin on proteins, and 90% is carried as bicarbonate ions in the plasma. The partial pressure of carbon dioxide ($PaCO_2$) in the capillaries is higher than that in the alveoli, thus CO_2 diffuses into the alveoli, from where it is exhaled.

In ideal gas exchange, ventilation (V) and perfusion (Q) should match perfectly, but even in

M. Elliott (✉) · D. Ghosh
Leeds Centre for Respiratory Medicine,
St James's University Hospital,
Leeds, West Yorkshire, UK
e-mail: mwelliott@doctors.org.uk

© Springer International Publishing AG, part of Springer Nature 2018
S. Hart, M. Greenstone (eds.), *Foundations of Respiratory Medicine*,
https://doi.org/10.1007/978-3-319-94127-1_9

normal physiology not all alveolar-capillary units have complete synchrony of ventilation and perfusion. Some perfectly ventilated alveoli might be under-perfused (large V/Q) and vice versa (low V/Q or shunt).

Alveolar Ventilation

In the steady state alveolar ventilation matches the carbon dioxide production in tissues according to:

PaCO₂ α CO₂ production (VCO₂)/Alveolar ventilation (V_A).

Hence, if there is a drop in alveolar ventilation, $PaCO_2$ will rise.

The sigmoid shape of the oxygen dissociation curve means that within the flat section of the curve a significant drop in PaO_2 will not cause a similar fall in oxygen saturation, making interpretation of blood gases as a whole more important that just focussing on one parameter. The respiratory efficiency of lungs can be assessed using the alveolar gas equation and the alveolar arterial (A-a) oxygen gradient. The alveolar oxygen tension (PAO_2) is dependent on various factors: atmospheric pressure (P_B), fractional inspired oxygen concentration (FiO_2), saturated vapour pressure, and respiratory rate.

The alveolar gas equation is as follows:

$$PA\ O_2 = FiO_2 \times (P_B - PH_2O) - PaCO_2/RQ.$$

RQ is the respiratory quotient, which is the balance between oxygen consumption (VO_2) and carbon dioxide production (VCO_2). At rest the ratio (R) of VCO_2 to VO_2 is approximately 0.8. At sea level, $P_B = 101$ kPa, at 37 °C and the partial pressure of water vapour $P_{H2O} = 6.2$ kPa breathing air, Fi $O_2 = 0.21$.

Hence the equation becomes

$$PA\ O_2 = 20 - PaCO_2/0.8.$$

The PaO_2 (arterial) is measured from the arterial blood gas tensions allowing calculation of the alveolar arterial (A-a) oxygen gradient (A-a gradient = $PAO_2 - PaO_2$). The normal A-a gradient for a 40-year-old non-smoking male is between 0.6 and 1.3 kPa. A gradient of more than 2.6 kPa indicates an abnormality of the lung as the cause

of hypoxaemia: this may be due to structural damage or alternatively transient and reversible abnormalities such as alveolar collapse leading to shunting.

Hypoxaemic Respiratory Failure

Type I or hypoxaemic respiratory failure happens due to V/Q mismatch and/or shunt, which leads to a widening A-a gradient. There is a mixture of low and high V/Q units depending on the disease process. The low units' contribution to hypoxaemia could be secondary to a decrease in ventilation due to airway or interstitial disease. It could also be due to excessive perfusion in normally ventilated areas due to diverted blood from areas with, for instance, a pulmonary embolus. The high V/Q units imply wasted ventilation but do not usually contribute to hypoxaemia, unless severe. Increasing FiO_2 to 100% will eliminate all low V/Q units, thus improving hypoxaemia. Failure to improve hypoxaemia by increasing inspired oxygen implies the presence of a shunt: deoxygenated blood bypasses the ventilated alveoli, leading to a reduction in arterial blood oxygen content. Such shunts can occur with pneumonia, collapse, or pulmonary oedema. They may also be anatomical.

Hypercapnic Respiratory Failure

Type II or hypercapnic respiratory failure is a consequence of ventilatory failure. The concept of ventilatory pump failure should be explored in the clinical context. There might not be enough drive for the pump to work, e.g. CNS depression, overdose with opiates, etc. The pump might fail if the work load is too high, e.g. severe bronchoconstriction in acute severe asthma. It might fail if the muscles are weak, e.g. neuromuscular conditions. There might be severe restriction of ventilation secondary due to a stiff chest wall or a fibrothorax. If hypoxaemia is due to hypoventilation, the A-a gradient stays normal. (NB there may be hypoxia and a widened A-a gradient because of alveolar collapse due to neuromuscular weakness or obesity even though the lungs are structurally normal). In COPD there is a rise in the dead space/tidal volume ratio of each breath, due to a rapid shallow breathing contributing to wasted ventilation and thereby to hypercapnia.

This breathing pattern results from adaptive physiological responses to reduce the risk of respiratory muscle fatigue and minimise breathlessness.

Both Type I and Type II respiratory failure can present acutely or chronically. Examples of conditions causing acute Type I failure include pulmonary oedema (either cardiogenic or non-cardiogenic as in ARDS), pneumonia, or acute asthma. Pulmonary fibrosis can present with acute Type I respiratory failure on a background of chronic Type I respiratory failure decompensated by acute pathology such as infection, or because of disease progression. Similarly, patients with neuromuscular conditions, kyphoscoliosis, or COPD can live with compensated Type II respiratory failure for long periods with decompensation occurring due to an acute event.

Non-invasive Ventilation (NIV) in Various Settings

NIV in Acute Type II Respiratory Failure (Fig. 9.1) [1]

COPD
The role of NIV is well established in acute exacerbations of COPD. A number of studies have shown reduction of mortality and intubation rate with NIV in acute decompensated acidotic Type II respiratory failure (pH < 7.35 and $PaCO_2 > 6$ kPa) following initial medical therapy.

Studies performed in the ICU showed a significant reduction in the need for endotracheal intubation, in-hospital mortality, length of stay, and complications with NIV. However, the YONIV study, a multicentre study in the UK, showed similar impact with early NIV use in mild and moderate acidotic patients on general respiratory wards [2]. Compared to standard treatment, treatment failure was less (15% versus 27%) as was in-hospital mortality (10% versus 20%). NIV led to a more rapid improvement in pH and greater fall in respiratory rate. A Cochrane review reported that mortality rates can be almost halved compared to standard treatment, with a number needed to treat (NNT) to save one life being 10 [3].

Immediate or standard medical treatment usually includes the following within the first hour:

controlled oxygen with a target saturation of 88–92%, nebulised Salbutamol and Ipratropium, prednisolone and antibiotic (if indicated). If the patient remains acidotic (pH < 7.35 ≥ 7.26, $PaCO_2 > 6$ kPa) at this point, NIV should be offered. There are very few absolute contraindications. These are mostly due to practical considerations of applying the mask, i.e. actively vomiting, facial deformity or trauma, uncontrolled agitation, etc. In patients who are comatose due to CO_2 narcosis, NIV can still be applied with success. There are, however, other situations requiring enhanced monitoring and special care, e.g. pneumothorax, haemodynamic instability, etc. [1].

A study looking at a group with more severe respiratory failure (mean pH 7.2) compared the use of NIV with conventional ventilation after failure of medical treatment. Even though the NIV group had similar length of ICU stay, ventilated days, overall complications, ICU mortality, and hospital mortality, 52% needed intubation, much higher than other studies with less severe acidosis. Hence if patients with pH < 7.26 are treated with NIV it should be in an environment where intubation can be performed without delay [1].

At the time of NIV initiation, pressures should be set at low levels (IPAP/EPAP of 15/5 cm H_2O) to allow patients to get acclimatised, but should be up-titrated by 2–5 cm H_2O every 10 min until a therapeutic response is achieved or the limit of tolerance is reached. In patients with more severe acidosis, a higher starting IPAP should be used. Generally, a full face mask should be used in the acute setting, as many patients mouth breath when very breathless. Oxygen should be added if necessary, aiming for saturations of 88–92% (Fig. 9.1).

Once a patient has been initiated on NIV it is important to continue close monitoring of both physiological and blood gas parameters. A drop in respiratory rate, heart rate, pCO_2, and improving pH indicate a good response to NIV. Patients should be monitored for level of alertness, patient ventilator synchrony, use of accessory muscles, and chest wall movements. The patient's comfort level should be monitored along with mask fit, leakage, and the skin in contact with mask. ABGs should be performed at 1, 4, and 12 h of initiation

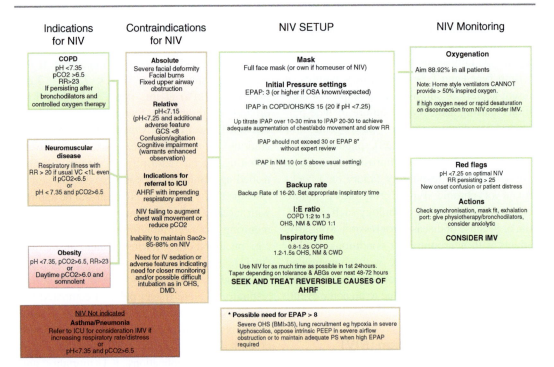

Fig. 9.1 NIV in acute Type II respiratory failure. Reprinted with permission; Copyright © 2017 BMJ Publishing Group Ltd. and British Thoracic Society. All rights reserved

of NIV, and thereafter guided by response until the acidosis is corrected. Patients who respond to NIV during the first few hours should have as much NIV as possible during the first 24 h. If improvement in both physiological and blood gas parameters continues, the amount of NIV usage should be gradually reduced over the next 48 h, starting with more breaks during daytime. NIV does not usually need to be continued beyond 72 h, unless clinically indicated.

Reasons for lack of improvement should be investigated. Possible reversible causes include inadequate pressure setting, leakage, asynchrony, inability to tolerate the mask, agitation, etc. Some of these factors can be addressed but, if in spite of that there is no improvement, NIV is deemed to have failed. It is important to differentiate between failure of "non-invasive" and of "ventilation" (Fig. 9.2). The former occurs primarily because of interface issues and is usually early: replacing one failing interface with a more invasive one (e.g. an endotracheal tube), and buying more time for medical therapies to work may lead to a successful outcome. By contrast, failure

of "ventilation," despite an adequate non-invasive interface, tends to occur later, after medical therapies have had a good chance of working. Furthermore, replacing one functioning interface with another is unlikely to lead to significant benefit. As a result, late failure is generally associated with a poor prognosis. A number of technical factors may lead to failure and these should be looked for and corrected if present (Fig. 9.3).

Sedation with short-acting agents may be considered in a controlled environment for agitated patients and may improve NIV tolerability. A clear plan for a situation of NIV failure should be made at the very outset, which should include the following potential scenarios: (1) intubation would be indicated; (2) intubation not indicated and NIV would be the ceiling of care; or (3) palliation.

NIV may help palliate breathlessness in the patient with severe advanced COPD who presents with an acute exacerbation. Unlike patients with malignancy, it is difficult to predict the timing of death in COPD. NIV gives the option of providing life-sustaining therapy while palliating

Fig. 9.2 Differentiating between failure of "non-invasive" and of "ventilation"

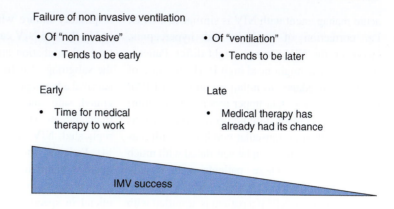

Failure of non invasive ventilation

- Of "non invasive"
  - Tends to be early

- Of "ventilation"
  - Tends to be later

Early

- Time for medical therapy to work

Late

- Medical therapy has already had its chance

IMV success

Failure because of the application of NIV – "poor tolerance"

Fig. 9.3 Trouble-shooting technical factors that may lead to failure of NIV. Reprinted with permission; Copyright © 2017 BMJ Publishing Group Ltd. and British Thoracic Society. All rights reserved

Problem	Cause(s)	Solution (s)
Ventilator cycling independently of patient effort	Inspiratory trigger sensitivity is too high	Adjust trigger Reduce mask leak
	Excessive mask leak	Change interface
Ventilator not triggering despite visible patient effort	Excessive mask leak	Reduce mask leak
	Inspiratory trigger sensivity too low	Adjust trigger For NM patients consider switch to PCV
Inadequate chest expansion despite apparent triggering	Inadequate Tidal volume	Increase IPAP. In NM or chest wall disease consider longer Ti
Chest/abdominal paradox	Upper airway obstruction	Avoid neck flexion Increase EPAP
Premature expiratory effort by patient	Excessive Ti or IPAP	Adjust as necessary

EPAP, expiratory positive airway pressure; IPAP, inspiratory positive airway pressure;NIV, non-invasive ventilation; NM, neuromuscular; PCV, pressure-controlled ventilation.

breathlessness, and allowing the patient to retain control over what is done for them. Withdrawal of treatment is also much easier than if the patient has been intubated and ventilated.

Other Conditions

There are other conditions in which patients can present with acute type II respiratory failure. Neuromuscular conditions should be considered in unexplained type II respiratory failure. Investigations for possible diaphragmatic weakness should include lying and sitting FVC, mouth pressures, a sleep study, and early morning blood gas. In motor neurone disease (MND) this may be the first presentation before a formal diagnosis has been made, and carries a high mortality irrespective of whether invasive ventilation or NIV is used.

Obesity hypoventilation syndrome (OHS) and other extrapulmonary restrictive conditions such as early onset kyphoscoliosis can present with acute type II respiratory failure, although symptoms suggesting nocturnal hypoventilation have usually been present for some time. The aim of acute management with NIV is similar to COPD, i.e. correction of acidosis and hypercapnia. However, the NIV settings might differ. Patients who are obese might need high IPAP (because of the high impedance to inflation) and high EPAP (because of coexistent upper airway obstruction) to achieve acceptable minute ventilation, whereas patients with neuromuscular conditions with normal underlying lungs can be ventilated with much lower pressures. These patients will usually require domiciliary ventilation, and it is reasonable to start acute NIV if a patient is admitted with an acute respiratory illness and hypercapnia but without acidosis. In patients with neuromuscular disease, NIV can be started if they have a markedly reduced vital capacity and are tachypnoeic. These patients may initially be normocapnic, but over time the increased respiratory rate cannot be sustained, they will fatigue and the CO_2 will rise.

NIV in Acute Type I Respiratory Failure

Acute Type I respiratory failure is a heterogeneous group, and the outcomes of NIV will depend on the aetiology. Positive pressure ventilator support, whether with CPAP or bilevel ventilation, can lead to a false sense of security. In contrast to hypercapnia, which develops over minutes to hours, hypoxia can develop over seconds to a minute or two. While the mask is in place, oxygen saturations are maintained, but if it is removed even for a short period, sudden hypoxaemia may result, and this may explain the trend towards an increase in cardiorespiratory arrests in patients with hypoxaemic respiratory failure treated with CPAP. It is recommended that any intervention with NIV in these patients should be in ICU, where patients can be very closely monitored and intubation can be performed without delay.

Pneumonia
The role of NIV in respiratory failure due to pneumonia remains controversial. A multicentre study in patients with severe pneumonia with acute

respiratory failure who were haemodynamically stable showed NIV can reduce the need for endotracheal intubation and duration of ICU stay. In the subgroup of patients with COPD there was a survival advantage at 2 months. NIV was well tolerated, safe, and did not compromise secretion management. This study has not been universally replicated; NIV failure is common in pneumonia [4]. Patients who fail with NIV and are subsequently ventilated have poorer outcomes and more complications. However, NIV might be beneficial in specific situations. A study looking at using NIV to avoid endotracheal intubation in recipients of solid organ transplantation with acute hypoxaemic respiratory failure showed NIV was associated with a significant reduction in intubation rate (20% versus 70%), fatal complications (20% versus 50%), length of ICU stay (5.5 versus 9 days), and ICU mortality (20% versus 50%), but no difference in hospital mortality [5]. "Sequential" NIV (1 h NIV every 3 h) was initiated at a much earlier stage than ventilatory support would usually be considered, and this is a key factor. NIV introduced at the point when intubation is being considered is unlikely to be successful.

Surgical Patients
Postoperative hypoxaemia following abdominal or thoracic surgery is common. Anaesthesia and postoperative pain cause hypoxemia, reduction in tidal volume, atelectasis, and diaphragm dysfunction. The use of NIV peri-operatively can reduce pulmonary dysfunction after thoracic surgery. Oxygenation and lung volumes are improved in patients receiving positive pressure; CPAP and NIV following abdominal surgery improve oxygenation, lung volumes, and atelectasis. In patients after bariatric surgery, NIV applied during the first 24 h improves FVC. Using CPAP postoperatively for hypoxaemia can also reduce intubation rate, pneumonia, and sepsis.

Acute Respiratory Distress Syndrome (ARDS) and Acute Lung Injury (ALI)
There have been few studies looking at impact of NIV in acute lung injury (ALI) and ARDS,

and as they are mostly small and the causes heterogeneous, the impact of NIV is difficult to interpret. The failure rate is high in advanced ARDS with haemodynamic instability, low admission pH, low PaO_2/FiO_2, and sepsis. Hence, the use of NIV as an alternative to invasive ventilation in severely hypoxemic patients with ARDS (i.e., $PaO_2(mmHg)/FIO_2 < 200$) is not generally advisable and should be limited to haemodynamically stable patients who can be closely monitored in an ICU.

High-flow nasal oxygen (HFNO) treatment is a new development that is an alternative to intubation and non-invasive ventilation in patients with type 1 respiratory failure due to ARDS, ALI, or in the postoperative setting. The system consists of a generator that can provide gas flow rates up to 60 L/min, active humidification that fully saturates the gas mixture, and an air/oxygen blender that can vary FiO_2 independent of gas flow. The gas flow is delivered through heated tubing to large-bore nasal prongs. Compared to standard oxygen delivery systems, oxygenation is enhanced because the high flow rate is closer to the patient's inspiratory flow rate (so reducing air entrainment), flushes out anatomical dead space, and provides a small amount of positive end-expiratory pressure (PEEP) to overcome auto-PEEP and reduce the work of breathing. Limited trial data suggest HFNO may be as effective as NIV in terms of avoiding intubation and improving oxygenation in the above settings, and is better tolerated.

Pulmonary Fibrosis

The outcome of patients with idiopathic pulmonary fibrosis (IPF) who develop acute respiratory failure is extremely poor. Invasive ventilation does not impact mortality, which remains very high. The studies are too small to draw any definite conclusions, but given that intubation has an almost 100% mortality, NIV might be considered in highly selected patients with IPF exacerbations; usually a purely palliative approach is more appropriate.

Summary of the Use of NIV in Patients with Respiratory Failure Due to Parenchymal Lung Disease

- Type 1 respiratory failure more usual
- If hypercapnic, disease is either very advanced (e.g. IPF) or severe (e.g. pneumonia), and palliation or intubation more appropriate
- Improvement in hypoxaemia because of non-invasive positive pressure may provide a false sense of security: when mask removed, sudden severe hypoxia may ensue
- NIV is generally only appropriate in a highly monitored environment with access to intubation within a very short time period, e.g. an ICU

Cardiogenic Pulmonary Oedema

The rationale for the use of NIV in acute cardiogenic pulmonary oedema (CPO) is largely based upon an understanding of the physiology of the effects of NIV in chronic heart failure. In addition to having beneficial effects upon ventilation, NIV has a beneficial effect upon cardiac function (see Table 9.1 below, "Physiological Effects of Ventilatory Support in Heart Failure").

Early studies of NIV showed a reduction in endotracheal intubation rate and in-hospital mortality [6]. No consistent advantage has been shown to bilevel ventilation over that achieved with CPAP, although there was a suggestion that a hypercapnic sub-group might benefit from bilevel ventilation, whereas another trial suggested an increased risk of myocardial infarction.

Two subsequent large trials (not included in the original meta-analyses), have given different results [7, 8]. Moritz et al. [7] recruited 120 patients from three French emergency departments. There was no standard therapy arm, but CPAP and NIV were compared. The primary endpoint was a combination of death, myocardial infarction, or intubation in the first 24 h. There was no difference between interventions on any outcome. Respiratory distress

Table 9.1 Physiological effects of ventilatory support in heart failure

Pulmonary effects
• Increase lung volume
• Bronchodilator
• Improved ventilation perfusion ratios
• Offloading of the respiratory muscles
• Reduce dead space
Cardiac effects
• Reduced afterload
• Reduced transmural pressure
• Reduced cardiac chamber size
• Reduce systemic blood pressure
• Reduce preload
Autonomic effects
• Attenuates sympathetic activity
• Improve parasympathetic activity

and physiology improved in both arms. Only 3% of patients required intubation, and only one person died within the first 24 h. The 3CPO trial recruited 1069 patients from 26 UK emergency departments [8]. This number is bigger than the sum of patients in all the trials entered into the meta-analyses. There was no difference in the primary outcome, 7-day mortality, between ventilation (NIV + CPAP) (9.5%) and standard therapy (9.8%). The combined endpoint of 7-day death or intubation was similar irrespective of ventilation modality. NIV was associated with a much greater reduction in the sensation of breathlessness and more rapid improvement in blood gas parameters and heart rate. There were no treatment-related adverse events and, in particular, no increase in myocardial infarction. NIV unquestionably leads to a more rapid physiological improvement and reduced dyspnoea, but the effects upon mortality are less clear. Approximately 90% of patients received nitrates, and it is possible that the cardiovascular effects of NIV in acute CPO were masked by nitrate treatment, working by the same mechanism.

In summary, the 3CPO trial showed that NIV was safe and the relief of dyspnoea, which was very intense, is reason enough to suggest a trial of NIV. It is important that this should not be at the expense of effective nitrate therapy. It is pertinent to note that the commonest reason for switching from the allocated treatment was clinical worsening in the control arm, and discomfort with the mask in the NIV arm. The relief of dyspnoea may therefore be at the expense of discomfort associated with the mask. Subsequent

meta-analyses, which included the data from the 3CPO trial, continue to show an advantage from positive airways pressure, and CPAP is recommended for patients with respiratory failure due to CPO [9].

NIV in Chronic Stable Type II Respiratory Failure

Slowly Progressive Neuromuscular Disease and Chest Wall Disorders

Despite a lack of randomised trials, NIV is established in the management of chronic respiratory failure due to neuromuscular disease and chest wall deformity. Two large case series and a number of smaller studies showed improvement in daytime arterial blood gases, quality of life, and survival, compared to that which would be expected without treatment.

Clinical Features

Symptoms of chronic hypoventilation (see Table 9.2 below, "Symptoms of Nocturnal Hypoventilation") are non-specific and may not immediately suggest the possibility of a respiratory disorder. They usually develop very insidiously and are often ignored by the patient or attributed to their "condition." It is important, therefore, that patients at risk are identified and alerted to key symptoms. Simple physiological monitoring indicates those at risk for nocturnal hypoventilation. Any intercurrent event, typically a chest infection, can precipitate respiratory failure at an earlier stage than would usually be the case, and this may resolve once the precipitating cause has been treated. Patients with motor neurone disease (MND) often have problems related to bulbar involvement, so swallowing difficulties, aspiration, and hypersalivation may be particularly problematic.

More Rapidly Progressive Neuromuscular Disease (e.g. Duchenne Muscular Dystrophy, Motor Neurone Disease)

NIV has been shown to prolong life and improve quality of life in motor neurone disease [10]. Patients with better bulbar function showed improvement in several measures of quality of

Table 9.2 Symptoms of nocturnal hypoventilation

- Morning headaches
- Disturbed sleep
- Daytime hypersomnolence
- Fatigue/lethargy
- Irritability
- Breathlessness/"bronchitis"
- Ankle oedema

life, and had a median survival benefit of 205 days with maintained quality of life for most of this period. NIV improved some quality of life indices in those with poor bulbar function, but conferred no survival benefit. Surprisingly, in patients with significantly impaired bulbar function, the survival in both the NIV and control arms was much better than in the group with normal or well-preserved bulbar function. This was probably because these patients could not perform the volitional tests properly, resulting in overestimated respiratory muscle impairment and randomisation at an earlier stage of their disease. Bulbar dysfunction should not preclude a trial of NIV, but patients may find treatment harder to tolerate.

Uncontrolled studies have shown excellent survival figures in Duchenne Muscular Dystrophy, with some groups reporting a 73% 5-year survival in patients with severe hypercapnic ventilatory failure.

In patients with rapidly progressive disease, there are a number of possible problems related to extending life by mechanical ventilation. These include life of marginal quality, loss of dignity, inability to communicate, disruption to the lives of other family members, and difficulty in stopping high-technology life-sustaining care once it has been started. Generally, patients and carers report significant symptomatic improvement and better quality of life.

Investigations

Spirometry, mouth and sniff nasopharyngeal pressures, and oximetry should be performed routinely in all patients, and are a useful way of monitoring progression. Nocturnal hypoventilation should be considered in patients with an FVC less than 50% predicted, and such patients

should have assessment of arterial blood gas tensions. Even if the patient is not hypercapnic by day, an elevated bicarbonate and base excess is suggestive of nocturnal hypoventilation. This should be complemented by overnight monitoring with pulse oximetry and ideally, transcutaneous CO_2. Full polysomnography is not required, but a respiratory variable sleep study may be helpful to exclude confounding upper airway obstruction. The assessment of respiratory muscle strength is difficult in MND patients with bulbar involvement because they are usually unable to cooperate with volitional tests. Assessment will need to be based upon symptoms, clinical evidence of reduced chest expansion, supplemented by arterial blood gas analysis and overnight monitoring [11].

Starting NIV

Daytime respiratory failure develops gradually. Hypoventilation initially occurs exclusively during REM sleep, then spills over into non-REM sleep, and then daytime respiratory failure ensues (Fig. 9.4). Seventy percent of patients with a normal daytime $PaCO_2$ but evidence of nocturnal hypoventilation require NIV within 1 year, and 90% within 2 years. NIV is best introduced at this time, and a traffic light analogy may be helpful in explaining this to patients. Red (hypercapnia) mandates institution of NIV. Amber (nocturnal hypoventilation but normal $PaCO_2$) indicates that the need for NIV is approaching, but is not yet mandatory. Green means that NIV is not required

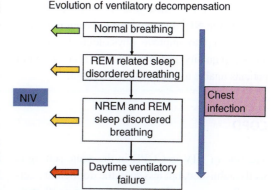

Fig. 9.4 Evolution of ventilatory failure

at the present time, but patients should be monitored and advised to report warning symptoms (see Symptoms of Nocturnal Hypoventilation in Table 9.2 above). The disadvantage of starting NIV before the patient has significant symptoms is that they have no symptomatic benefit, yet still experience all the inconvenience of NIV. The major advantage of earlier introduction of NIV is that there is more opportunity to acclimatise themselves to treatment. Some patients, however, are more symptomatic than they realise and feel better once NIV has been started. Orthopnoea responds particularly well to treatment.

The same principles apply in patients with MND, but once they enter the "red" zone they are in a very precarious situation, and NIV should be instituted without delay. If the patient is hypercapnic, NIV should be started within 24–48 h.

Whereas the role of NIV is firmly established, further data are still needed about the timing of initiation of NIV and the appropriate therapeutic goals (see below). There are no firm guidelines, but NIV should be considered when symptoms of hypoventilation develop with a FVC < 1 L or abnormal overnight oximetry or daytime hypercapnia with or without hypoxia. Patients admitted as an emergency with an episode of acute respiratory failure should also be considered for long-term domiciliary ventilation.

Patients receiving domiciliary ventilation often report an improved sense of well-being and better quality sleep even if there are only small changes in arterial blood gas tensions. Severe sleep disruption occurs in patients with both COPD and neuromuscular/chest wall deformity, and is improved during NIV. NIV withdrawal studies confirm that sleep fragmentation recurs quickly even if daytime gases remain stable.

However, NIV does not have to be administered during sleep to improve physiological variables and sleep quality, and daytime NIV is an option in patients unable to sleep with a ventilator.

COPD

The role of NIV in COPD in the acute setting is well established, but less so in the domiciliary setting. Previous smaller studies showed conflicting results on survival and quality of life (QoL). One study showed that domiciliary NIV might improve survival, but at the cost of QoL [12]. A Cochrane review in patients with COPD with stable hypercapnia failed to show a consistent improvement in gas exchange, 6-min walking distance, health-related quality of life, lung function, respiratory muscle strength, and sleep efficiency [13]. It has been argued that some of the studies failed to address the fundamental physiological abnormality (hypercapnia), and inadequate pressure settings failed to correct the alveolar hypoventilation. Home NIV in highly selected patients with hypercapnic COPD with a history of recurrent admissions may reduce hospital admissions and total bed days. Ventilation strategies targeting a reduction of $PaCO_2$ have shown positive results. High-intensity ventilation (higher pressures and back-up rate) can be helpful to some stable COPD patients and reduces daytime $PaCO_2$ [14] without interfering with sleep quality. Using more aggressive ventilation strategies in trial settings have produced conflicting results, with some studies showing reduced mortality and improved QoL [15], whereas others failed to show any improvement in mortality or hospital admission in spite of a reduction in $PaCO_2$ [16]. The difference is probably explained by patient selection and the timing of when persistent hypercapnia was identified: the negative study recruited mildly hypercapnic patients 48 h after discontinuing acute NIV, whereas the positive study recruited patients with more severe hypercapnia at least 4 weeks after stopping NIV. Following treatment of an acute exacerbation, hypercapnia gradually improves, so persistent hypercapnia may identify a particularly subset of stable hypoventilating COPD patients who have more to gain from regular nocturnal NIV. Further support for this comes from HOT-HMV, [17] which selected recently exacerbated COPD patients with persistent hypercapnia at least 2 weeks after acidosis had resolved, and showed a delay in hospital readmission, but no improvement in 12-month mortality.

On current evidence, NIV should not be initiated immediately following an acute exacerbation of COPD. Patients should be reassessed for hypercapnia when stable 2–6 weeks following the event. If they remain hypercapnic with a

$PaCO_2 > 7$ kPa, then NIV should be considered. The titration of NIV should aim to control nocturnal hypoventilation and/or reduce spontaneously breathing $PaCO_2$ by 20% from baseline. NIV should be considered in stable patients, e.g. attending for long-term oxygen assessment, if $PaCO_2 > 7$ kPa. Motivation is key: The patient who is poorly tolerant of NIV during an acute episode or who does not comply with aspects of their therapy (e.g. oxygen therapy) is unlikely to cope with NIV.

Obesity

There are no controlled trials assessing mortality in patients with respiratory failure due to obesity. Improvement in physiological variables and a reduction in days in hospital have been seen in uncontrolled studies. There is usually a choice to be made between bilevel NIV or CPAP [18]. Selection of patients can be based on their initial response to a night on CPAP. If obstructive events are prevented and adequate oxygenation achieved, then CPAP would be reasonable for long-term treatment. It seems intuitively logical that bilevel NIV may be preferable in patients with a predominance of hypoventilation over obstructive events. Patients with a large number of apnoeas are more likely to respond to CPAP than those with few apnoeas in whom CO_2 retention is due to other mechanisms. CPAP be started at 4 cm H_2O and gradually increased until apnoeas disappear and flow limitation resolves. Patients unresponsive to CPAP are likely to be more obese, with a higher $PaCO_2$ and lower nocturnal oxygen saturation, than responsive patients. If there is evidence of persisting hypoventilation based upon oximetry, or preferably transcutaneous CO_2, pressure support can be added to optimise nocturnal hypoventilation. Modern "smart" ventilators can do this automatically, but to date there are no trials which have shown that they are superior to expert manual titration.

Conclusion

The domiciliary use of NIV in patients with chest wall deformity and slowly progressive neuromuscular disease is well established, but further data are needed about the optimal timing of its introduction. In patients with more rapidly progressive neuromuscular disease, timing is less of an issue because the interval between when NIV might be introduced and when it has to be is usually relatively short; the major concern relates to the appropriateness of intervention in an individual patient. Clarity is emerging about the indications of long-term domiciliary NIV in COPD and obesity. The exact aim of NIV is not yet clearly defined, but on the basis of current knowledge, should be targeted to control nocturnal hypoventilation, reduce respiratory muscle activity, and improve sleep quality. Fortunately, these goals are not mutually exclusive.

Indications for Domiciliary NIV

Slowly progressive neuromuscular disease and chest wall deformity (traffic light classification)

- Reduced vital capacity and respiratory muscle strength
- Evidence of nocturnal hypoventilation
- Daytime hypercapnia
- Symptoms of nocturnal hypoventilation

Rapidly progressive neuromuscular disease (MND)

- As above but with a lower threshold
- Orthopnoea a particularly important symptom

COPD

- Not during hospitalisation following an AECOPD
- $PaCO_2 > 7$ kPA when stable (at least 2 weeks after acute NIV)
- Obesity
- Coexistent obstructive sleep apnoea

Obesity hypoventilation

- CPAP should usually be tried first unless high baseline $PaCO_2$
- "Pure" REM related hypoventilation

References

1. Davidson AC, Banham S, Elliott M, Kennedy D, Gelder C, Glossop A, et al. BTS/ICS guideline for the ventilatory management of acute hypercapnic respiratory failure in adults. Thorax. 2016;71(Suppl 2):ii1–35.

2. Plant PK, Owen JL, Elliott MW. Early use of non-invasive ventilation for acute exacerbations of chronic obstructive pulmonary disease on general respiratory wards: a multicentre randomised controlled trial. Lancet. 2000;355:1931–5.

3. Ram FS, Picot J, Lightowler J, Wedzicha JA. Non-invasive positive pressure ventilation for treatment of respiratory failure due to exacerbations of chronic obstructive pulmonary disease. Cochrane Database Syst Rev. 2004;3:CD004104.

4. Antonelli M, Conti G, Moro ML, Esquinas A, Gonzalez-Diaz G, Confalonieri M, et al. Predictors of failure of noninvasive positive pressure ventilation in patients with acute hypoxemic respiratory failure: a multi-center study. Intensive Care Med. 2001;27(11):1718–28.

5. Antonelli M, Conti G, Bufi M, Costa MG, Lappa A, Gasparetto A, et al. Noninvasive ventilation for treatment of acute respiratory failure in patients undergoing solid organ transplantation: a randomized trial. JAMA. 2000;283:235–41.

6. Masip J, Roque M, Sanchez B, Fernandez R, Subirana M, Exposito JA. Noninvasive ventilation in acute cardiogenic pulmonary edema: systematic review and meta-analysis. JAMA. 2005;294(24):3124–30.

7. Moritz F, Brousse B, Gellee B, Chajara A, L'Her E, Hellot MF, et al. Continuous positive airway pressure versus bilevel noninvasive ventilation in acute cardiogenic pulmonary edema: a randomized multicenter trial. Ann Emerg Med. 2007;50(6):666–75.

8. Gray A, Goodacre S, Newby DE, Masson M, Sampson F, Nicholl J, et al. Noninvasive ventilation in acute cardiogenic pulmonary edema. N Engl J Med. 2008;359(2):142–51.

9. Vital FM, Ladeira MT, Atallah AN. Non-invasive positive pressure ventilation (CPAP or bilevel NPPV) for cardiogenic pulmonary oedema. Cochrane Database Syst Rev. 2013;5:CD005351.

10. Bourke SC, Tomlinson M, Williams TL, Bullock RE, Shaw PJ, Gibson GJ. Effects of non-invasive ventilation on survival and quality of life in patients with amyotrophic lateral sclerosis: a randomised controlled trial. Lancet Neurol. 2006;5(2):140–7.

11. Motor neurone disease: the use of non-invasive ventilation in the management of motor neurone disease. NICE clinical guideline 105. London: National Institute for Health and Clinical Excellence; 2010. Version: July 2010 PMHID: PMH0033019.

12. McEvoy RD, Pierce RJ, Hillman D, Esterman A, Ellis EE, Catcheside PG, et al. Nocturnal non-invasive nasal ventilation in stable hypercapnic COPD: a randomised controlled trial. Thorax. 2009;64(7):561–6.

13. Struik FM, Lacasse Y, Goldstein R, Kerstjens HM, Wijkstra PJ. Nocturnal non-invasive positive pressure ventilation for stable chronic obstructive pulmonary disease. Cochrane Database Syst Rev. 2013;6:CD002878.

14. Dreher M, Storre JH, Schmoor C, Windisch W. High-intensity versus low-intensity non-invasive ventilation in patients with stable hypercapnic COPD: a randomised crossover trial. Thorax. 2010;65(4):303–8.

15. Kohnlein T, Windisch W, Kohler D, Drabik A, Geiseler J, Hartl S, et al. Non-invasive positive pressure ventilation for the treatment of severe stable chronic obstructive pulmonary disease: a prospective, multicentre, randomised, controlled clinical trial. Lancet Respir Med. 2014;2(9):698–705.

16. Struik FM, Sprooten RT, Kerstjens HA, Bladder G, Zijnen M, Asin J, et al. Nocturnal non-invasive ventilation in COPD patients with prolonged hypercapnia after ventilatory support for acute respiratory failure: a randomised, controlled, parallel-group study. Thorax. 2014;69(9):826–34.

17. Murphy PB, Rehal S, Arbane G, Bourke S, Calverley PMA, Crook AM, et al. Effect of home noninvasive ventilation with oxygen therapy vs oxygen therapy alone on hospital readmission or death after an acute COPD exacerbation: a randomized clinical trial. JAMA. 2017;317(21):2177–86. https://doi.org/10.1001/jama.2017.4451.

18. Howard ME, Piper AJ, Stevens B, Holland AE, Yee BJ, Dabscheck E, et al. A randomised controlled trial of CPAP versus non-invasive ventilation for initial treatment of obesity hypoventilation syndrome. Thorax. 2016;72:437–44. https://doi.org/10.1136/thoraxjnl-2016-208559.

Pneumonia

10

10

Thomas P. Hellyer, Anthony J. Rostron,
and A. John Simpson

Background

Pneumonia is common, affecting up to 1% of adults in the UK each year. Although most patients with pneumonia make a complete recovery with antibiotics and supportive care, pneumonia remains a common cause of death. Mortality among adults admitted to hospital with pneumonia is approximately 10%, with around half of deaths occurring in patients aged 85 years or older. Pneumonia has been classified according to the location and circumstances in which it develops, distinguishing community-acquired pneumonia (CAP), hospital-acquired pneumonia (HAP), aspiration pneumonia, and pneumonia in the immunocompromised host. Within the category of HAP, most is known about ventilator-associated pneumonia (VAP), which is pneumonia arising de novo in intubated and mechanically ventilated patients. This pragmatic classification indicates the most likely range of causative pathogens, thus guiding empirical antibiotic therapy.

While this classification system has been helpful in guiding treatment, some confusing aspects of terminology have arisen, some of which are worth considering. In particular, strictly speaking, aspiration *pneumonitis* is a chemical injury induced by non-infective liquid entering the lung (for example gastric acid in a patient whose conscious level has deteriorated rapidly, perhaps due to alcohol intoxication, and who cannot protect his/her airway and is vomiting). This scenario is usually witnessed and the aspiration is of moderate volume. Aspiration *pneumonia* entails repeated, clinically silent and usually unwitnessed entry of small volumes of infected material into the lung, usually from the oropharynx, in patients with chronically impaired swallow and/or consciousness (for example in patients with neurological conditions such as stroke, motor neurone disease, or multiple sclerosis). The distinction is important because, at least initially, aspiration pneumonitis does not require antibiotic treatment. Unfortunately, the two terms are often used interchangeably, and the situation is further confused in that a true bacterial pneumonia can complicate aspiration pneumonitis a few days after the initial aspiration. Similarly, the reader may encounter terms such as "healthcare-associated pneumonia" (HCAP), which seeks to distinguish HAP from pneumonia acquired in healthcare organisations other than hospitals (e.g. nursing homes), but the range of organisms implicated are not sufficiently different for us to make the distinction here. Finally, as VAP becomes increasingly used as a marker of healthcare standards, a bewildering and confusing array of new terms (e.g. ventilator-associated events, ventilator-associated conditions, infective

T. P. Hellyer (✉) · A. J. Rostron · A. J. Simpson
Institute of Cellular Medicine, Newcastle University,
Newcastle upon Tyne, UK
e-mail: t.p.hellyer@ncl.ac.uk

© Springer International Publishing AG, part of Springer Nature 2018
S. Hart, M. Greenstone (eds.), *Foundations of Respiratory Medicine*,
https://doi.org/10.1007/978-3-319-94127-1_10

ventilator-associated conditions) has emerged. The key point here is that these are terms employed to aid epidemiological surveillance, and not terms that should be used to make diagnoses in real time. They will therefore not appear again in this chapter.

In recent years excellent, comprehensive guidelines have been published for the management of community-acquired pneumonia (CAP) in adults [1, 2]. The key recommendations from these guidelines are readily accessible, and firmly embedded in the knowledge base of the medical community.

The chapter will focus on adult pneumonia. Very good guidelines on childhood pneumonia can be found elsewhere [3]. Parapneumonic effusion and empyema are important complications of pneumonia, and are considered briefly in this chapter, with greater detail found in the chapter on Pleural Diseases. Before we consider pneumonia in more detail, it is also worth reflecting that John Bunyan's identification (in the seventeenth century) of tuberculosis as "the captain of all these men of death" remains pertinent today. Therefore, the most historically resilient and important global cause of pneumonia deserves a chapter all of its own.

Pathological-Clinical Correlates in Pneumonia

In the strictest pathological sense, pneumonia is defined as inflammation of the gas exchanging regions of the lung. Because infection is the commonest cause of alveolar inflammation, pneumonia is regarded here as *infective* inflammation of the alveolar regions. It is worth noting, however, that the strict definition of pneumonia leads, sometimes confusingly, to terms like usual interstitial pneumonia (UIP) and non-specific interstitial pneumonia (NSIP) in the interstitial lung disease literature (as both are characterised by inflammatory infiltrates in alveolar walls and so, in the true pathological sense, are "pneumonias").

It is generally believed that if pathogenic bacteria evade the multitude of innate immune defences in the conducting airways, alveolar macrophages (AMs) are capable of removing low-level alveolar inoculation. Very occasionally these defences are overwhelmed, and AMs signal recruitment to the alveolus of a cellular inflammatory exudate, predominantly composed of neutrophils. Neutrophils are avidly phagocytic cells, recruited to engage, ingest, and kill bacteria. Bacteria are packaged into phagolysosomes inside neutrophils, within which reactive oxygen species and high concentrations of proteolytic enzymes are generated, leading to bacterial death. It is generally believed that the cytokines generated locally and systemically to recruit neutrophils contribute to the fever, malaise, loss of appetite, weight loss, confusion, and delirium experienced by patients. In severe pneumonia, a significant contribution to lung destruction may come from toxic contents of neutrophils being spilled extracellularly and "attacking" the host, although there may be a contribution from bacterial virulence factors also.

During the battle between bacteria and neutrophils, the alveolar spaces become packed with neutrophils and exudate (consolidation), while alveolar walls are expanded by engorged capillaries. Each involved alveolus is therefore effectively contributing to "shunt," with perfusion but no ventilation. Dyspnoea, and ultimately hypoxaemia, ensues if sufficient alveoli are involved. Because adjacent bronchi are not involved, if enough alveolar tissue is consolidated the chest X-ray (CXR) or CT scan often reveals the classical "air bronchogram" (Fig. 10.1). Similarly, air flows down a bronchus unimpeded in pneumonia, but breath sounds are distorted and amplified by the consolidated alveoli, which leads to bronchial breathing on auscultation, and whispering pectoriloquy. In practice, however, pneumonia is more commonly a patchy process (Fig. 10.2, *left* panel), with foci of infected alveoli rather than one large contiguous area of consolidation. Therefore, inspiratory crackles (as inspired air opens partly consolidated alveoli) are a far more common auscultatory finding than bronchial breathing. The relatively rare presentation with lobar pneumonia still provides valuable clinical information, as it is almost always caused by *Streptococcus pneumoniae* or (far less com-

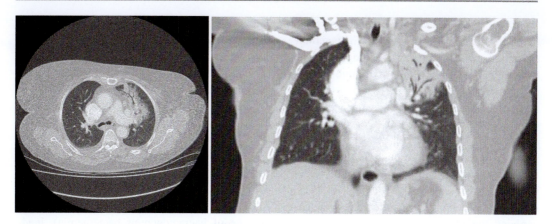

Fig. 10.1 CT scan illustrating left upper lobe pneumonia, with a transverse view in the left panel and a coronal view in the right panel. The air bronchogram is shown as an air-filled (black) line among the solid, consolidated (white) lung tissue

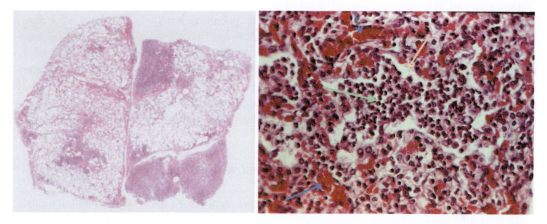

Fig. 10.2 Left-hand panel is a low-power histological section of lung, stained with haematoxylin and eosin (H&E). The dense pink areas show pneumonia, in a characteristically patchy distribution. The right-hand panel shows a histological section, stained with H&E, demonstrating pneumonia. The green arrow points to a collection of neutrophils in an alveolar space. The orange arrow points to a white area that would have been filled with protein-rich liquid exudate filling the alveolus. The blue arrows point to the ghostly outline of alveolar capillaries, in alveolar walls, significantly engorged with prominent red blood cells

monly) *Klebsiella pneumoniae*, usually in an expanded, consolidated right upper lobe.

Much of our understanding of the macroscopic pathology of pneumonia is derived from post-mortem specimens of lobar pneumonia from the pre-antibiotic era. Classical studies describe a congestive phase quickly followed by "red hepatisation" where the lobe appears macroscopically like liver on cut section, the alveolar walls being expanded by capillaries engorged with erythrocytes (many of which spill out into the alveolus itself) and neutrophils, and the alveolar spaces filling with exudate from those capillaries

(Fig. 10.2, *right* panel). Exudate fluid is rich in plasma proteins including fibrinogen. Fibrin strands formed in the alveolus may serve to limit the spread of infection, localise bacteria to areas where host defences are concentrated, and provide a scaffold for alveolar repair. However, excessive fibrinous reaction in severe pneumonia may potentially lead to fibrotic scar formation.

A striking finding in pneumonia, and particularly in lobar pneumonia, is that the process can completely resolve, with restoration of entirely normal alveolar architecture. Indeed, a feature of histological pneumonia is that alveolar walls are recognisable in the consolidation, as shown in the right hand panel of Fig. 10.2. This remarkable feat of resolution was recognised long before the widespread use of antibiotics. The process seems to be characterised by a carefully regulated process that depends on neutrophils clearing bacteria efficiently, then undergoing apoptosis (programmed cell death) without disgorging their toxic contents. Macrophages ingest erythrocytes and apoptotic neutrophils, as well as scavenging extracellular debris, and migrate to regional lymph nodes. This sequence explains the classical macroscopic phases of "white hepatisation" as capillaries become less engorged and macrophages predominate over erythrocytes and neutrophils in the still-packed alveoli.

For bacterial killing, neutrophils produce myeloperoxidase, which imparts a green colour to sputum. Patchy pneumonia rarely impinges on the pleura. Pneumonia only causes pain when the inflammation involves the pleura, and the pain of pneumonia is almost always pleuritic in nature. Pleural involvement commonly results in an effusion and, if infection penetrates from the alveolar space into the pleural space, may lead to empyema. Inflammation of the diaphragmatic pleura (especially on the right) can cause pain referred to the right iliac fossa and mimic appendicitis.

Complications of Pneumonia

The causes of death from pneumonia are usually progression to septic shock and/or progression to acute respiratory distress syndrome. Rarely, aggressive lung necrosis may complicate pneumonia, as for example when pneumonia is caused by *Staphylococcus aureus* producing the Panton-Valentine leukocidin (PVL) virulence factor. Pneumonia has been associated with cardiovascular complications, which may account for some early deaths but also, potentially, for the observation that mortality is increased in the year following apparently good recovery from pneumonia. A growing literature has characterised

features of CAP requiring admission to the intensive care unit and, perhaps not surprisingly, severity of illness on admission, bilateral pulmonary infiltrates, and ventilator support are all independently associated with increased mortality. Severe pneumonia is more common in patients with co-morbidities.

In the post-antibiotic era, initial presentation with lung abscess is uncommon. It is more common in homeless patients and in patients with alcohol dependence, perhaps through a combination of poor dental hygiene (increasing the rate of haematogenous bacteraemia), inadequate nutrition, late presentation, and relative immunosuppression.

Failure of all consolidated alveoli to re-aerate after pneumonia may leave minor atelectasis, seen as fine linear scars on CXR. Severe pneumonia leading to necrosis and/or acute respiratory distress syndrome (ARDS) is commonly accompanied by more widespread scarring, which may produce a restrictive ventilatory defect detected on lung function testing.

Pleural Effusion

In practical terms, the most common complication to consider is pleural effusion. A separate chapter on pleural diseases provides greater detail, but briefly pleural effusion is a frequent accompaniment of pneumonia. Frequency estimates vary widely, but in general around one-third of patients hospitalised with pneumonia have some evidence for associated pleural effusion. These effusions are divided into "parapneumonic" effusions (in which the pleura produces a reactive exudate in response to inflammation but the pleural space is not itself infected), and empyema (in which the pleural space is infected). Parapneumonic effusions usually resorb and resolve spontaneously with clearance of the pneumonia, and scarring is rare. However, effusions are occasionally large, and may have compressive effects on the adjacent consolidated lung, adding to breathlessness.

Empyemas

Empyemas complicate approximately 1% of pneumonias managed in hospital, and have far more serious consequences. Bacteria may be identified on Gram stain or via culture, but absence of an identifiable pathogen does not exclude empyema if the clinical and biochemical features support the diagnosis. Importantly, fibrinogen is rapidly converted to insoluble fibrin, usually leading to walled off locules of pus, such that the pleural space no longer has a single, drainable collection, but multiple small, unconnected collections (Fig. 10.3). Once empyemas become loculated, they can wall off chronic pockets of infection, which consume enormous amounts of energy, cause pain, and make chest drain insertion

futile in that one tube will only drain one single locule. In the pre-antibiotic era, empyemas were well recognised to form painful sinuses through to the skin, though this is rare now.

The characteristics described dictate management of effusions associated with pneumonia. If there is sufficient fluid to aspirate easily and safely under ultrasound guidance, a 10–20 mL sample will be sufficient to test pH, protein, lactate dehydrogenase, differential white cell count, Gram stain, and bacterial culture. Light's criteria can be used to determine exudate from transudate (the latter is not associated with pneumonia), and the gross appearance, pH, LDH, differential count, and microbiology can help distinguish empyema from parapneumonic effusion. Ultrasound can determine whether loculation has started.

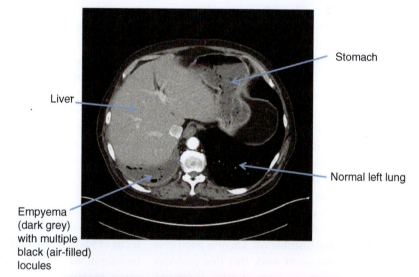

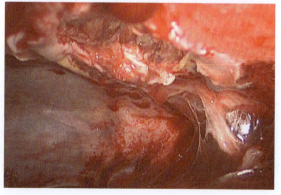

Fig. 10.3 Upper panel: Transverse CT scan showing a dense effusion in the right lower thorax. Aspiration revealed pus, and the aspirated material had low pH, low glucose, and high LDH concentrations. The multiple black holes in the dense effusion imply there are air-filled "pockets." The implication is that the empyema has become complicated by fibrinous strands walling off separate collections. The lower panel shows a thoracoscopic appearance of a subacute empyema. Image courtesy of Mr. Malcolm Will

Labels on figure: Stomach; Liver; Normal left lung; Empyema (dark grey) with multiple black (air-filled) locules

Small parapneumonic effusions usually require no drainage. Large parapneumonic effusions causing breathlessness are usually managed with an intercostal drain. Empyema that has not loculated must be drained with an intercostal tube. Prompt pleural drainage can prevent the complications of empyema. Empyemas complicated by the development of loculation may require surgical intervention in order to break down fibrinous bands, creating one collection, which can then be drained. Clearly these recommendations are in the context of the pneumonia also being managed with antibiotics and other measures, as detailed below.

Aetiology and Pathogenesis

Community-Acquired Pneumonia

CAP is estimated to have an incidence of just below 10 per 1000 of the population in Western countries, though this figure hides a skew towards increasing incidence with age. Approximately a quarter of patients require hospitalization, and the in-hospital mortality is approximately 10%. The figures described reflect the adult population in the West, and simply aim to give a sense of the magnitude of the problem. As an important aside, the seminal paper by Black et al. [4] is recommended to the reader, which describes five million deaths annually under the age of five, and charts their global distribution. There is good evidence from subsequent work that this problem persists, and that the majority of these deaths are from pneumonia or the combination of pneumonia and gastroenteritis. Death from pneumonia in children, and in adults not admitted to hospital, remains rare in the West.

In CAP, by far the predominant pathogen is *Streptococcus pneumoniae*, which accounts for between 70% and 90% of cases. *S. pneumoniae* is a Gram-positive coccus with a thick capsule, decorated with antigens that distinguish different serotypes. These antigens lend themselves to the development of vaccines and diagnostic tests. The beta-lactam ring of penicillin binds and inhibits the cross-linking of peptidoglycan, a pro-

cess crucial to cell wall formation in bacteria such as *S. pneumoniae*. The dominant place of *S. pneumoniae* in producing CAP (and the fact that some rarer pathogens that cause CAP are susceptible to penicillin) explains why penicillins such as amoxicillin are at the core of CAP treatment. However, three sets of organisms require special attention in this context.

Soon after the widespread use of penicillin dramatically reduced mortality from CAP, it became apparent that some forms of CAP were "atypical" in not being susceptible to penicillin, generally occurring in younger patients, and having a tendency to extra-pulmonary manifestations alongside the pneumonia. The pathogens responsible for these "atypical pneumonias" were soon characterised as having no cell wall (and hence being inherently resistant to penicillin). These include *Mycoplasma pneumoniae*, *Coxiella burnetii*, *Chlamydophila pneumoniae*, and *Chlamydophila psittaci*, which generally cause self-limiting infections, but can produce severe pneumonia. The major concern in this group relates to *Legionella pneumophila*, which can cause severe and life-threatening pneumonia, and a range of extrapulmonary manifestations including cardiac, neurological and renal disease; diarrhoea; hyponatraemia; hypophosphataemia; and muscle pains with high serum creatine kinase. Legionnaire's disease is transmitted by droplets from contaminated water in cooling towers or air conditioning systems, and has been the focus of high-profile outbreaks and public health investigations. Because *L. pneumophila* can cause moderate and severe pneumonia, guidelines recommend that macrolides are added to penicillin in these scenarios.

The second important caveat relates to influenza. During influenza pandemics, mortality from CAP increases, most dramatically seen in the infamous 1917 outbreak, which is thought to have killed more people than both world wars combined. Some patients undoubtedly died from influenza pneumonia, but equally there is no doubt that influenza increases susceptibility to secondary bacterial pneumonia.

This leads to the third caveat, surrounding *Staphylococcus aureus*. The incidence and severity of *S. aureus* pneumonia is markedly increased during influenza pandemics. *S. aureus* pneumonia carries a high mortality, and almost all UK strains produce penicillinases. As a consequence, if severe CAP is acquired in an influenza season, flucloxacillin (or other penicillinase-resistant penicillins) are prescribed. It is a common misconception that *S. aureus* is the only pathogen that complicates influenza. *S. pneumoniae* behaves more aggressively after influenza, and *Haemophilus influenzae* (which is usually associated with mild CAP) can cause severe pneumonia when secondary to influenza.

S. pneumoniae itself can cause severe pneumonia, and as it is responsible for most CAP, it is not surprising that *S. pneumoniae* is consistently found to be the organism most associated with severe pneumonia in ICU series.

Collectively these observations explain why mild CAP is treated with amoxicillin, and moderate to severe CAP with amoxicillin and a macrolide (with flucloxacillin added during influenza outbreaks). These combinations cover most pathogens most of the time. Occasional clinical clues can suggest specific pathogens, but they are rarely pathognomonic. As discussed earlier, right upper lobe pneumonia with lobar expansion suggests *S. pneumoniae* or *K. pneumoniae*. Cavitation suggests *S. aureus*, *K. pneumoniae*, or tuberculosis. The presence of chronic obstructive pulmonary disease (COPD) increases the likelihood of *H. influenzae* pneumonia, though *S. pneumoniae* remains the commonest pathogen in CAP secondary to COPD, and some cases of pneumonia in patients with COPD may be caused by *Moraxella catarrhalis* (which produces beta-lactamase and so is resistant to amoxicillin) and *Pseudomonas aeruginosa* (also resistant to penicillin). Return from foreign travel with pneumonia raises the possibility of Legionnaire's disease (especially after a stay in hotels with air conditioning systems in warm countries), and some particular pneumonias have associations with particular geographical locations (for example melioidosis in South East Asia and Northern Australia, and the Middle East Respiratory Syndrome coronavirus [MERS-CoV] outbreaks).

Hospital-Acquired Penumonia

HAP is defined as new pneumonia arising two or more days after admission to hospital, and which was not evolving in the community prior to admission. It has been estimated that the prevalence of HAP is around 1%. Most patients in whom HAP is suspected are elderly and frail. Differentiation of true HAP from a range of other hospital-acquired thoracic pathologies is difficult, and obtaining microbiological samples from the alveolar regions is harder still—bronchoalveolar lavage (BAL) is rarely justified or likely to be tolerated, good-quality sputum sampling reflective of the alveolar regions is rare, and antibiotics are frequently started empirically. HAP occurring in the first week of a hospital admission is likely to be caused by *S. pneumoniae*, *S. aureus*, *H. influenzae*, or coliforms, but with passing time the range of potential pathogens becomes wider, with greater representation of more virulent and antibiotic-resistant pathogens.

Ventilator-Associated Pneumonia

VAP is new pneumonia arising at least 48 h after intubation and mechanical ventilation. Although estimates vary considerably, VAP appears to occur in about 20% of intubated and mechanically ventilated patients, and to have a crude mortality rate of around 30% (though the attributable mortality over and above that of patients in ICU with equivalent severity of illness without pneumonia is far smaller) [5].

In contrast to CAP, a quite different set of pathogens is implicated in HAP. VAP is the best-characterised form of HAP. VAP occurring early in an intensive care unit (ICU) stay is more likely to be caused by organisms such as *S. pneumoniae*, methicillin-sensitive *S. aureus*, *H. influenzae*, and Gram-negative bacilli. However, late-onset VAP (>7 days) can be caused by a plethora of organisms that are generally more virulent and more likely to be antibiotic-resistant. Gram-negative bacilli including *P. aeruginosa*, bacteria of the Enterobacteriaceae family, and the Gram-positive *S. aureus* are the dominant pathogens. Empirical therapy for late-onset VAP should take this into account. It is vital to have good microbiological surveillance and epidemiology, such that hospitals know the most likely pathogens in their institution, as the microbiological epidemiology of HAP and VAP varies considerably between hospitals (and often in different units within the same hospital).

Aspiration Pneumonia

The bacterial aetiology of aspiration pneumonia is less well understood. There is a widely held belief that anaerobic bacteria are disproportionately represented in aspiration pneumonia, but other studies have implicated Gram-negative coliforms. Part of the problem in studying aspiration pneumonia relates to practical difficulties in obtaining high-quality, representative alveolar samples. Patients with suspected aspiration pneumonia are often too frail to cough well enough to produce adequate sputum samples (or may have no sputum production), and may be too unwell for bronchoscopy.

Central to the pathophysiology of pneumonia is the bacterial inoculum reaching the lung. Some of the most important lower respiratory tract infections, such as tuberculosis, influenza, and Legionnaire's disease are undoubtedly acquired by direct inhalation of airborne droplets. In contrast, it seems likely that VAP is caused by "micro-aspiration" of small volume inocula from a colonised oropharynx. This is supported by effective subglottic suction drainage (removal of potentially infected secretions sitting just about the cuff of an endotracheal tube) being associated with significantly reduced VAP, and by the close correlation between colonising oropharyngeal bacteria and pathogens later isolated from the pneumonic lung.

With regard to aspiration pneumonia, witnessed, large-volume aspiration is a relatively rare occurrence, and far more common is repeated, low-volume aspiration in elderly patients with reduced conscious level and/or impaired laryngeal protection reflexes. It is therefore likely that most aspiration pneumonia follows the same pathogenesis as VAP, with altered colonisation profiles emerging in the oropharynx

in a hospital or nursing home environment, with repeated aspiration of small inocula into the lung.

Which of these routes of inoculation (direct droplet/aerosol inhalation or microaspiration) is predominantly responsible for CAP caused by *S. pneumoniae* is harder to determine. Colonisation of the oropharynx with *S. pneumoniae* is relatively common in the healthy population, and higher in hospitalised cohorts, who are known to have a high frequency of micro-aspiration. However aerosol spread of *S. pneumoniae* is well known to occur. There is, therefore, fairly persuasive evidence that *S. pneumoniae* can reach the alveolar spaces through either route. This situation may well apply to other pathogens implicated in CAP.

Principles of Diagnosis

When faced with a patient with possible pneumonia it is important to determine if (1) pneumonia is the most likely diagnosis on clinical grounds, and if so, (2) what is the most likely organism?

Many illnesses mimic pneumonia (Table 10.1) and the diagnosis is not always straightforward. Furthermore the "gold standard" diagnosis of pneumonia (using histology and culture of lung biopsy material to confirm infected, inflamed alveolar tissue) is unachievable and undesirable in most patients, and the surrogate clinical tools for diagnosis are inadequate. These difficulties in diagnosis tend to encourage the overuse of antibiotics. Clinicians generally would rather overtreat than miss a potentially curable condition. This is clearly a logical and justifiable stance when considering an individual patient, but it does have two broad consequences. The first is that, especially in hospitals, this increases evolutionary pressure for the emergence of antibiotic-resistant pathogens, at a time when the lack of new antibiotics is well recognized. The second consequence of having a low threshold for "false positives" is that the true (non-infective) cause of the patient's presentation will often remain undiagnosed. We remain some way short of the optimal situation in which accurate diagnostics give sufficiently high sensitivity and specificity to target antibiotics only to those patients who require them.

Table 10.1 Non-infective mimics of community-acquired pneumonia

	Discriminating clinical features
Congestive heart failure	History of orthopnoea or paroxysmal nocturnal dyspnoea. Peripheral oedema, cardiomegaly, elevated jugular venous pressure, third or fourth heart sounds. Markedly elevated brain natriuretic peptide (BNP) CXR: Cardiomegaly, pulmonary oedema, bilateral pleural effusions
Exacerbation of COPD	CXR: Absence of consolidation, evidence of emphysema
Pulmonary embolism	Risk factors for venous thromboembolism (VTE), including previous VTE, prolonged immobility, malignancy, congestive heart failure, trauma/surgery, pregnancy. Lack of leukocytosis on full blood count CXR: Hampton's hump, Westermark's sign. ECG changes indicative of right heart strain
Exacerbation of asthma	Wheeze CXR: Hyperinflation, no consolidation
Primary or secondary pulmonary neoplasm	More gradual onset of constitutional symptoms (weight loss, fatigue, decreased appetite). Lack of fever. Persistent or severe haemoptysis CXR: Masses without air bronchograms, lymphadenopathy
Collagen vascular disease (e.g. systemic lupus erythematosus, rheumatoid arthritis)	Evidence of extra-pulmonary symptoms and signs (e.g. synovitis, rash, iritis)
Drug-induced pneumonitis	Candidate drug in medication history. Scant expectoration. Few abnormalities on clinical examination
Sarcoidosis	History of fatigue and weight loss, evidence of extra-pulmonary disease. Lymphadenopathy on chest imaging
Eosinophilic pneumonia	Symptom duration of weeks to months. Female preponderance. Association with atopy. Scant expectoration. Eosinophilia on full blood count
Pulmonary vasculitides	History of rash, arthritis, sinusitis. CXR: Diffuse alveolar infiltrates or cavitation. Renal insufficiency. Positive anti-neutrophil cytoplasmic antibodies
Cryptogenic organising pneumonia	Symptom duration of weeks to months. Lack of response to antibiotics. Previous imaging shows consolidation in a different site
Acute hypersensitivity pneumonitis	Exposure to relevant potential allergen (e.g. pigeons). History of malaise and myalgia. Scant expectoration. Diffusely abnormal pulmonary shadowing on CXR
Radiation pneumonitis	Recent course of radiotherapy

Clinical acumen, radiology, and microbiological sampling have their limitations. The careful consideration of all three together allow a reliable diagnosis of CAP much of the time, but the level of diagnostic confidence is lower when considering HAP/VAP.

A history of breathlessness, productive cough, fever, fatigue, and pleuritic chest pain evolving over a few days, along with signs of tachypnoea, bronchial breathing, and whispering pectoriloquy make a diagnosis of probable pneumonia easy, and diagnostic confidence can be confirmed with a compatible CXR. However, this constellation of features rarely occur, and some patients with pneumonia have no cough or breathlessness, and many do not have sputum production.

The history must be considered in the context of the background level of function and immune competence. Co-morbidities (such as COPD, diabetes mellitus, renal impairment, liver disease, chronic heart disease, or malignancy) and immunosuppressant medications all predispose to pneumonia. The history should include questions about smoking and alcohol consumption (*K. pneumoniae* is associated with alcohol dependency) and foreign travel (*L. pneumophila* and return from areas where particular pneumonias are endemic). Enquiry should also be made about recent flu-like symptoms and relevant contacts (*S. pneumoniae*, *S. aureus*, *H. influenzae*, and even primary influenza pneumonia may cause pneumonia in influenza seasons), occupation and contact with animals (avian exposure suggests possible psittacine pneumonia, but generally zoonoses are rare). The sexual and substance history is also important, and HIV testing should be considered in all patients with pneumonia. A history of dysphagia and choking is also relevant, as these features are clearly associated with an increased risk of pneumonia, particularly right lower lobe and middle lobe pneumonia.

Myalgia, diarrhoea, and headache may alert clinicians to the possibility of Legionnaire's disease in patients with moderate to severe pneumonia, and abdominal pain (while obviously deserving full attention in its own right) can occasionally represent referred pain from diaphragmatic pleurisy.

In addition to the physical signs on chest examination previously described, significant dental decay suggests oral pathogens (especially anaerobes) obtaining a haematogenous route from the gums to the lungs. In frail, elderly patients with impaired swallowing, this raises the possibility of repeated aspiration.

History and examination are rarely conclusive, so radiology is crucial. Air bronchograms in a well-centred, postero-anterior CXR on deep inspiration are pathognomonic, but rarely achieved in the slumped, frail elderly. This situation is magnified in the context of suspected HAP, while on the ICU, CXRs in semi-recumbent patients are notoriously hard to interpret and, it is well recognised that even good-quality CXRs often miss consolidation that may be detected on computed tomography (CT) scanning.

Microbiological sampling is of crucial importance in the diagnosis of pneumonia and for guiding treatment. While in the appropriate clinical context, a Gram stain from a high-quality sputum sample revealing (for example) strings of Gram-positive cocci consistent with *S. pneumoniae*, would confirm diagnosis and guide treatment, this is rarely possible. There are three main problems to consider in relation to microbiological sampling of the respiratory tract. The first is that many patients with pneumonia have no sputum production. Secondly, patients are commonly already taking empirical antibiotics on presentation to hospital, and it is recognised that sputum culture is less likely to give an accurate reflection of pneumonia in that setting. Thirdly, as pneumonia is infection of the alveolar regions of the lungs, it is often hard to be certain that the sample is derived from the relevant part of the respiratory tract. In the context of CAP, the main challenge is to disregard contaminants or colonising bacteria from the upper respiratory tract. In general, however, a good-quality expectorated sputum sample is considered representative of alveolar pathology in patients with CAP.

Unfortunately, the situation in HAP and VAP is starkly different. In suspected HAP, high-quality sputum production in an antibiotic-naïve patient is a rare occurrence, as is a clearly diagnostic CXR. In this setting empirical antibiotics are usually given. Suspected HAP is notoriously poorly studied, but at a conservative estimate, an alternative diagnosis to pneumonia is likely to be present in over 50% of patients.

Suspected VAP presents a uniquely different set of circumstances. Here, patients are already critically ill, and the additional burden of pneumonia seems to confer an appreciable attributable mortality. The risk of "missing" pneumonia here adds further to the pressure to prescribe empirical antibiotics. Studies consistently show true pneumonia to be present in only around one-third of patients with suspected VAP. Because mucus production in the conducting airways is markedly increased in mechanically ventilated patients, tracheal aspirates are poorly reflective of alveolar pathology, and contribute significantly to false positive diagnoses of pneumonia. Unlike in most cases of CAP or HAP, the clinician has potential access to the alveolar space in that bronchoscopy and bronchoalveolar lavage (BAL) can be performed under controlled circumstances via the endotracheal tube, and high-quality BAL specifically samples the relevant region. The clinician must choose between empirical treatment (in the knowledge that the correct diagnosis may not be VAP in two-thirds of cases) and an invasive diagnostic procedure. One large randomised controlled trial (RCT) suggested better outcomes with a bronchoscopic approach, but another showed no difference [6, 7]. It is argued that image-directed bronchoscopic

BAL (and the culture of >10^4 colony forming units/ml) is strongly suggestive of VAP.

Blood cultures are strongly recommended in patients with suspected moderate or severe pneumonia, particularly when the patient is febrile. Similarly, it is worthwhile culturing pleural fluid if this can be easily, quickly, and safely obtained.

A plethora of antigenic and molecular tests are becoming available. The exquisite sensitivity of PCR-based tests further increases the absolute requirement for high-quality sampling before performing microbiology. A clearly predominant organism in a high-quality sample greatly increases the likelihood that it is the responsible pathogen. Low-level identification of multiple organisms from low-quality samples is more likely to indicate contamination or colonisation. The concern is that increasingly sensitive tests, if not used judiciously, may exacerbate the problem of over-prescription of antibiotics.

Prognosis and Stratification

The CAP/HAP/aspiration/immunocompromised host classification has ensured better empirical antibiotic selection for pneumonia generally. In parallel, management has been improved through introduction of prognostic risk stratification scores. These are applicable to CAP, and the most commonly used are the CURB65 and Pneumonia Severity Index scores [8, 9]. The CURB65 score (Table 10.2) is simple to use and derived from UK cohorts. Guidelines propose that patients with CAP and CURB65 scores of 0–1 can be managed at home, a score of 2 should be managed in hospital, and scores of 3–5 should prompt consideration of a higher level of care (for example in an ICU).

Three very important caveats must be noted. The first is that the CURB65 score must not replace clinical judgment. It provides a prognostic estimation with wide confidence intervals, and clinical judgment and experience should always "trump" the CURB65, which should be viewed as a supporting guide. The second caveat around CURB65 is that it is a tool applied at a single point in time (usually at presentation) yet deterioration can occur rapidly. The third caveat is that CURB65 performs less well at predicting those patients who require management in an intensive care environment, again emphasising the primary role of clinical judgment in assessing prognosis in patients with CAP.

If patients are discharged from hospital with mild pneumonia (CURB65 0–1), a general practitioner or district nurse should be able to confirm appropriate progress in the ensuing period. In all other settings, hospital wards can monitor progress to detect any clinical deterioration or the development of complications.

Principles of Treatment

The mainstays of treatment in pneumonia can be divided into general measures and antibiotic therapy.

General Measures

Patients are often hypoxaemic, but the optimal level of PaO_2 to improve outcomes in pneumonia is undefined; supplemental oxygen is generally used to maintain a PaO_2 ≥8 kPa, or for oxygen saturations to be maintained at 94–98%. Insensible fluid loss is often underestimated and requires correction. As with all systemic inflammatory processes, pneumonia generally promotes venous thrombus formation, which is compounded by immobility. Patients should have thromboprophylaxis unless specifically contra-indicated, and mobilised from bed as quickly as is feasible.

Table 10.2 CURB65 score for mortality risk assessment in hospital[a]

| Confusion (abbreviated mental test score 8 or less, or new disorientation in person, place or time) |
| Blood **u**rea of over 7 mmol/L |
| Respiratory **r**ate of 30 breaths per minute or more |
| Low **b**lood pressure (diastolic 60 mmHg or less, or systolic less than 90 mmHg) |
| Age **65** years or more |

[a]CURB65 score is calculated by giving 1 point for each of the prognostic features

Pneumonia induces a significant catabolic effect that is multifactorial and is probably responsible for systemic upset and muscle wasting. Physiotherapy and dietetic input is important to maintain muscle tone and independent mobility, and to increase calorific intake. Anti-emetics can obviously help in allowing better calorific intake. The profound fatigue of pneumonia can persist for weeks or months after an otherwise full recovery. The pleurisy that accompanies about 15% of cases of pneumonia should be treated with analgesics, and opioids may be required to relieve pain and allow more effective aeration of the affected side, but there is no evidence for their use as antitussives.

If a patient with pneumonia fails to respond to apparently good treatment, the most likely explanation is that the diagnosis of pneumonia is incorrect, or that the underlying medical condition that predisposed to pneumonia is dictating the tempo of the illness. Failure to respond should lead to consideration of complications such as empyema. Other possibilities (particularly in HAP/VAP, aspiration, and severe CAP) include inadequate or inappropriate antibiotic coverage for the responsible pathogen(s), or the involvement of an antibiotic-resistant organism(s).

On discharge, patients must be followed up, as pneumonia can occasionally be the first declaration of a tumour occluding a bronchus, and so a repeat CXR at 6–8 weeks is generally advised, particularly in smokers and in patients aged over 50. Complete radiographic resolution is age-dependent and lags well behind clinical improvement, but all CXRs should be improving by 6–8 weeks, and failure of resolution should prompt further investigation, usually with CT in the first instance.

Antibiotic Therapy

Community-Acquired Pneumonia

The consensus on treatment in the UK for patients who have adequate social circumstances, who can safely have oral intake, and have no medication allergies, outside of an influenza pandemic, are as follows:

- CURB65 score 0–1: manage at home with oral amoxicillin.
- CURB65 score 2: manage in a hospital ward with oral amoxicillin and oral clarithromycin (because there is a low but appreciable risk of *L. pneumophila* being responsible).
- CURB65 score 3–5: manage in hospital and consider management in a critical care area such as an ICU, keeping in mind that CURB65 is less effective in predicting which patients require critical care (a pragmatic approach combining clinical judgment, CURB65, and arterial blood gas results is advised).

In terms of antibiotics, combinations such as intravenous co-amoxiclav and clarithromycin should be used for CURB65 3-5. If *L. pneumophila* is strongly suspected, additional cover should be considered (e.g. using levofloxacin), and if there is a known flu pandemic and/or the patient has had flu-like symptoms preceding the pneumonia, consider adding intravenous flucloxacillin to cover *S. aureus*. The exact choice of antibiotics, particularly when drug allergies are present, is best guided by discussion with hospital microbiologists and consult with the most recent updates on the British Thoracic Society and NICE websites.

Guidelines generally recommend that patients hospitalised with CAP (particularly of CURB65 score 3–5) should receive antibiotics within 4 h of clinical suspicion, on the basis of evidence that delayed antibiotics are associated with higher mortality. This emphasises the observation that in CAP, diagnostic sampling should not delay prescribing. In general, if clinical assessment and CXR are compatible with CAP, then as the antibiotic medication is being prescribed and prepared for administration, an attempt should be made to obtain: blood cultures; sputum (for culture, including Legionella culture, and for PCR to cover atypical pathogens and respiratory viruses as appropriate); and ultrasound-guided pleural aspirate, if appropriate. Urine should be obtained for pneumococcal and Legionella antigen testing, which can be very useful as "rule in" tests. Blood can be sent for serological tests if atypical pathogens or viral pathologies are particularly expected.

The duration of antibiotics required for uncomplicated CAP has been a subject of considerable debate. The general trend in pneumonia care is for shorter courses of antibiotics, and recent NICE guidelines recommend 5 days for mild CAP managed in the community, and 7–10 days for moderate and severe CAP. Treatment may be extended according to clinical judgement, particularly if *S. aureus* or Gram-negative enteric bacilli are confirmed. Longer antibiotic courses are often required if complications such as empyema or abscess ensue.

One particular controversy that continues to arise is whether the antibiotics recommended in the UK guidelines increase the risk of *Clostridium difficile* colitis. This divides opinion significantly, and many hospitals have adjusted their own CAP guidelines to recommend antibiotics less commonly associated with *C. difficile*. It currently seems reasonable to apply the national guidelines, unless local microbiological epidemiology suggests a clear association between the antibiotics in question and *C. difficile* colitis.

A further interesting development has been the use of blood C-reactive protein (CRP) concentrations to monitor response to therapy. In patients with moderate and severe pneumonia, it is generally recognised that CRP should be falling after 3 days of adequate antibiotic therapy, and if it is not, an explanation for the lack of response should be sought.

NICE guidelines have also made recommendations on antibiotic initiation based on CRP for patients in the community with suspected lower respiratory tract infection. Antibiotics should not be offered if CRP is <20 mg/L; a delayed course can be given if CRP is 20–100 mg/L and symptoms worsen; and antibiotics should be initiated if CRP concentrations are >100 mg/L.

Hospital-Acquired Pneumonia (with Particular Focus on Ventilator-Associated Pneumonia)

Guidelines for the management of VAP (and HAP more generally) advise that antibiotic therapy be dictated by the severity of the patient's illness, the likelihood of multi-drug resistant pathogens, and the time spent in hospital [10–13]. At the time of writing, updated European guidelines on VAP are pending. A broad amalgamated interpretation of the various guidelines would suggest that if the patient with VAP has been in the intensive care unit for under 5 days, if they are not considered to be at high risk of a multi-drug resistant pathogen (Table 10.3), and if they are not severely unwell (for example no evidence for severe sepsis), then monotherapy with a limited-spectrum antibiotic (e.g. co-amoxiclav) for approximately 8 days seems appropriate.

The guidelines take slightly differing views on management if the patient has been in hospital for more than 5 days and/or is at risk of a multi-drug resistant (MDR) pathogen(s) and/or is severely unwell. However, if an organism has been confidently isolated, the general consensus is to use a single antibiotic to which it is fully sensitive for around 8 days. If no organism is isolated, then the North American view is generally to give two antibiotics with different modes of action, with the aim of covering a range of Gram-negative pathogens (most importantly

Table 10.3 Risk factors for multi-drug resistant pathogens in the aetiology of ventilator-associated pneumonia

Recent episode of hospital admission (≥2 days in the previous 90 days)
Nursing home resident
Recent exposure to antibiotics (within previous 90 days)
Recent wound care
Recent immunosuppression or chemotherapy
≥5 days since ICU admission
Duration of mechanical ventilation
Dialysis
Family member with multi-drug resistant pathogen
Endemic multi-drug resistant bacteria in local ecology

P. aeruginosa), *S. pneumoniae,* and MSSA, with the addition of cover for MRSA if it is known to be prevalent on the ICU in question. UK guidelines give less-specific advice, but favour monotherapy where possible, making use of local microbiological epidemiology. Treatment is again recommended to be for approximately 8 days. The figure of 8 days is based on a trial that compared 15 versus 8 days of treatment, and found no difference in outcomes [14]. Interestingly, a recent paper suggests that adherence to previous American Thoracic Society and Infectious Diseases Society of America guidelines for the empirical treatment of VAP in patients at risk of MDR pathogens was associated with increased mortality [15]. The precise interpretation of these findings is difficult, but one tentative suggestion would be to seek a pathogen wherever possible in the hope of reducing the antibiotic load.

The guidelines generally recommend that, where possible, respiratory samples be obtained when VAP is suspected, with empirical antibiotics started immediately afterwards, according to published guidelines. If standard cultures (typically 2–3 days later) suggest a responsible organism, then antibiotics can be de-escalated and rationalised at that stage. If good-quality cultures return with no growth, and if the patient is not deteriorating, then antibiotics can potentially be withdrawn. This approach seems very sensible, but clinically it often proves challenging. Clearly this approach is irrelevant in patients in whom no respiratory samples are obtained, or in patients in whom there is an ongoing extra-pulmonary indication for antibiotics. Some centres seek to improve antibiotic stewardship by considering early withdrawal of antibiotics if procalcitonin levels are clearly decreasing in parallel with clinical improvement, or if the "Clinical Pulmonary Infection Score" (a relatively cumbersome scoring system with a range from 0 to 12) [16] remains at ≤6 over days 0–3 of empirical treatment.

The urgency of antibiotic prescription in VAP is also less clear-cut than for CAP. Delayed prescription of appropriate antibiotics is associated with increased mortality in VAP, but the evidence that the increased mortality begins before 4 h of the clinical suspicion of VAP is weak. Nevertheless, when VAP is suspected, it seems eminently sensible to obtain a good-quality BAL sample within the next 4 h if possible, then start empirical monotherapy immediately, and refine the antibiotics based on clinical course and culture results.

Aspiration Pneumonia

As for HAP, the true prevalence, microbiological aetiology, and optimal management strategy for aspiration pneumonia are hard to define.

The microbiology of aspiration pneumonia is gradually shifting from being predominantly a disease caused by anaerobic bacteria to one more akin to early HAP, with perhaps an over-representation of Gram-negative bacilli. In longer-term residents of nursing homes, *P. aeruginosa* may complicate aspiration pneumonia.

It seems reasonable to treat patients with a high likelihood of aspiration pneumonia who are admitted from home as though they have CAP or early HAP. As *L. pneumophila* is not implicated, it seems reasonable to treat these patients with co-amoxiclav, but to be guided by local microbiological epidemiology, and to have a low threshold for broadening Gram-negative cover if there is deterioration. If the patient has been admitted from a nursing home or hospital facility, it may be advisable to give Gram-negative cover, either with a cephalosporin or (if nursing home or hospital residence has been long-term) with an antipseudomonal antibiotic.

Prevention

Smoking cessation, influenza vaccination, and pneumococcal vaccination all appear to reduce the risk of pneumonia in susceptible populations (Table 10.4).

The evidence base for measures to prevent VAP is vast. There is persuasive evidence that

Table 10.4 Vaccination recommendations for the prevention of community-acquired pneumonia

Vaccination	Pneumococcal polysaccharide vaccine	Inactivated influenza vaccine	Live attenuated influenza vaccine
Route of administration	Intramuscular	Intramuscular	Intranasal
Recommended groups	All persons >65 years of age Persons aged 2–64 years with chronic cardiovascular, pulmonary, renal or liver disease, diabetes mellitus, cerebrospinal fluid leaks, alcohol dependence, asplenism, taking immunosuppression, or in long-stay care facilities	All persons ≥50 years Persons aged 6 months—49 years with chronic cardiovascular, pulmonary, renal or metabolic disease, haemoglobinopathies, taking immunosuppression, pregnancy, or people in long-term care facilities Household contacts of the above groups Patients ≤18 years taking aspirin therapy Children aged 6–23 months Health care professionals	Healthy children aged between 2 and 7 years. Children aged between 8 and 17 years with chronic conditions
Revaccination schedule	Only required once after 5 years in: 1. Adults who received first dose ≤65 years 2. Asplenism 3. Immunocompromise	Annual	Annual

general infection control measures like good hand hygiene reduce the incidence of nosocomial infection, and this probably extends to VAP. Risk factors for VAP are well described, and form the basis for a plethora of preventive strategies. The biggest risk factors for VAP are intubation and inappropriate use of antibiotics, although avoidance of either may be impossible. Effective preventive measures appear to include managing the patient in a semi-recumbent (rather than supine) position of 30–45°, daily interruption of sedation as a prelude to weaning, and subglottic drainage. Controversy continues over whether oral chlorhexidine and selective digestive decontamination are advantageous preventive strategies.

Future Challenges in Pneumonia

There are endless ways in which management and prevention of pneumonia could be improved. In concluding this chapter, we shall consider four important aims that will be difficult to achieve, but where success could make a major difference to outcomes. The first is obviously the generation of novel ways to eradicate pathogens efficiently without toxicity to the host. The dearth of new antibiotics emerging for use in clinical practice is well documented, though intensive research continues into new ways of disrupting key bacterial survival mechanisms. In this context, increasing interest is focusing on ways to boost host innate immune mechanisms that clear bacterial pathogens, and these may begin to suggest novel, non-antibiotic-based approaches.

The improvement of diagnostic accuracy in pneumonia clearly also presents a challenge for the future. This is particularly true in elderly, hospitalised patients, given that frailty and extensive co-morbidity broadens the differential diagnosis considerably, impairs the diagnostic precision of CXR, and reduces realistic chances of obtaining microbiological samples representative of the alveolar space. The ideal scenario is generation of a rapid, near-patient blood test that discriminates pneumonia from other causes of lung inflammation. This remains a distant aspiration, but there is much activity and interest in finding truly diagnostic biomarkers. There is also considerable interest in obtaining microbiological diagnoses from less-invasive specimens. Some caution needs to be exercised here. There has been an explosion of interest in the microbiome, and in whole genome sequencing of pathogens. This has fundamentally re-positioned our understanding of the normal and disease-associated microbiome deep in the lung. However, the relationship between detailed molecular microbiology of pneumonia and effective change of management is far from being worked out. Until it is, one concern is that the extreme sensitivity of molecular diagnostics may lead to detection of harmless commensals that are misinterpreted as pathogens, in turn leading to overuse of antibiotics.

A third area of interest attracting increasing interest (particularly in sepsis research) is the contribution of the host innate response to outcomes in severe infection. There is an intriguing body of literature suggesting that an over-active or under-active innate immune response to serious infective or non-infective insults may dictate clinical outcomes to a greater extent than the infection itself. A prolonged state of relative immunosuppression in response to sepsis may be particularly important in this regard. While improved understanding of the innate immune response to pneumonia is required, early indications suggest that the identification of key pathways regulating the magnitude of the innate immune response may provide targets for therapeutic intervention.

The previous areas highlighted would have major implications for improving pneumonia care in healthcare systems such as the UK's. The far greater challenge facing medicine is to harness sufficient political will and organisation of clinical infrastructures to address the appalling ongoing incidence of pneumonia, particularly at the extremes of life, in developing countries.

Acknowledgements The authors are very grateful to Drs Anna Beattie, Fiona Black, and Joaquim Majo (all Newcastle upon Tyne Hospitals NHS Foundation Trust) for supplying images, and to Dr. Wendy Funston, Newcastle University, for help in reviewing the manuscript.

References

1. National Institute for Health and Care Excellence. Pneumonia in adults: diagnosis and management. Clinical guideline [CG191] Published date: December 2014. Available at: https://www.nice.org.uk/guidance/cg191.
2. Lim WS, Baudouin SV, George RC, Hill AT, Jamieson C, Le Jeune I, et al. BTS guidelines for the management of community acquired pneumonia in adults: update 2009. Thorax. 2009;64(Suppl 3):iii1–55.
3. Harris M, Clark J, Coote N, Fletcher P, Harnden A, McKean M, et al. British Thoracic Society guidelines for the management of community acquired pneumonia in children: update 2011. Thorax. 2011;66(Suppl 2):ii1–23.
4. Black RE, Morris SS, Bryce J. Where and why are 10 million children dying every year? Lancet. 2003;361(9376):2226–34.
5. Chastre J, Fagon JY. Ventilator-associated pneumonia. Am J Respir Crit Care Med. 2002;165:867–903.
6. Fagon JY, Chastre J, Wolff M, Gervais C, Parer-Aubas S, Stéphan F, et al. Invasive and noninvasive strategies for management of suspected ventilator-associated pneumonia. Ann Intern Med. 2000;132(8):621–30.
7. Canadian Critical Care Trials Group. A randomized trial of diagnostic techniques for ventilator-associated pneumonia. N Engl J Med. 2006;355:2619–30.
8. Lim WS, van der Eerden MM, Laing R, Boersma WG, Karalus N, Town GI, et al. Defining community acquired pneumonia severity on presentation to hospital: an international derivation and validation study. Thorax. 2003;58(5):377–82.
9. Fine MJ, Auble TE, Yealy DM, Hanusa BH, Weissfeld LA, Singer DE, et al. A prediction rule to identify low-risk patients with community-acquired pneumonia. N Engl J Med. 1997;336(4):243–50.
10. Masterton RG, Galloway A, French G, Street M, Armstrong J, Brown E, et al. Guidelines for the management of hospital-acquired pneumonia in the UK: report of the working party on hospital-acquired pneumonia of the British Society for Antimicrobial Chemotherapy. J Antimicrob Chemother. 2008;62:5–34.
11. Rotstein C, Evans G, Born A, Grossman R, Light RB, Magder S, et al. Clinical practice guidelines for hospital-acquired pneumonia and ventilator-

associated pneumonia in adults. Can J Infect Dis Med Microbiol. 2008;19:19–53.

12. Kalil AC, Metersky ML, Klompas M, Muscedere J, Sweeney DA, Palmer LB, et al. Management of adults with hospital-acquired and ventilator-associated pneumonia: 2016 clinical practice guidelines by the Infectious Diseases Society of America and the American Thoracic Society. Clin Infect Dis. 2016;63:e61–e111.

13. Torres A, Ewig S, Lode H, Carlet J, European HAP Working Group. Defining, treating and preventing hospital acquired pneumonia: European perspective. Intensive Care Med. 2009;35(1):9–29.

14. Chastre J, Wolff M, Fagon JY, Chevret S, Thomas F, Wermert D, et al. Comparison of 8 vs 15 days of antibiotic therapy for ventilator-associated pneumonia in adults: a randomized trial. JAMA. 2003;290:2588–98.

15. Kett DH, Cano E, Quartin AA, Mangino JE, Zervos MJ, Peyrani P, et al. Implementation of guidelines for management of possible multidrug-resistant pneumonia in intensive care: an observational, multi-centre cohort study. Lancet Infect Dis. 2011;11:181–9.

16. Pugin J. Clinical signs and scores for the diagnosis of ventilator-associated pneumonia. Minerva Anastesiol. 2002;68:261–5.

Bronchiectasis

11

Adam Hill

What Is Bronchiectasis?

Bronchiectasis is defined pathologically as inflamed, permanently damaged, and dilated airways. This leads to a break in the primary host defences, alteration of the mucociliary escalator, and allows chronic infection of the airways. In the inflamed airways there is excess neutrophilic airways inflammation and despite this inflammatory response, there is chronic infection. The neutrophil products are thought to perpetuate the inflammatory response and, in particular, neutrophil elastase release causes both chronic bronchitis and emphysema. A vicious cycle of infection, inflammation, and damage occurs.

Diagnosis

The minimum criteria for diagnosing clinically significant bronchiectasis are regular cough and sputum production, and radiological confirmation with computed tomography (CT) of the chest. Plain chest radiography cannot be relied on, as it is both insensitive and non-specific. The minimum radiological criteria are based on CT appearances, namely bronchial dilatation with the internal diameter of the bronchus being larger than the diameter of the adjacent artery. Patients who meet this criterion but have no symptoms have isolated radiological bronchiectasis, but which is not thought to be clinically relevant.

Prevalence

A UK study has examined the prevalence of bronchiectasis as a diagnosis coded by primary care over the period 2004–2013 [1]. The point prevalence has increased in women from 0.3% to 0.6%, and from 0.3% to 0.5% in men.

Regarding hospitalisation, data from 12 U.S. states over the period 1993–2006 demonstrate an average annual age-adjusted hospitalisation rate of 16.5 hospitalisations per 100,000 population. This was increasing, with an average annual percentage increase of 2.4% in men and 3.0% in women. Women and those aged over 60 years had the highest rate of hospitalisations. Further U.S. data from 30 health-care plans reported a prevalence increasing from 4.2 per 100,000 for those aged 18–34 years to 271.8 per 100,000 in those aged >75 years. The prevalence was again higher among women, a consistent finding across studies.

A. Hill
Royal Infirmary and University of Edinburgh,
Edinburgh, UK
e-mail: adam.hill@ed.ac.uk

© Springer International Publishing AG, part of Springer Nature 2018
S. Hart, M. Greenstone (eds.), *Foundations of Respiratory Medicine*,
https://doi.org/10.1007/978-3-319-94127-1_11

Prognosis

A UK study noted the age-adjusted mortality rate for women with bronchiectasis to be 1438 per 100,000 against 636 for the general population (comparative mortality odds ratio of 2.26) and, in men, the age-adjusted mortality rate for bronchiectasis population was 1915 per 100,000 compared to 895 for the general population (comparative mortality odds ratio of 2.14) [1].

Loebinger et al. reported the factors associated with decreased survival in 2009 in a cohort of 91 patients over 13 years [2]. The factors independently associated with reduced survival were increasing age, worsening St. George's Respiratory Questionnaire activity score, *Pseudomonas* colonisation, reduced total lung capacity, increased residual volume/total lung capacity, and reduced gas transfer.

Two clinical scoring systems, the Bronchiectasis Severity Index (BSI) and FACED scores have been designed to predict future events, including hospitalisations (BSI score only) and mortality in patients with bronchiectasis (BSI and FACED scores).

FACED includes FEV_1 (<50% predicted, 2 points), Age (≥70 years, 2 points), *Pseudomonas* chronic colonisation (1 point), extent of bronchiectasis (>2 lobe involvement on CT, 1 point), and dyspnoea (modified MRC scale ≥3 (breathless walking 100 m), 1 point). All the variables are dichotomised and scored 0 vs. 1 or 2. The total FACED score predicted 5-year all-cause mortality in mild, moderate, and severe disease (defined as a score of 0–2, 3–4 and 5–7 points respectively) of 4%, 25%, and 56%.

The BSI combines age, body mass index, FEV_1, previous hospitalisation, exacerbation frequency, colonisation status, and radiological appearances (see Table 11.1). The score was designed to predict future exacerbations and hospitalisations, health status, and death over 4 years. An online calculator is available at www.bronchiectasisseverity.com.

Table 11.1 Bronchiectasis severity index (BSI)

BSI factor	Score points
Age (years)	50–69 years 2; 70–79 years 4; 80+ years 6
Body mass index <18.5 (kg/m²)	2
FEV_1% predicted	50–80% 1; 30–49% 2; <30% 3
Previous hospital admission in 2 years prior to study	5
≥3 exacerbations in last 1 year	2
MRC score Score 4 = stops due to breathlessness after walking 100 m Score 5 = house bound due to breathlessness, or breathless on dressing or undressing	4 = 2; 5 = 3
Chronic colonisation with *Pseudomonas aeruginosa*	3
Chronic colonisation with other potential pathogenic organisms	1
≥3 lobes or cystic bronchiectasis on CT chest	1

A score of 0–4 (mild bronchiectasis) is associated with 0–2.8% mortality and 0–3.4% hospitalisation rate over 1 year, and 0–5.3% mortality and 0–9.2% hospitalisation rate over 4 years. Score 5–8 (moderate bronchiectasis) is associated with 0.8–4.8% mortality and 1.0–7.2% hospitalisation rate at 1 year, and 4–11.3% mortality and 9.9–19.4% hospitalisation rate at 4 years. A score of 9 or over (severe bronchiectasis) was associated with 1-year 7.6–10.5% mortality, and 16.7–52.6% hospitalisation rate, and 4-year 9.9–29.2% mortality and 41.2–80.4% hospitalisation rates

Main Causes of Bronchiectasis from Cases Series

Secondary Care Studies [3]

In up to 53% of adult patients, no cause can be identified, and are labelled as idiopathic. The most common identified causes are past infection such as pneumonia, whooping cough, mycoplasma, viral pneumonia (adenovirus, measles, influenza and respiratory syncytial virus), or tuberculosis, occurring in 29–42% adults. If symptoms develop soon after the infectious insult, there is supportive evidence that the cause is post-infectious. The longer the lag period to symptoms developing, the less clear is the causal relationship.

Studies suggest specific immune defects in 1–8% of adults, and include primary and secondary immunodeficiencies. The commonest primary immunodeficiencies identified are common variable immunodeficiency, X-linked agammaglobulinaemia, and IgA deficiency. There are four IgG subclasses (1–4), but the clinical significance of isolated IgG subclass deficiencies is not known in the presence of normal total IgG concentrations. Specific antibody deficiency can be identified investigating antibody production to peptide antigens (such as tetanus) and polysaccharide antigens (such as *S. pneumoniae* and *Haemophilus influenzae* type B) at baseline and 21 days post-vaccination, with a failure of antibody response indicating a primary antibody deficiency.

In case series, bronchiectasis has been shown to be associated with connective tissue disease in 2–6% in adult studies. There have been associations with rheumatoid arthritis, systemic sclerosis, systemic lupus erythematosus, ankylosing spondylitis, relapsing polychondritis, Sjogren's, Marfan's syndrome, and Ehlers-Danlos syndrome.

Asthma was identified in 0–4%, and allergic bronchopulmonary aspergillosis is found from 0–7% in adult studies. As asthma is one of the diagnostic criteria for allergic bronchopulmonary aspergillosis, this implies an under-diagnosis of asthma in these case series.

Less common associations include: ciliary defects, found in 0–2% in adult studies but up to 15% in paediatric studies; cystic fibrosis found in 0–4% in adult studies and up to 17% in paediatric studies; congenital or airway abnormalities found in 0–1% in adult studies and up to 15% in paediatric studies (examples include Williams-Campbell syndrome with bronchial cartilage deficiency and tracheobronchomegaly (Mounier-Kuhn syndrome)); inflammatory bowel disease in 0–2% in all age groups; obstruction/foreign body 0–10% in all age groups; aspiration or inhalation 0–4% in adults and up to 18% in paediatric studies. In adults, bronchial obstruction can be due to aspiration of foreign material or due to endobronchial benign or malignant tumours. Foreign body aspiration in adults is usually related to neurological impairment. There is a longstanding debate whether gastro-oesophageal reflux disease is associated with bronchiectasis related to acid or gaseous reflux. Current opinion is to only investigate and treat patients with bronchiectasis who have symptoms of oesophageal reflux.

A diagnosis of primary ciliary dyskinesia is suggested in adults by the presence of one or more of the following features: history going back to infancy; continuous productive cough; upper respiratory tract symptoms with regular nasal discharge, sinusitis, anosmia, hearing impairment, chronic otitis media and grommets; dextrocardia; infertility; bronchiectasis worse in the lower and middle lobes.

The diagnosis of cystic fibrosis should be considered in bronchiectasis occurring before the age of 40, persistent isolation of *Staphylococcus aureus*, or unusual organisms usually associated with cystic fibrosis such as *Burkholderia cepacia*, features of malabsorption, male primary infertility, and predominant upper lobe bronchiectasis on CT scanning.

Primary Care [1]

From a large UK primary care database study of bronchiectasis, the following were associated with bronchiectasis: asthma 42.5%; COPD 36.1%; HIV 6.9%; rheumatoid arthritis 6.2%; other connective tissue disease 5.2%; allergic bronchopulmonary aspergillosis 1.8%; inflammatory bowel disease 2.8%; hypogammaglobulinaemia 0.9%; bone marrow transplant 0.1%. There is increased interest in the relationship of COPD and bronchiectasis. In a recent meta-analysis of six observational studies with 881 patients, [4] the mean prevalence of bronchiectasis in patients with COPD was 54.3%, ranging from 25.6% to

69%. Coexistence of bronchiectasis and COPD occurred more often in male patients with longer smoking histories. Patients with COPD and comorbid bronchiectasis had greater daily sputum production, more frequent exacerbations, poorer lung function, higher level of inflammatory biomarkers, more chronic colonization by potential pathogenic microorganisms, and higher rate of *Pseudomonas aeruginosa* isolation.

Microbiology

Colonisation vs. Infection

With conventional microbiological culture methods, about 75% of patients with bronchiectasis are chronically infected with potential pathogenic organisms. Colonisation implies that the pathogen is present in the sputum but not causing a local or systemic inflammatory response, whereas infection implies the pathogen is pathogenic, inducing an inflammatory response. Patients with pathogens at 10^5 colony-forming units/mL or more have airways inflammation, which rises with rising bacterial load, and is therefore an infecting pathogen [5]. Systemic inflammation occurred at bacterial loads $\geq 10^7$ colony-forming units/mL or more associated with raised serum levels of the vascular endothelial marker intercellular adhesion molecule 1 (ICAM-1).

Neither quantitative microbiology nor direct measures of airways inflammation are routinely available, but sputum purulence is an adequate marker of bronchial airway inflammation.

The isolation of a pathogen two or more times in the preceding year whilst clinically stable, and mucopurulent or purulent phlegm when clinically stable, should be regarded as an infection.

Spectrum

There is a wide spectrum of bacteria isolated, but the most frequent pathogens identified are *Haemophilus influenzae* and *Pseudomonas aeruginosa*. *Haemophilus influenzae* is present in about 40% of patients and *Pseudomonas aeruginosa* in 20–25% of bronchiectasis patients in the UK. There are, however, a large number of potential pathogenic organisms, which highlights the importance of sending sputum for microbial culture and sensitivity testing on a routine basis, both when clinically stable and in exacerbation.

In a UK study of 385 patients, 38.6% had *Haemophilus influenzae*, 21% *Pseudomonas aeruginosa*, 12.4% *Staphylococcus aureus*, 11.4% *Moraxella catarrhalis*, 9.7% *Streptococcus pneumoniae*, and 9.3% mixture of other bacteria [5].

Using anaerobic culture and 16S rDNA pyrosequencing molecular techniques, the bacteria that have been found to be most abundant in bronchiectasis include *P. aeruginosa*, and *H. influenzae*, but also the anaerobic bacteria *Prevotella* and *Veillonella* [6]. The clinical significance of anaerobes is not known. Further work using 16S has shown that with exacerbations there is loss of microbial diversity.

Fungal isolation can be seen in patients with allergic bronchopulmonary aspergillosis, and aspergillus species are increasingly isolated in patients receiving long-term inhaled antibiotic therapy. This isolation is not thought to be pathogenic, and currently these patients are not thought to require treatment with anti-fungal therapy. Environmental mycobacteria occur in 9% of the bronchiectasis population, although rates up to 30% have been reported in the United States [7]. The commonest species identified is *Mycobacterium avium* complex (MAC).

Which Technique?

In the NHS conventional non-quantitative culture is currently the only means of receiving a timely result from sputum microbiology testing. Quantitative bacteriology is not routinely carried in sputum samples that would allow an assessment of bacterial load, akin to that received for urinary tract infections.

As described above, there are molecular methods available using 16S rDNA pyrosequencing, but such tests are, however, costly, take a long time for analysis, and the interpretation particularly challenging in view of the multiplicity of pathogens identified. There are also specific PCR

DNA probes that can identify individual bacterial pathogens, but it is not known whether such techniques are superior to conventional culture methods. Currently these molecular techniques remain research tools.

Investigations

Treatable Causes

It is important to carry out investigations in all patients to identify treatable causes of bronchiectasis (see Table 11.2). The conditions which are particularly important to investigate include allergic bronchopulmonary aspergillosis, common variable immunodeficiency, cystic fibrosis, and environmental mycobacterial infection, as there are disease-specific treatments - allergic bronchopulmonary aspergillosis (oral corticosteroids ± antifungal agents such as itraconazole), common variable immunodeficiency (immunoglobulin replacement therapy), and environmental mycobacterial infection (a triple antimycobacte-

rial regimen for 18–24 months, such as Rifampicin or Ethambutol, and Clarithromycin for 2 years for MAC). In inflammatory bowel disease, it is recognised that some patients can have purulent phlegm and not grow any pathogens. These patients have been shown to respond to inhaled or oral corticosteroid therapy.

Other Routine Investigations

This depends on the severity of bronchiectasis. For mild bronchiectasis, annual spirometry and sputum for routine microbial culture when clinically stable and at the start of exacerbations are recommended. For advanced bronchiectasis sputum, routine and mycobacterial culture and repeat the sputum microbiology for conventional culture at each clinic visit (usually three to six monthly) and at the start of exacerbations. At each visit there should be spirometry, oxygen saturations, and an annual chest radiograph. Repeat CT scanning of the chest is reserved for the deteriorating patient.

Table 11.2 Investigations for treatable causes in bronchiectasis

Condition	Investigations	Results
Allergic broncho-pulmonary aspergillosis (ABPA)	FBC, IgE, IgE to aspergillus (alternatively skin prick tests to aspergillus), CXR, CT	Peipheral blood eosinophilia Elevated total IgE Increased IgE to aspergillus Positive skin prick test to aspergillus Positive IgG to aspergillus Fleeting infiltrates on CXR or CT chest Proximal bronchiectasis
Common variable immunodeficiency (CVID)	IgG, IgA and IgM	Reduced total IgG; no paraprotein identified
IgG subclass deficiency	IgG1, IgG2, IgG3 and IgG4	Reduced IgG subclasses
Inflammatory bowel disease	Faecal calprotectin; colonoscopy	Results in keeping with ulcerative colitis or Crohn's disease
Gastro-oesophageal reflux disease (GORD)	Upper GI endoscopy/barium meal ±24 h pH monitoring	Results in keeping with gastro-oesophageal reflux disease
Cystic fibrosis	Sweat test + CF Cytogenetics	Sweat chloride >40 nmol/L and CF genetic mutation
Non-tuberculous mycobacterial disease	CT chest; three spontaneous or induced sputum samples for mycobacterial culture; broncho-alveolar lavage	Environmental mycobacteria cultured on at least two sputum samples or one lavage sample and CT scanning showing nodular bronchiectasis or fibrocavitatory disease
Primary ciliary dyskinesia	High-speed video microscopy analysis, genotyping, transmission electron microscopy and nasal nitric oxide are used to investigate PCD	Nasal NO production <30 nL min^{-1} cut-off has good sensitivity and specificity (91% and 96%, respectively) and is a good preliminary screening tool for *ruling out* PCD

Table 11.3 Assessing severity of bronchiectasis

Characteristic	Mild	Moderate	Severe
Sputum colour	Mucoid	Mucopurulent	Purulent
24 h sputum volume	<5 mL	In between	≥20 mL
Exacerbation frequency	<2/year	In between	≥3/year
Exacerbation severity	Oral Ab responding well to outpatient treatment	In between	Often poor response to oral antibiotics and often intravenous antibiotics needed, sometimes requiring hospitalisation
Sputum bacteriology when stable	Mixed normal flora	Mixed normal flora or potential pathogenic organisms (*Haemophilus influenzae, Streptococcus pneumoniae, Moraxella catarrhalis, Staphylococcus aureus*)	*Pseudomonas aeruginosa*, enteric gram-ve non fermenters, methicillin resistant *Staphylococcus aureus*
Affected lobes on CT scanning	<3 lobes		≥3
Degree of bronchial dilatation	Tubular	Varicose	Cystic

Assessing Severity in Bronchiectasis

The assessment of severity of bronchiectasis can be split into mild, moderate, and severe (see Table 11.3) based on clinical, microbiological, and radiological criteria. Examples of tubular, varicose, and cystic bronchiectasis are shown (Fig. 11.1). The assessment of severity as highlighted below is useful in clinical practice. The FACED and BSI scores are used for assessing prognosis [8, 9].

Treatment

Because of impaired mucociliary clearance, chest clearance techniques are recommended to keep the airways free of secretions.

The techniques used most commonly are the active cycle of breathing, autogenic drainage, and use of positive expiratory pressure devices. Positive expiratory pressure devices such as the acapella, flute and flutter valves are helpful to facilitate airways clearance. All patients should be reviewed by a respiratory physiotherapist and taught the appropriate airways clearance technique. The frequency should be dependent on the severity of the bronchiectasis and, in more advanced disease, chest clearance should be carried out at least twice daily.

Adjuncts to Chest Clearance

There has been long-standing interest in muco-active therapy. Inhaled beta-agonists accelerate mucociliary clearance in a variety of conditions, and there is limited evidence to suggest they increase sputum volume when added to standard physiotherapy techniques in patients with bronchiectasis. There is still a lack of randomised controlled trial evidence in muco-active therapy to support or refute the use of inhaled hypertonic saline. Inhaled mannitol did not reduce overall exacerbations, and inhaled DNAase was potentially harmful, and so these agents should not be routinely used in patients with bronchiectasis. There is no evidence to support or refute the use of oral agents such as carbocysteine or similar drugs.

Anti-inflammatory Therapy

Inhaled Corticosteroids

Inhaled corticosteroids have been shown—in high dosage (Fluticasone 500 mcg bd) for 1 year—to reduce sputum volume and improve sputum inflammatory markers, but have not been shown to reduce exacerbation frequency. There are, however, concerns about their long-term safety, in particular adrenal suppression, skin

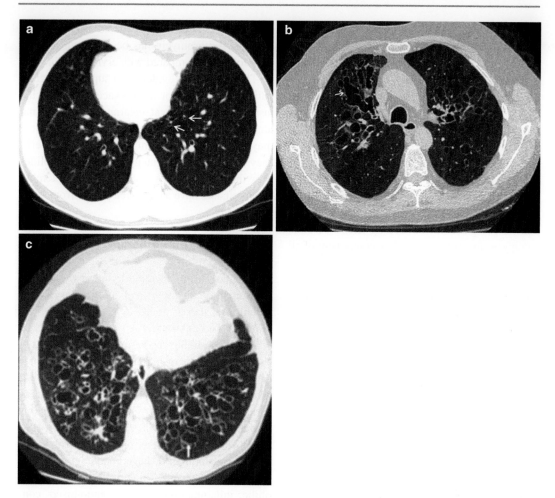

Fig. 11.1 Examples of appearances of bronchiectasis as seen on CT scanning. (**a**) Tubular (cylindrical) bronchiectasis is the mildest form, where there is loss of the normal tapering of the airways, which are enlarged and cylindrical. The bronchus and accompanying branch of the pulmonary artery are normally the same calibre, but in tubular bronchiectasis dilatation of the bronchus leads to the "signet ring" sign when seen in cross section. In varicose bronchiectasis (**b**), the affected bronchus is irregularly narrowed and dilated. (**c**) In cystic bronchiectasis, the bronchi exhibit saccular dilatation, which when aggregated, lead to a "bunch of grapes" appearance. Different forms of bronchiectasis may coexist

thinning, cataract formation, local side effects, haemoptysis, and a potential to increase pneumonia risk. Overall, there is a lack of randomised controlled trial evidence to support or refute the benefit of inhaled cortico steroids for bronchiectasis, so are not routinely recommended, unless there is co-existent asthma.

Macrolide Therapy

Recent systematic reviews and meta-analysis confirm the benefit of long-term macrolide therapy in reducing the frequency of exacerbations in stable bronchiectasis. It is not known whether the beneficial effect of macrolides is due to their anti-infective properties, anti-inflammatory properties, or a combination. In a meta-analysis of nine randomised controlled trials (recruiting 530 patients) long-term macrolides significantly reduced the risk of the exacerbations, SGRQ, dyspnoea, sputum volume, and decline in FEV1. Eradication of pathogens, overall rate of adverse events, and emergence of new pathogens were not improved, while gastrointestinal adverse events increased significantly with macrolides, and there was increased macrolide resistance in the oropharyngeal streptococci [10].

Before embarking on long-term macrolide therapy the benefit:risk ratio needs careful consideration. Risks that need to be considered are: (1) the effects on macrolides on hearing and balance as the majority of patients eligible will be middle aged or elderly; (2) the effects on Streptococcal resistance to macrolides—studies up to 1 year in bronchiectasis show no deleterious effect, but long-term studies are needed; (3) concern about losing a potential therapy for environmental mycobacteria. It is essential that environmental mycobacterial infection is excluded in patients being considered for long-term macrolide therapy, as macrolides are a key component of all drug regimens. There is a concern, in addition, that long-term macrolides promote mycobacterial infection, as macrolides have been shown to impair autophagy, [11] which is essential for clearance of mycobacteria; (4) concern from microbiome studies that macrolides may affect the normal microbiome and promote the development of colonisation with *Pseudomonas aeruginosa*, but further long-term studies are needed to explore this.

In the BLESS trial of 1 year of therapy with erythromycin in bronchiectasis patients with baseline airway infection dominated by *Pseudomonas aeruginosa*, erythromycin did not change microbiota composition significantly. In those with infection dominated by organisms other than *P. aeruginosa*, erythromycin caused a significant change in microbiota composition with a reduced relative abundance of *Haemophilus influenzae* and increased abundance of *P. aeruginosa*. There are increased GI side effects, but none of the studies to date show this leads to patients not being able to tolerate long-term treatment. In patients on concomitant statins, it is important a statin is used that macrolides do not interact with, such as pravastatin, fluvastatin, or rosuvastatin.

Several macrolide studies showed evidence of reduced exacerbations, which is a key endpoint to achieve in bronchiectasis. Positive trials used azithromycin 500 mg three times weekly for 6 months, azithromycin 250 mg daily for 1 year, and erythromycin 250 mg twice daily for 1 year. From UK Bronchiectasis National Audits, azithromycin seems to be the preferred agent, and the three times weekly regimen is popular with patients. Azithromycin has been known for less GI intolerance compared with erythromycin.

There is strong evidence to support selecting patients with three or more exacerbations in the last year despite chest clearance. The optimal length of therapy is not known, but treatment may be needed long-term for its continued efficacy. One potential strategy is to use macrolides over the worst months, usually from September to March, and have a drug-free period from April to September.

Experimental Anti-inflammatory Therapies

There has been increased interest in anti-inflammatory therapy, and preliminary trials include oral statins, oral CXCR2 antagonists, and oral elastase inhibitors.

A double-blind randomised controlled trial showed that atorvastatin therapy 80 mg once daily for 6 months reduced cough and improved neutrophil apoptosis in patients with moderately severe bronchiectasis [12]. No patients in this study were infected with *Pseudomonas aeruginosa*. The improved neutrophil apoptosis is the mechanism thought to have beneficial effects in bronchiectasis by enhancing resolution of neutrophilic inflammation. Larger randomised controlled trials are needed to assess the impact on reducing exacerbations and also whether it is beneficial in patients infected with *Pseudomonas aeruginosa*.

CXCR2 is one of the chemokines that activates inflammatory cell recruitment, and its antagonist AZD5069 reduces sputum neutrophil counts without reducing the number of exacerbations. An oral neutrophil elastase inhibitor (AZD9668) had a mild bronchodilator effect, but no effect on sputum neutrophilia.

Long-Term Oral vs. Inhaled Antibiotic Therapy

Inhaled antibiotic therapy has the benefit of targeting therapy to the site of infection. In addition, it allows high concentration of antibiotics in the airways in comparison to intravenous antibiotic therapy, and may therefore work in patients with apparent resistance patterns on *in vitro* sensitivity testing. Side effects include bronchospasm, which occurs in about 10% of patients despite a negative challenge test to the inhaled antibiotic [13]. Another issue is the high cost compared with oral therapy. Oral therapy has the benefit of ease of administration, but leads to increased systemic activity, and up to 30% have GI side effects such as abdominal pain and diarrhoea.

Long-Term Oral Antibiotic Therapy

Early studies in the 1950s conducted by the Medical Research Council showed the benefit of long-term tetracycline taken twice weekly over 1 year in improving symptoms and having less time off work. Eight months of high-dose amoxicillin (3G twice daily) led to improved symptoms and less severe exacerbations, but no overall effect on exacerbations. There is a distinct lack of randomised controlled trial evidence investigating targeted oral antibiotic therapy. In practice, long-term amoxicillin can be used for of patients with recurrent exacerbations (three or more per year) and chronic infection with *Haemophilus influenzae* that is beta lactamase negative. Alternative long-term treatments commonly used are amoxicillin with clavulanic acid and doxycycline.

Long-Term Inhaled Antibiotic Therapy

A meta-analysis of inhaled antibiotic therapy showed a consistent sizeable effect of reducing the bacterial load by nearly 3 log units at 28 days [13]. Previous research has shown that bacterial load drives airways and systemic inflammation, and is linked to out-patient and in-patient exacerbations [5]. A reduction in bacterial load should therefore be of significant benefit to patients.

There has been considerable debate whether treatment should be intermittent (e.g. 28 days on and 28 days off) or continuous. Inhaled ciprofloxacin taken twice daily for 6 months (28 days on and off) in patients chronically infected with *Pseudomonas aeruginosa* improved time to next exacerbation in a per protocol analysis, but recent large RCTs have yielded conflicting results. The

largest international trial studied inhaled aztreonam three times daily for 4 months (28 days on and off) in patients predominantly chronically infected with *Pseudomonas aeruginosa*. Aztreonam reduced the bacterial load, but failed to reach its primary endpoint of improving respiratory symptoms in the Quality of Life Bronchiectasis questionnaire.

Trials for 6 months or longer have shown that continuous inhaled colomycin 1 MU twice daily for 6 months in patients chronically infected with *Pseudomonas aeruginosa* prolonged time to next exacerbation in patients who took their therapy 80% of the time or more. In a single-blind study, long-term nebulised gentamicin over 1 year (80 mg twice daily) in patients chronically infected with any potential pathogenic organism and two or more exacerbations annually improved time to next exacerbation and reduced overall exacerbations. There was also improved bacterial clearance, sputum colour, health-related quality of life, and exercise tolerance.

Currently we select patients with three or more exacerbations per year and chronic infection with *Pseudomonas aeruginosa* for continuous therapy with either inhaled colomycin or inhaled gentamicin.

Stepwise Approach to Management

Step 1 Pertinent to all patients with bronchiectasis. Treat underlying cause if identified. All should see a specialist respiratory physiotherapist to be taught airways clearance techniques + pulmonary rehabilitation if there is significant breathlessness. All should have an annual influenza vaccination and receive the pneumococcal vaccination. There should be prompt treatment for exacerbations. For exacerbations, a sputum sample should be sent for microbial culture and then empirically treatment started with oral antibiotics, and not await the culture results, as this would delay therapy. The antibiotics chosen should be based on previous microbiology and sensitivity results, or if not available, amoxicillin 500 mg three times daily. The BTS guidelines recommend 14 days antibiotics for all exacerbations [3] but the length of treatment can be reduced to 7 days in mild bronchiectasis. Some patients clinically respond despite *in vitro* resistance, so only failure to respond requires a change in treatment. Intravenous antibiotics are reserved for either deteriorating patients who have failed appropriate oral antibiotic therapy based on sensitivity testing, or have pathogens where there are no oral treatments available (for example in patients with *Pseudomonas aeruginosa* resistant to ciprofloxacin). Patients may respond despite *in vitro* resistance, so a brief trial of oral treatment should still be considered, but timely escalation to intravenous treatment should be considered if deteriorating. All patients should have a written self-management plan.

In a systematic review, patients with *Pseudomonas aeruginosa* had more exacerbations, worse health-related quality of life, increased hospitalisation, and increased mortality. There is ongoing debate whether there should be an attempted eradication of *Pseudomonas aeruginosa* on its first isolation. The reason for the debate is that isolation depends on frequency of testing, the culture method used, whether molecular methods are used, and the fact that in a proportion of patients *Pseudomonas aeruginosa* is intermittently isolated. If eradication is attempted, the optimal regimen is not known. A trial of eradication with oral ciprofloxacin is recommended for 14 days, and if this fails, to receive a 14-day course of an intravenous anti-pseudomonal antibiotic. Some centres will treat with an inhaled anti-pseudomonal antibiotic for 3 months.

Step 2 If patients have three or more exacerbations despite Step 1, it is key that patients are reassessed by the physiotherapist to check that they are carrying out regular chest physiotherapy, and there should be a consideration of a personalised trial of a muco-active treatment.

Step 3 If patients have three or more exacerbations despite Step 2, then starting a long-term antibiotic should be considered. The definition of chronic infection with a pathogen is the isolation of a pathogen two or more times in the preceding year whilst clinically stable. If patients are chronically infected with *Pseudomonas aeruginosa*, then a long-term inhaled anti-pseudomonal antibiotic or a long-term macrolide should be considered. If infected with other potential pathogenic bacteria, long-term macrolides or, alternatively, long-term oral or inhaled targeted antibiotics, are options. If no pathogen is identified, a long-term macrolide should be considered. Long-term macrolides should only be used if patients do not have environmental mycobacteria, as monotherapy would be contraindicated in such patients.

Step 4 If three or more exacerbations despite Step 3, consider combination therapy with a long-term inhaled antibiotic with a long-term macrolide. The hypothesis for using combination therapy is that macrolides may have anti-inflammatory properties and could therefore be additive to inhaled antibiotics.

Step 5 If there are five or more exacerbations despite Step 4, consider regular intravenous antibiotics every 2–3 months.

Major Complications of Bronchiectasis

Haemoptysis

Major haemoptysis more than 20 mL is a complicating factor, and often accompanies acute exacerbations. First-line therapy should be treating the exacerbation. If the major haemoptysis persists despite antibiotic therapy, bronchoscopy can localise the site of bleeding and bronchial angiography used to identify the ectatic bronchial arteries, which can then be embolised. This is now the first-line management for major haemoptysis in preference to surgical intervention.

Vascular Disease

There is increasing evidence that bronchiectasis is an independent risk factor for systemic vascular disease. In light of this, in patients with more advanced bronchiectasis, it seems sensible that attention is paid to modifiable risk factors such as smoking, hypertension, and hypercholesterolemia if present.

Respiratory Failure

This is managed using the same guidelines as for COPD. Long-term oxygen therapy for 15 h or longer is recommended in those that meet the requirements for long-term oxygen therapy. Non-invasive intermittent positive pressure ventilation (NIV) should be considered if there are recurrent admissions with acidosis or symptomatic carbon dioxide retention despite long-term oxygen therapy. Lung transplantation should follow international recommendations, but will require a double lung transplant. Patients considered are usually patients under the age of 60, those with recurrent infections, and respiratory failure requiring long-term oxygen therapy.

Management of the Deteriorating Patient

A deteriorating patient may present with significant and prolonged deterioration of symptoms, increased frequency or severity of exacerbations, frequent hospital admissions, early relapse after treatment of an exacerbation, or a rapid decline in lung function.

Assessment
- Ensure patient understanding
- Assess disease progression: oxygen saturations room air and arterial blood gases if appropriate; spirometry and consider lung volume and gas transfer measurement; CT Chest (contrast if pulmonary embolism suspected).
- Reassess pathogens: sputum C + S (routine bacteriology and fungal culture); three sputum samples for mycobacterial culture; If no sputum, consider induced sputum or broncho-alveolar lavage.
- Reassess aetiology: check specific aetiologies have been excluded, in particular cystic

fibrosis, allergic bronchopulmonary aspergillosis, gastro oesophageal reflux disease, common variable immunodeficiency and inflammatory bowel disease.
- Consider comorbidities: consider echocardiogram to assess LV function and for pulmonary hypertension; assess if have rhinosinusitis and whether treated; exclude pulmonary embolism if suspected.

Optimisation
- Airways clearance: check compliance; to see respiratory physiotherapist to check on optimum regimen ± pulmonary rehabilitation; consider muco-active treatment.
- Exacerbations: check patients are receiving prompt and appropriate antibiotics; check receiving correct antibiotic duration; check not meeting the requirements for intravenous antibiotic therapy.
- Assess oxygenation: give long term oxygen therapy if meets criteria.

Further Management
- Treat identified cause or underlying aetiology if found
- Consider intravenous antibiotic course
- Consider long term antibiotic
- Consider NIV
- Consider surgery: surgery is rarely carried out in bronchiectasis patients except in the context of a foreign body/endobronchial tumour with subsequent bronchiectasis. Surgery can be used in patients with localised disease unresponsive to medical therapy, but in practice this is very rare; consider transplantation
- Consider end-of-life care

Follow-Up

The following are indications for continuing secondary care managed by a multidisciplinary team led by a respiratory physician: patients with chronic *Pseudomonas aeruginosa* infection, opportunistic mycobacteria or MRSA; deteriorating bronchiectasis with declining lung function; three or more exacerbations a year; receiving long-term antibiotic treatment; bronchiectasis associated with rheumatoid arthritis, immune deficiency, inflammatory bowel disease, primary ciliary dyskinesia, ABPA; advanced disease and/or considering lung transplantation.

References

1. Quint JK, Millett ER, Joshi M, Navaratnam V, Thomas SL, Hurst JR, et al. Changes in the incidence, prevalence and mortality of bronchiectasis in the UK from 2004 to 2013: a population-based cohort study. Eur Respir J. 2016;47(1):186–93.
2. Loebinger MR, Wells AU, Hansell DM, Chinyanganya N, Devaraj A, Meister M, et al. Mortality in bronchiectasis: a long-term study assessing the factors influencing survival. Eur Respir J. 2009;34(4):843–9.
3. Pasteur MC, Bilton D, Hill AT. British Thoracic Society Bronchiectasis (non CF) Guideline Group. British Thoracic Society guideline for non-CF bronchiectasis. Thorax. 2010;65(Suppl 1):i1–58.
4. Ni Y, Shi G, Yu Y, Hao J, Chen T, Song H. Clinical characteristics of patients with chronic obstructive pulmonary disease with comorbid bronchiectasis: a systemic review and meta-analysis. Int J Chron Obstruct Pulmon Dis. 2015;10:1465–75.
5. Chalmers JD, Smith MP, McHugh BJ, Doherty C, Govan JR, Hill AT. Short- and long-term antibiotic treatment reduces airway and systemic inflammation in non-cystic fibrosis bronchiectasis. Am J Respir Crit Care Med. 2012;186(7):657–65.
6. Tunney MM, Einarsson GG, Wei L, Drain M, Klem ER, Cardwell C, et al. Lung microbiota and bacterial abundance in patients with bronchiectasis when clinically stable and during exacerbation. Am J Respir Crit Care Med. 2013;187(10):1118–26.
7. Chu H, Zhao L, Xiao H, Zhang Z, Zhang J, Gui T, et al. Prevalence of nontuberculous mycobacteria in patients with bronchiectasis: a meta-analysis. Arch Med Sci. 2014;10(4):661–8.
8. Martinez-Garcia MA, de Gracia J, Vendrell Relat M, Girón RM, Máiz Carro L, de la Rosa Carrillo D, et al. Multidimensional approach to non-cystic fibrosis bronchiectasis: the FACED score. Eur Respir J. 2014;43(5):1357–67.
9. Chalmers JD, Goeminne P, Aliberti S, McDonnell MJ, Lonni S, Davidson J, Poppelwell L, et al. The bronchiectasis severity index. An international derivation and validation study. Am J Respir Crit Care Med. 2014;189(5):576–85.
10. Wu Q, Shen W, Cheng H, Zhou X. Long-term macrolides for non-cystic fibrosis bronchiectasis: a systematic review and meta-analysis. Respirology. 2014;19(3):321–9.
11. Renna M, Schaffner C, Brown K, Shang S, Tamayo MH, Hegyi K, et al. Azithromycin blocks autophagy and may predispose cystic fibrosis patients to mycobacterial infection. J Clin Invest. 2011;121(9):3554–63.
12. Mandal P, Chalmers JD, Graham C, Harley C, Sidhu MK, Doherty C, et al. Atorvastatin as a stable treatment in bronchiectasis: a randomised controlled trial. Lancet Respir Med. 2014;2(6):455–63.
13. Brodt AM, Stovold E, Zhang L. Inhaled antibiotics for stable non-cystic fibrosis bronchiectasis: a systematic review. Eur Respir J. 2014;44(2):382–93.

Cystic Fibrosis

Daniel Peckham and Paul Whitaker

Introduction

Cystic Fibrosis (CF) is a multisystem disease characterised by recurrent lower respiratory tract infections, high sweat chloride, pancreatic insufficiency and male infertility. It is one of the most common life limiting genetically inherited conditions affecting Caucasians. It is an autosomal recessive disease with an incidence between 1:2000 and 1:90,000 births, varying between populations. In the UK, the incidence is about 1:2500 live births and the carrier frequency is 1:25.

With improvement in early diagnosis and treatment, many patients are living into adulthood and middle age. Median survival is around 40 years with median age at death being around 30 years [1]. Registry data shows that successive cohorts are progressively living longer, and it is anticipated that children born today will live well over 50 years. The introduction of effective new therapies which correct the underlying defect are likely to significantly change the long-term outlook.

The high prevalence of carrier status in the western hemisphere may be linked to selective advantages. For example, carrier status may provide partial protection from gastrointestinal infections such as cholera and typhoid and a reduced risk of salt and water depletion in more temperate climates. Studies have shown that cystic fibrosis transmembrane conductance regulator (CFTR) protein acts as a cellular receptor for the transport of *Salmonella typhi* across the intestinal wall and can be activated by cholera and bacterial enterotoxins.

Genetics

The CF gene was localised in 1985 to the long arm of chromosome 7. This was followed by identification of the gene sequence in 1989, which encoded a 1480 amino acid protein called the cystic fibrosis transmembrane conductance regulator [2]. The first mutation to be identified was p.Phe508del, which occurs in 75% of patients with CF in the UK. It results from a three base-pair deletion in exon 10 of the CFTR gene, resulting in the omission of phenylalanine at position 508, resulting in abnormal folding, retention in the endoplasmic reticulum, and degradation of the CFTR protein.

Over 2000 mutations have now been identified, with only a handful being responsible for the majority of cases of CF. CFTR mutations are now categorised into seven classes according to the mechanisms by which they produce quantitative or qualitative changes in CFTR function (Fig. 12.1).

D. Peckham (✉) · P. Whitaker
Leeds Centre for Respiratory Medicine,
St James's University Hospital, Leeds, West Yorkshire, UK
e-mail: D.g.peckham@leeds.ac.uk

© Springer International Publishing AG, part of Springer Nature 2018
S. Hart, M. Greenstone (eds.), *Foundations of Respiratory Medicine*,
https://doi.org/10.1007/978-3-319-94127-1_12

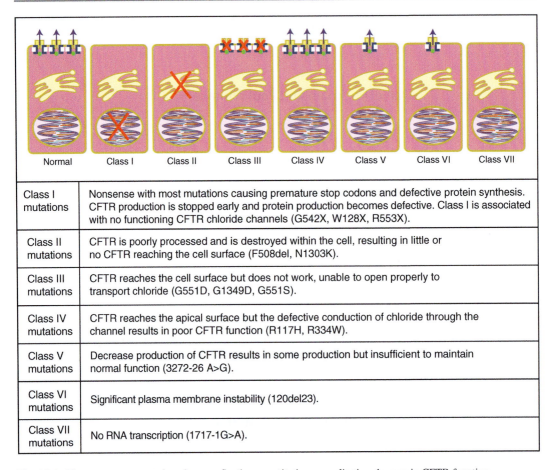

Class I mutations	Nonsense with most mutations causing premature stop codons and defective protein synthesis. CFTR production is stopped early and protein production becomes defective. Class I is associated with no functioning CFTR chloride channels (G542X, W128X, R553X).
Class II mutations	CFTR is poorly processed and is destroyed within the cell, resulting in little or no CFTR reaching the cell surface (F508del, N1303K).
Class III mutations	CFTR reaches the cell surface but does not work, unable to open properly to transport chloride (G551D, G1349D, G551S).
Class IV mutations	CFTR reaches the apical surface but the defective conduction of chloride through the channel results in poor CFTR function (R117H, R334W).
Class V mutations	Decrease production of CFTR results in some production but insufficient to maintain normal function (3272-26 A>G).
Class VI mutations	Significant plasma membrane instability (120del23).
Class VII mutations	No RNA transcription (1717-1G>A).

Fig. 12.1 There are seven mutation classes reflecting quantitative or qualitative changes in CFTR function

The Cystic Fibrosis Transmembrane Conductance Regulator

The CFTR protein is an ATP-binding cassette transporter that functions as a ligand-gated anion channel. It comprises two membrane-spanning domains and two nucleotide binding domains separated by a regulatory domain. The two membrane-spanning domains form a low conductance chloride channel which is regulated by the binding and hydrolysis of ATP at the nucleotide binding domains following initial phosphorylation of the R domain. CFTR conducts chloride and bicarbonate and regulates sodium and water absorption across the airway epithelium.

The presence of the CFTR protein throughout the body including the lung, submucosal glands, pancreas, liver, sweat ducts, and reproductive tract explains the multisystem nature of CF. The amount of functioning CFTR appears to be related to clinical status with some "milder" mutations presenting with congenital absence of vas deferens with or without mild respiratory disease. However, the spectrum of mutations in the CFTR gene gives rise to variable clinical phenotypes that may not be predictable from the genotype alone, due to the influences of other factors such as the environment and modifier genes. It has been hypothesised that less than 10% of functioning CFTR results in mild phenotypes, while absent expression causes "classical" disease. Variation in CFTR function can exist within the same genotype, and this may have implication for phenotype. For example, CFTR expression in nasal p.Phe508del epithelium appears to correlate with lung disease. A more personalised, functional assay of CFTR has recently been developed using epithelial organoids from the intestine. This model can assess CFTR function between individuals and assess personalised responses to different drug therapies.

Pathophysiology

Mucus clearance is a primary defence mechanism in the human airways and acts as a physical barrier and escalator for removing inhaled microorganisms and particles from the lower airways. In healthy lungs, ciliary movement is protected by a periciliary layer of fluid with the tips of the cilia just touching the mucus layer. As the cilia beat, they move the mucus layer towards the pharynx.

CFTR is situated in the apical airway epithelial cell membrane where it functions as a chloride and bicarbonate channel and a regulator of other channels. In CF there is an absence or reduction in chloride and bicarbonate efflux and up-regulation of sodium absorption across the epithelial sodium channels (ENaC). Studies in mouse models with heightened ENaC activity have shown features which are similar to those seen in CF lung disease, supporting the role of abnormal sodium and water transport in CF airways.

The airway epithelium in CF exhibits a combination of defective chloride and bicarbonate secretion and increased sodium absorption (Fig. 12.2) that leads to a loss of the osmotic equilibrium, dehydrated airway surface liquid

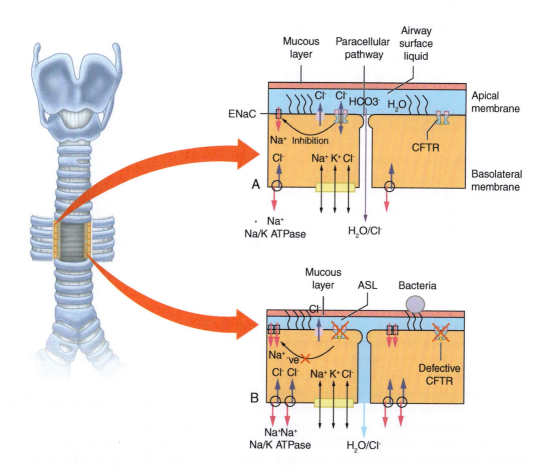

Fig. 12.2 (**a**): normal airways epithelium showing normal CFTR channel function and negative inhibition of sodium absorption. (**b**) CF airway epithelium (Class III) with defective CFTR function, reduced airway surface liquid height and pH, and increase sodium and water absorption

(ASL), and predisposes the lung to chronic pulmonary infection and bronchiectasis.

These changes alter the biophysical properties of mucus, reduce the depth of airway surface liquid, and impair mucociliary clearance. Reduced bicarbonate secretion will also decrease ASL pH and impairs the bacteria-killing ability of naturally occurring antimicrobial peptides.

Infection and Inflammation

Defective CFTR function is associated with increased bacterial adhesion and loss of bacterial internalization. Bacterial colonization promotes auto-inflammation and triggers a perpetuating cycle of infection and inflammation, which result in lung damage and progressive bronchiectasis. This neutrophil-driven inflammatory response is associated with high levels of cytokines such as interleukin (IL)-8, IL-1β, IL-6, IL-17, IL18, and tumour necrosis factor-alpha, which increase neutrophil recruitment into the lungs. Lung damage develops as a result of leakage of neutrophil proteases, oxygen radicals, and DNA. In particular, neutrophil elastase destroys the proteins involved in maintaining the structural integrity of the lungs, as well as inactivating molecules such as complement and IgG that are important in phagocytosis of bacteria. DNA released from dying neutrophils increases sputum viscosity and leads to oxidative stress.

Sweat Glands

In 1953 following a heat wave in New York, an excess number of patients with CF were noted to have developed heat prostration. This phenomenon led to the discovery by both Darling and Di Sant Agnes that CF patients had a high sodium and chloride concentration in sweat. The sweat test has now become a gold standard diagnostic test for CF worldwide. Sweat chloride concentration is also used as a biomarker of CFTR activity in clinical trials and to monitor adherence to new therapies such as ivacaftor.

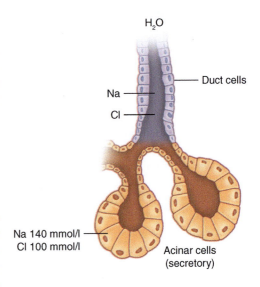

Fig. 12.3 The sweat gland

The abnormality in sweat ion concentration occurs following defective absorption of chloride and, secondarily, sodium from the sweat duct (Fig. 12.3). Unlike respiratory epithelium, the ducts are impermeable to water absorption and in healthy individuals will result in sweat excretion, which is hypotonic to the plasma.

CFTR in Other Organs

CFTR is expressed throughout the intestinal tract and plays a key role in chloride and bicarbonate secretion. Abnormal CFTR function leads to mucosal dehydration, defective CFTR-dependent bicarbonate secretion and abnormal formation and release of mucus from the gut. The successful creation of CF animal models including the mouse, pig, and ferret has provided great insight into the pathophysiology of CF. For example, it had been presumed that the high incidence of CF-related diabetes was solely related to pancreatic endocrine damage. More recent data from the CFTR-knockout ferret model has shown abnormal insulin secretion prior to the development of structural pancreatic damage. This reflects the role of CFTR in the normal regulation of glucose-induced insulin secretion.

Learning Points

- Cystic Fibrosis (CF) is one of the most common life-limiting, genetically inherited conditions affecting Caucasians.
- The CF gene is localised on the long arm of chromosome 7 and encodes a 1480 amino acid protein called the cystic fibrosis transmembrane conductance regulator (CFTR).
- Over 2000 mutations have been identified, with only a handful being responsible for the majority of cases
- CFTR mutations are now categorised into seven classes according to the mechanisms by which they produce quantitative or qualitative changes in CFTR function.
- Defective CFTR expression in the airways results in a reduced depth of airway surface liquid, altered biophysical properties of mucus, and impaired mucociliary clearance.
- In CF, defective CFTR function results in reduced or absent Na and Cl absorption, which results in excessive salt concentrations.
- Abnormal CFTR function leads to mucosal dehydration, defective CFTR-dependent bicarbonate secretion, and abnormal formation and release of mucus from the gut.
    CFTR is involved in regulating glucose-induced insulin secretion.

Diagnosis

A diagnosis of CF is made from the clinical picture in combination with a high sweat chloride and/or two positive CF-causing mutations. If genetic mutations cannot be documented, the diagnosis must be supported by two sweat test results. In the event of equivocal results, nasal or rectal electrophysiological measurements can be undertaken.

Screening

In the UK all babies are offered screening for CF using the standard heel prick test to measure immunoreactive trypsinogen (IRT), which is ele-vated two to fivefold in the blood of affected newborns [3]. Elevated IRT occurs in response to trypsin leakage from the pancreas into the blood. While the test is sensitive, it is not specific enough to make a diagnosis of CF. If the first IRT test is equal to or above the 99.9th centile then a second IRT test is undertaken on a repeat dried blood spot at day 21. A positive second IRT will trigger mutation analysis using a panel of the four most common alleles. If a subject is identified as a carrier, then further mutation analysis is undertaken against a larger panel of mutations. Despite screening, a small proportion of patients with CF will remain undiagnosed until adulthood. These late diagnosis are often, but not always, associated with pancreatic sufficiency and milder mutations.

Sweat Test

The measurement of sweat sodium (Na) and chloride (Cl) electrolyte concentrations has long been the mainstay of diagnosis of CF [4]. The procedure should be undertaken by qualified individuals who regularly do the test. Sweat testing should not be undertaken before 2 weeks of age, to avoid a false-positive test. Sweat testing should be delayed in subjects who are dehydrated, underweight, or systemically unwell. Older patients often report developing salt deposits on the skin surface after intense exercise and/or heat exposure (Fig. 12.4). False-positive sweat

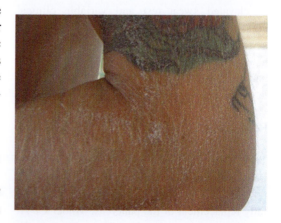

Fig. 12.4 Salt crystals on the surface of the skin

tests can occur in various conditions, including Shwachman-Diamond syndrome.

A sweat chloride concentration over 60 mmol/l is characteristic of CF, and the chloride concentration is usually higher than sodium. A sweat chloride between 30 and 60 mmol/l is equivocal and is associated with milder genotypes [5]. The Cystic Fibrosis Foundation (CFF) consensus regards a sweat chloride which is less than 40 mmol/l as being normal as long as the individuals are over 6 months of age. A normal sweat test can occur rarely in patients with CF .

Mutations

Over 2000 CF causing mutations have been identified. The diagnosis is initially based on screening using a panel of up to 50 of the most common CFTR mutations, which will vary according to patient's ethnicity. Extended mutation analysis can be undertaken at reference centres if further characterisation is required. Some mutations will have variable expression, such as R117H, which is influenced by the polythymidine sequence of intron 8. The presence of R117H + p.Phe508del on a background of 5T is associated with elevated or borderline sweat test, moderate lung disease, pancreatic exocrine sufficiency, and male infertility. In contrast, R117H/ p.Phe508del in association with 7T is associated with a normal, borderline, or elevated sweat test and variable clinical presentation.

Extended genetic screening should be undertaken in family members, including siblings and partner, especially prior to conception.

Pancreatic Function

The majority of patients with CF are pancreatic insufficient; ultrasound and computed tomography will demonstrate increased echogenicity and fatty replacement of the pancreas. Milder CFTR mutations are associated with pancreatic suffi-

ciency. Pancreatic status can be assessed by measuring faecal elastase in the stool, and the test is unaffected by enzyme therapy. The test can also be used to monitor the onset of pancreatic insufficiency in pancreatic sufficient patients.

Lung Function

The typical lung function picture is obstructive with reduced Forced Expiratory Volume in 1 s (FEV1) and FEV1/FVC ratio. There is often significant small airways disease with a reduced FEF 25–75. Lung function tends to decline by 2–3% each year, although this varies significantly between patients and birth cohorts. Increased variation and decline in lung function is seen in patients with poor adherence. Large sudden falls in lung function are also seen following segmental and or total lobar collapse due to retained secretions, usually associated with allergic bronchopulmonary aspergillosis (ABPA).

Radiology

The characteristic chest X-ray changes of CF include accentuated bronchial markings, small ring shadows, nodular shadows, and more extensive confluent consolidation (Fig. 12.5a–c). The CXR is an insensitive marker of mild disease and seldom reflects severe lung involvement and disease progression.

Computed tomography (CT) is a lot more sensitive in identifying progression and characterising the extent of mucus plugging, bronchiectasis, and gas trapping (small airways disease), as seen in Fig. 12.5. CT is also used to guide bronchoscopy and help identify atypical infection in patients not responding to conventional treatment.

Fleeting shadows, mucus impaction, tree in bud, and segmental or lobar collapse are seen in ABPA.

Features of echogenic bowel on antenatal ultrasound can be associated with a diagnosis of CF and should trigger further investigations.

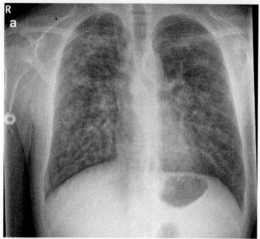

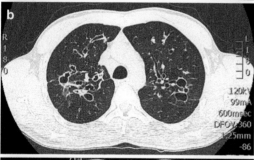

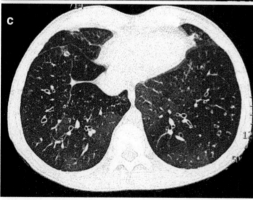

Fig. 12.5 (**a–c**) Radiological features of cystic fibrosis. (**a**) CXR: Extensive bronchiectasis in a patient with cystic fibrosis. P.A.S port in right arm. (**b**) Chest computed tomography demonstrating extensive cystic bronchiectasis. (**c**) Chest CT demonstrating bronchiectasis with marked air trapping reflecting small airways disease (black areas)

Semen Analysis

The majority of male patients with CF are infertile. Screening for azoospermia should be considered in difficult diagnoses. A minority of men with CF are fertile, especially those with the 3849-10 kb C-T mutation. Therefore it is essential that sperm analysis is routinely offered in conjunction with reproductive health education.

Nasal Potential Difference and Intestinal Current Measurements

Nasal potential difference (NPD) and intestinal current measurements using Ussing chambers can be used to characterise CFTR function in patients with milder phenotypes where the diagnosis is uncertain [6]. NPD is more commonly used, and examines the different ion channels involved in transepithelial ion transport. The procedure involves introducing a small catheter into the nose with the tip positioned along the nasal floor or inferior turbinate. Following baseline measurements, responses of the various channels can be measured in response to topical infusions of amiloride (ENAC blocker), chloride free solution (increases CFTR Cl efflux), isoprenaline (stimulates cAMP mediated CFTR Cl efflux), and ATP (non CFTR Cl channel efflux) (Fig. 12.6). In CF the baseline nasal PD is significantly more negative, with a greater inhibition by amiloride and little or no response to chloride-free and isoprenaline solutions.

Learning Points

- A diagnosis of cystic fibrosis is made from the clinical picture, in combination with two positive CF-causing mutations and /or two high sweat chloride levels.
- Neonatal screening is now part of the routine heel prick test and uses immunoreactive trypsinogen with or without DNA analysis.
- A small proportion of patients with CF remain undiagnosed until adulthood.
- A sweat chloride concentration >60 mmol/l is characteristic of CF. Levels between 30 and 60 mmol/l are equivocal and occur in patients with milder mutations.

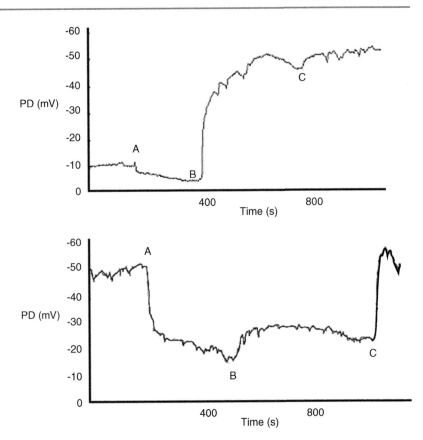

Fig. 12.6 A nasal PD profile of a control (top) and CF subject (bottom). The baseline PD is higher in CF due to two to threefold increase in sodium absorption across the cells. A: PD falls following addition of the ENAC blocker amiloride. B: CFTR efflux following addition of low chloride solution followed by isoprenaline. C: perfused with ATP which activates non CFTR Cl channels. The response is heightened in CF

- The majority of patients with CF are pancreatic insufficient, which can be assessed using faecal elastase in the stool.
- CT a sensitive tool for identifying progression and characterising the extent of mucus plugging, bronchiectasis, and gas trapping.
- The majority of male patients with CF are infertile. Semen analysis can be a useful diagnostic tool in more complicated cases.
- Nasal potential difference and intestinal current measurements are used to characterise CFTR function in patients with milder phenotypes where the diagnosis is uncertain.

Clinical Features

CF is a multisystem disease and the diverse signs and symptoms reflect the presence of CFTR throughout the body (Table 12.1, Fig. 12.7). Increased survival has also given rise to new challenges in CF care, including the emergence

of complications such as diabetic vasculopathies, renal failure, and malignancy.

Respiratory Tract

CF is characterised by repeated respiratory tract infections, airway inflammation, progressive bronchiectasis, and small airway disease. Pulmonary disease accounts for the majority of morbidity and mortality, with respiratory failure accounting for 85% of deaths. During the early stages of disease, patients are often asymptomatic with little clinical evidence of the disease, but bronchoscopy and CT surveillance studies in asymptomatic infants have demonstrated evidence of early airway inflammation, infection, and lung damage.

The progression of respiratory symptoms is associated with finger clubbing, chest hyperinflation, and bronchiectasis. Clinical signs can

Table 12.1 Examples of clinical manifestations seen in patients with cystic fibrosis

Body organ	Common manifestations
Lung	Bronchiectasis
	Repeated respiratory tract infections
	Haemoptysis
	Pneumothroax
	Allergic bronchopulmonary aspergillosis
	Aspergillus bronchitis
	Aspergilloma
	Respiratory failure
Nose and sinuses	Nasal polyps
	Chronic sinusitis
	Epistaxis
Liver	Fatty liver/elevated liver function test
	Focal biliary cirrhosis
	Biliary strictures and lithiasis
	Gallbladder disease
	Portal hypertension
	Oesophageal varices
Bowel	Gastro-oesophageal reflux
	Gastroparesis
	Small bowel overgrowth
	Meconium ileus
	Distal intestinal obstruction syndrome
	Intussusception
	Volvulus
	Fibrosing colonopathy
	Rectal prolapse
	Inflammatory bowel disease
	Malignancy
Pancreas	Pancreatic insufficiency
	Pancreatitis
	Pseudocyst
Reproductive	Male infertility
	Amenorrhea
	Delayed puberty
Bone/joints	Osteoporosis
	Hypertrophic osteoarthropathy
	Fractures
	CF related arthritis
Metabolic	Pseudo Bartter's syndrome
Central nervous systems	Chiari I malformation

include coarse crepitations and wheeze. Wheeze may be due to concomitant asthma or as a result of mucus retention, endobronchial inflammation, ABPA, or aspiration. It is not infrequent for wheeze to resolve following physiotherapy and intravenous antibiotic therapy. With disease progression, the prevalence of pneumothorax and haemoptysis increases.

Nasal symptoms are very common as a result of nasal polyps, rhinitis, and chronic sinusitis.

Infections

Pulmonary exacerbations in patients with CF accelerate deterioration of lung function and cause increased morbidity and mortality. Viral infections are common in both children and adults, and are frequently associated with pulmonary exacerbations. Rhinovirus is by far the most common virus isolated, and in adults may result in a heightened inflammatory response and worse clinical outcome [7]. The second commonest virus is influenza, highlighting the importance of annual flu vaccination.

Both viral and bacterial infections, with *Staphylococcus aureus* and *Haemophilus influenzae*, predominate in younger children. Chronic colonisation with *Pseudomonas aeruginosa* is common in many patients by their late teens, although this can be delayed by effective surveillance and intense treatment of the first isolate. *P. aeruginosa* is ubiquitous, with the majority of acquisitions occurring from environmental sources, although multiple transmissible strains have been reported. It is associated with an increase in pulmonary exacerbations and significant morbidity and mortality. Most cases of chronic infection with *P. aeruginosa* involve the mucoid form, which produces a large amount of a polysaccharide. This mucoid matrix allows the creation of protected biofilm microcolonies, which make the bacteria more resistant to killing, and is associated with a worse prognosis and a more rapid decline in lung function [8]. Lung damage is largely a result of the host inflammatory response to *P. aeruginosa* and other infections. Chronic *P. aeruginosa* infection can be defined according to the Leeds Criteria, where positive isolates occur in more than 50% of months in the previous 12-month period.

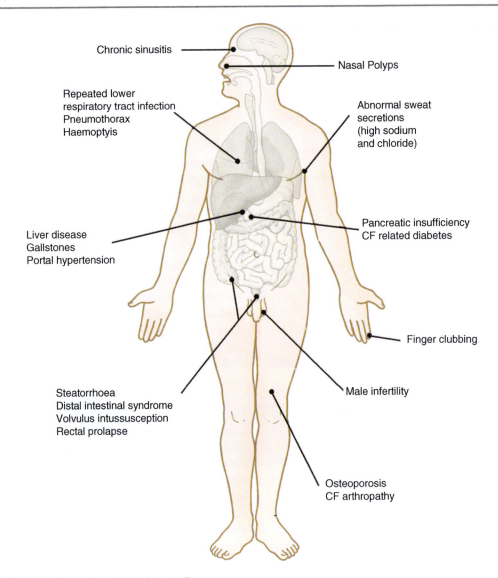

Chronic sinusitis

Nasal Polyps

Repeated lower
respiratory tract infection
Pneumothorax
Haemoptyis

Abnormal sweat
secretions
(high sodium
and chloride)

Liver disease
Gallstones
Portal hypertension

Pancreatic insufficiency
CF related diabetes

Finger clubbing

Steatorrhoea
Distal intestinal syndrome
Volvulus intussusception
Rectal prolapse

Male infertility

Osteoporosis
CF arthropathy

Fig. 12.7 Cystic fibrosis is a multisystem disease

Other opportunistic bacteria associated with evolution of airway disease in CF include methicillin-resistant *Staphylococcus aureus* (MRSA) and gram-negative bacteria including the various genomovars of the *Burkholderia cepacia* complex, *Achromobacter xylosoxidans*, *Stenotrophomonas maltophilia*, and *Pandoraea apista*. Polymerase chain reaction and deep sequencing has further changed our understanding of the CF microbiome, leading to the identification of numerous organisms not previously isolated, including the anaerobes and *Streptococcus milleri*. Within the microbiome, complex interactions between organisms takes place. For example *P. aeruginosa* can suppress the growth and virulence of other bacteria such as *Burkholderia multivorans*, *Burkholderia cenocepacia*, and *Pandoraea apista*.

The *Burkholderia cepacia* complex (BCC) is a group of gram-negative organisms that established themselves as major pathogens in the 1980s as a result of both misidentification and poor infection control. Cross-infection became a major problem, with some centres having a colonisation rate of up to 40%. The commonest genomovars to affect patients with CF are *B. multivorans* and *B. cenocepacia*. They are highly transmissible bacteria and usually resistant to multiple antibiotics. *B. cenocepacia* is associated with the highest mortality [9] and is a contraindication to lung transplantation.

Stenotrophomonas maltophilia is a gram-negative bacillus first identified in CF sputum in the 1970s. It is acquired from environmental sources, and *in vitro* sensitivities show that this is a highly resistant organism. Using data from the CFF patient registry Goss et al. found that patients acquiring *S. maltophilia* are in general older, female, and have worse baseline lung function. Chronic colonisation is present in 12.5% of patients with CF. Studies do not show an increased mortality with *S. maltophilia,* but there is a significantly increased risk of pulmonary exacerbation compared to a non-*S. maltophilia* cohort.

Achromobacter xylosoxidans is an aquatic gram-negative bacillus. It can cause chronic colonisation, although much less commonly than *P. aeruginosa* and *S. maltophilia.* Acquisition can result in a more rapid decline in pulmonary function and a more pronounced inflammatory response.

Nontuberculous Mycobacteria

There has recently been an increased prevalence of nontuberculous mycobacteria (NTM) in the CF population. This may reflect patient-to-patient transmission, more intensive sampling, the use of long-term macrolide antibiotics, and intensive antibiotic usage. The commonest NTM in patients with CF are *Mycobacterium abscessus* complex and *Mycobacterium avium* complex (MAC). Infection can be transient, and the diagnosis must be confirmed as per the ATS/IDSA criteria. The subspecies of *M. abscessus* have different levels of virulence, and infection can herald a more rapid decline in lung function, increased mortality, and a relative contraindication to lung transplantation. Management is

challenging, with limited evidence to support treatment options.

Fungus

There is a high prevalence of fungal colonisation and infection in patients with CF. *Aspergillus fumigatus* remains the most common fungal species and can be isolated in up to 58% of sputum samples. The fungus results in a spectrum of conditions ranging from hypersensitivity to frank infection. These include bronchopulmonary aspergillosis (ABPA), aspergillus bronchitis, aspergilloma, and in post-transplant recipients, invasive aspergillosis. ABPA is due to an IgE mediated hypersensitivity reaction that leads to wheeze, mucus plugging, and pulmonary infiltrates on chest X-ray. It can be identified by elevated total IgE (> 500 IU/ml), eosinophilia, and elevated specific antibodies against *A. fumigatus.* Corticosteroids are the mainstay of ABPA treatment although anti-fungal drugs may reduce the antigen load and be steroid sparing. Aspergillus bronchitis is a term which refers to patients who have respiratory symptoms, an elevated Aspergillus IgG, and *A. fumigatus* in their sputum but do not meet the criteria for ABPA. This is more of a subacute infection where *A. fumigatus* acts as a pathogen and symptoms often respond to anti-fungal drugs without the need for steroids. Unfortunately, immunology can be difficult to interpret in fungal disease in CF, and treatment trials with clinical and physiological monitoring are often needed.

Other fungi such as *Scedosporium apiospermum* and *S. exophiala* have also been implicated in pulmonary exacerbations.

Gastrointestinal Tract

A combination of pancreatic malabsorption and abnormal secretions can lead to partial or complete bowel obstruction of the intestinal lumen. In younger patients this can lead to rectal prolapse and intussusception. Some patients suffer from constipation, and up to 10% of older patients suffer distal intestinal obstruction syndrome

(DIOS). It is more common in patients who had previous meconium ileus and more severe mutations. In DIOS patients present with progressive colicky abdominal pain, nausea, and anorexia. This is due to either partial or complete bowel obstruction due to an accumulation of viscous mucofaeculant material in the terminal ileum and ascending colon. Fortunately, most patients can be managed by hydration and high doses of laxatives. On abdominal examination a palpable faecal mass can sometimes be felt, even in asymptomatic individuals. Patients with CF have an increased risk of volvulus, bowel obstruction secondary to adhesions, and GI malignancy.

Pancreas

CFTR is expressed in the pancreatic ducts, where it facilitates the transport of chloride and bicarbonate and facilitates fluid secretion. Defective CFTR results in physiological changes causing fatty replacement of the pancreas, fibrosis, and reduced exocrine parenchyma. Approximately 95% of patients in Northern Europe are pancreatic insufficient. This is due to acinar damage and atrophy following obstruction of the pancreatic ducts. Pancreatic insufficiency is related to genotype, and some patients with milder mutations can remain pancreatic sufficient. Loss of exocrine function leads to loose fatty stools, abdominal discomfort, weight loss, and deficiency of fat-soluble vitamins. Patients who are pancreatic insufficient are treated with pancreatic enzyme supplements. Patients who are pancreatic sufficient may present with acute or chronic pancreatitis.

Cystic Fibrosis-Related Diabetes

The prevalence of CF-related diabetes (CFRD) increases with age, and affects up to 50% of adults. It is a result of pancreatic destruction and CFTR dysfunction. Early diagnosis and intervention with insulin has a profound impact on patient well-being and survival, and patients over 13 years of age should undergo routine screening with OGTT, HbA1c, and/or blood glucose moni-

toring. Impaired glucose tolerance is common and reflects both structural damage and the role of CFTR in the normal regulating of insulin secretion. CFRD is distinct from Type 1 and Type 2 diabetes, and in the absence of screening can be heralded by significant decline in lung function and weight several years before diagnosis. CFRD is associated with complications such as retinopathy, nephropathy, and neuropathy.

Liver

CF liver disease is the third commonest cause of death after pulmonary disease and complications of transplantation. CFTR is expressed in cholangiocytes and gallbladder epithelial cells, and plays an important role in bile duct secretion. It is not expressed in hepatocytes and other liver cells. The CFTR contributes to Cl/HCO_3 exchange and, when defective, results in dehydrated secretions and plugging of intrahepatic ducts leading to focal biliary cirrhosis. Liver disease is usually diagnosed in childhood, especially in the first decade of life, although it can rarely present in adulthood. The prevalence of liver disease is estimated to be around 40% in children at 12 years of age. Of those children with liver disease, around 20% have features suggestive of cirrhosis and portal hypertension. For severe liver disease, liver transplantation is considered, but benefits need to be weighed against the risk of surgery.

Biliary manifestations are seen in 5–33% of patients and include abnormalities of intra- and extrahepatic bile ducts, gallbladder thickening and contraction, micro gallbladder, and cholelithiasis. Biliary tract abnormalities are found in up to 50% of patients, and 25% have asymptomatic gallstones or atrophic gallbladders.

Renal

Hyperoxaluria, nephrocalcinosis, and nephrolithiasis occur relatively commonly in patients with CF. The incidence of renal stones ranges from 2 to 6.3% and results from pancreatic insufficiency, intestinal malabsorption, and a reduction in the levels of *Oxalobacter formigenes* in the gut flora following antibiotic therapy. With improved survival, drug-induced acute and chronic kidney injury is becoming more prevalent. It results from the frequent use of drugs such as the aminoglycosides.

Fertility

Almost all men with CF are infertile as a result of obstructive azoospermia, but sexual performance remains unaffected. Women with CF are fertile, but the increase thickness of cervical mucus can make conception difficult. FEV1 of more than 60% predicted is generally accepted as an indicator that pregnancy will not adversely affect the woman's health.

Osteoporosis and Joint Disease

CF is associated with an increased incidence of osteoporosis, osteopenia, and fractures. The aetiology of low bone density is multifactorial, and relates to a combination of inadequate peak bone mass during puberty and increased bone losses in adults. Risk factors include hypogonadism, delayed puberty, CFRD, lung disease, malabsorption, and relative inactivity. It is now recognised that CFTR itself plays an important part in bone formation and regeneration. As a result, most centres undertake routine screening for reduced bone mineral content by dual energy X-ray absorptiometry.

Learning Points

- Lung disease accounts for the majority of morbidity and mortality in patients with CF, with respiratory failure accounting for 85% of deaths.
- Airway inflammation, infection, and lung damage occurs in asymptomatic infants.
- Viral infections are common in both children and adults, occurring in up to 40–60% of pulmonary exacerbations.

- *Staphylococcus aureus* and *Haemophilus influenzae* predominate in younger patients, with chronic *Pseudomonas aeruginosa* infection increasing with age.
- Up to 10–20% of patients will develop distal intestinal obstruction syndrome.
- Approximately 95% of patients are pancreatic insufficient. The diagnosis can be confirmed by measuring stool faecal elastase.
- CF-related diabetes occurs in up to 50% of adults. Early diagnosis and insulin therapy have a profound impact on patient well-being and survival.
- CF liver disease is the third commonest cause of death after pulmonary disease and complications of transplantation.
- Nephrolithiasis occurs relatively commonly in patients with CF.
- There is an increased incidence of osteoporosis, osteopenia, and fractures

Management

Treatment of CF is aimed at protecting the airways through early and effective intervention to reduce disease progression. This involves a multidisciplinary approach, including close monitoring combined with conventional therapies such as pancreatic replacement, nutritional support, regular aerobic exercise, physiotherapy, mucolytics, antibiotics, and psychosocial support. This holistic approach has proved successful in improving quality of life and long-term outcome. Key treatments are discussed below.

Physiotherapy

Chest physiotherapy with regular airway clearance is an important part of the treatment of CF. Commonly used approaches include autogenic drainage, active cycle of breathing, positive expiratory pressure masks, and vibrating vest. The techniques used should be guided by patient preference, as adherence is often poor. Regular aerobic exercise can also improve lung function and self-image, but is complementary to physiotherapy and is not an alternative. Noncompliance results in retained secretions, which in some cases leads to segmental atelectasis and lobar collapse.

Mucolytics

Infected bronchial secretions in patients with CF become viscous and difficult to clear, partly because of the presence of high levels of extracellular DNA released by degrading leucocytes. These long strands of DNA can be broken up using once-daily nebulized rhDNase. Treatment is safe, well established, and effective for patients with CF, and should be considered first-line in patients with mild, moderate, and severe respiratory disease [10]. A formal trial should be undertaken with pre- and post-lung function to ensure that it is well tolerated and does not cause bronchospasm. Treatment is associated with reduced pulmonary exacerbations and improved lung function, downregulation of airway inflammation, and helps preserve small airway function in children with good lung function. A dose of 2.5 mg is nebulised daily, not less than an hour before chest physiotherapy. While there is no evidence that increasing the dose achieves greater therapeutic effect, it is sometimes administered twice daily as a short-term measure, with intense physiotherapy for patients with very tenacious secretions and an acute pulmonary exacerbation. Direct installation into the segmental bronchi at bronchoscopy can be undertaken in cases of resistant lobar or segmental collapse due to retained secretions.

Nebulised hypertonic saline temporarily increases the hydration of airway surface liquid by increasing the ion concentration in the ASL and osmotically drawing fluid into the airway lumen. Inhalation aids mucus clearance by stimulating large shear stresses and promoting the separation of mucus plaques from the airway walls. Treatment results in a sustained increase in mucociliary clearance, a slight increase in respiratory function, less frequent respiratory exacerbations, and improved quality of life [11].

Mannitol works as an osmotic agent drawing water into the ASL. Initial concerns regarding the sugary nature of mannitol encouraging bacterial growth have not been demonstrated in clinical trials. Inhaled mannitol is an alternative therapy but its relative efficacy against other mucolytic therapies is unclear.

Respiratory Infections

Antibiotics remain the mainstay of treatment and are used to treat, prevent, eradicate, and control pulmonary infection.

Acute Infections

If new respiratory symptoms do not settle after oral antibiotics, then treatment with intravenous antibiotics is recommended. It is important to remember that significant new infection may be present even when careful listening with the stethoscope does not reveal any new added sounds in the chest, and in the absence of any new chest X-ray changes. There may be only a persistent or new cough. Neglect of early signs and symptoms may result in permanent damage to the respiratory tract and the onset of a slowly progressive deterioration in respiratory function.

Respiratory exacerbations are loosely defined in terms of more breathlessness, increased cough, change in sputum colour to more yellow or green, changes on chest X-ray, and loss of appetite and weight.

Common signs and symptoms of exacerbations include:

- Increased productive cough
- Increased breathlessness
- Change in sputum colour or volume
- Poor appetite
- Fever
- New signs on respiratory examination
- New radiological signs, indicating infection

The initial choice of antibiotics depends on the bacterial sensitivity pattern, although there is dispute about whether *in vitro* laboratory sensitivities equate to *in vivo* activity. Treatment is usually for 2 weeks, and a combination of two classes of antibiotics is usually used in an attempt to reduce resistance and improve outcome. In patients with chronic *P. aeruginosa,* a 2-week course of a beta-lactam (piperacillin-tazobactam, ceftazidime, meropenem, aztreonam) with either tobramycin or colistin is often prescribed.

Staphylococcus aureus

Recurrent or persistent isolation of *S. aureus* in routine throat swabs or sputum is usually treated with long-term oral antibiotics (flucloxacillin) at least for the first few years of life. Some units treat all patients from diagnosis with antistaphylococcal antibiotics, reducing the need for hospitalisation and improving clinical status in early life. Others treat each staphylococcus isolate with a course of oral antibiotics.

Pseudomonas aeruginosa

P. aeruginosa causes chronic persistent infection requiring regular administration of intravenous antibiotics for episodes of respiratory exacerbations. Although oral antibiotics are useful in the early stages of *Pseudomonas* infection, resistance often occurs rapidly, and intravenous antibiotics are then the only alternative. Regular elective intravenous antibiotics were recommended in the 1980s, when they were shown to significantly improve 5-year survival for patients with chronic *P. aeruginosa* infection. Many centres have moved away from routine therapy in an attempt to reduce the risks of hypersensitivity reactions, toxicity (renal function, hearing, balance), and the emergence of resistance.

Current treatment guidelines recommend that all patients with chronic *P. aeruginosa* should receive long-term inhaled anti-pseudomonas antibiotic therapy, as long as the drugs are tolerated. The aim is to suppress infection and reduce the decline in lung function and number of pulmonary exacerbations. The inhalation route has the added benefit of delivering the drug at high concentrations while minimizing systemic toxicity. The launch of dry powder tobramycin and colomycin for inhalation provides a speedy alternative to nebulization. Inhaled antibiotics are also used in the long-term management of *Burkholderia cepacia* complex, *Achromobacter,* and *Mycobacterium abscessus* infection.

Inflammation

Chronic inflammation in the lung develops following repeated infective exacerbations and chronic infection. Certain classes of drugs have been shown to have anti-inflammatory and immunomodulatory properties. Despite an incomplete understanding of the underlying mechanism of actions, several agents including high-dose NSAIDs, steroids, macrolides, and leukotriene antagonists are routinely used in clinical practice to slow down the progression of CF-related lung disease. NSAIDs are not routinely used in the UK due to the high adverse effect profile and risk of renal disease. Even low-dose NSAIDs should be avoided in combination with aminoglycosides and colistin.

The macrolides are a group of antibiotics which have been widely used in CF as conventional antibiotics and anti-inflammatory agents. Macrolide use in CF was stimulated by the success of long-term erythromycin in the treatment of diffuse panbronchiolitis (DPB), a condition that shows some similarities to CF in that it is associated with chronic sinusitis, mucoid *P. aeruginosa* colonisation, and bronchiectasis. Several large multi-centre studies have demonstrated that macrolide therapy can result in fewer courses of intravenous antibiotics, improvement or maintenance of lung function, reduction in median CRP levels, and improvement in quality-of-life scores [12]. Patients receiving long-term azithromycin show an increased prevalence of macrolide-resistant strains of *S. aureus* and *H. influenzae*. Macrolides have been associated with prolongation of cardiac repolarisation, and a baseline ECG is advised to exclude a prolonged QT interval. There is little data on long-term use of macrolides and whether the described benefits are maintained.

Pancreatic Enzyme Replacement Therapy (PERT)

The majority of patients with CF have pancreatic malabsorption and will require routine pancreatic enzyme replacement therapy. Appropriate pancreatic enzyme replacement should be given and reviewed regularly. In infants and children, high-dose pancreatic enzyme supplements have been associated with colonic strictures, but there does not seem to be a similar risk in adults. Due to individual variation in dose requirements, treatment should be titrated according to fat intake and gastrointestinal symptoms, including stool frequency and consistency. The total dose of enzymes should not usually exceed 10,000 IU lipase/kg/day due to the potential risk of fibrosing colonopathy. Pancrease HL and Nutrizym 22 should be avoided in children aged 15 and under.

Fat-Soluble Vitamins

Pancreatic insufficiency leads to malabsorption of fat-soluble vitamins. Supplements of the fat-soluble vitamins such as vitamin A, D, and E are therefore required by most patients with CF. There are different preparations, and doses should be titrated according to fasting blood levels. Vitamin A deficiency is associated with night blindness and xerophthalmia and may play an import role as an antioxidant and affect mucus secretion. Fasting blood levels should be measured annually together with zinc, retinal binding protein, and C-reactive protein to aid accurate interpretation. Vitamin D deficiency is associated with rickets, osteomalacia, and low bone mineral density. Vitamin K deficiency is associated with a prolonged prothrombin time and increased risk of bleeding. The majority of individuals with Vitamin K deficiency will have a normal clotting, and subclinical presentation may be associated with the development of CF-related low bone mineral density, but further studies are needed.

Liver Disease

Patients with abnormal liver function tests and hyperechogenicity on ultrasonography are usually given ursodeoxycholic acid with or without taurine due to the increased demand of the latter for bile acid conjunction. This hydrophilic bile acid improves liver function tests and may reduce progression of CF-related liver disease. It is important to recognise that even in established cases of cirrhosis, serum liver enzymes may be completely normal. Early consideration/referral of liver transplantation for patients with severe liver cirrhosis should be considered. Portal hypertension and oesophageal varices and should be treated conventionally.

Nutrition

Patients who are well nourished have better outcomes. The energy requirements of patients with CF vary widely, and generally increase with age and disease severity. Poorly controlled absorption of dietary fat and increased energy expenditure both increase energy requirements. To meet energy needs, all patients should be seen regularly by a dietitian experienced in the management of CF, who will monitor growth and tailor dietary advice to the individual. Dietary fat is not generally restricted as this nutrient is essential to achieve a good calorie intake. Changes in dietary advice are likely to occur over the next decade, as patient survival increases and new risk factors develop. In patients with inadequate weight gain or poor appetite, dietary supplements should be considered as they will help improve energy intake. Some patients will still be unable to achieve or maintain adequate energy intake, and in these cases, early intervention with more invasive forms of nutritional support such as nasogastric or gastrostomy feeding should be considered.

CF-Related Diabetes

Insulin therapy is the treatment of choice in CFRD and is associated with improved respiratory function and nutritional status [13]. Many patients only show significant hyperglycaemia after meals, and ketoacidosis does not tend to occur unless there is underlying type 1 diabetes. All patients should receive individualised dietary review and advice at the time of the diagnosis of CFRD. They should usually maintain a high-energy diet, and the insulin dose should be tailored to their individual requirements. They should not have a low-carbohydrate diet, but should be encouraged to eat regular meals with appropriate carbohydrate content each day.

Distal Intestinal Obstruction Syndrome

DIOS is a relatively common complication of CF, and can present with nonspecific abdominal discomfort, right iliac fossa (RIF) pain, or symptoms mimicking other pathologies such as acute appendicitis. There is often tenderness with or without a faecal mass in the RIF. The symptoms are often recurrent and can be related to dehydration and poor adherence to pancreatic enzyme supplementation. Patients presenting with acute DIOS should be kept well hydrated, given appropriate analgesia, and treated with high-dose oral Gastrografin or a balanced electrolyte solution such as Klean-Prep. This can be administered either orally or via nasogastric tube. *N*-acetylcysteine can also be used as an additional therapy with the aim of breaking up the inspissate. If symptoms do not improve, or signs of peritoneal irritation or complete obstruction develop, then a surgical opinion should be sought without delay. In refractory cases either caecostomy with manual evacuation and right hemicolectomy and partial small bowel resection are needed.

Bone Disease

CF is associated with an increase incidence of osteoporosis, osteopenia, and fractures. It is important to ensure that patients with CF take adequate exercise, and have good nutritional status, with appropriate calcium, vitamin D, and vitamin K supplementation.

Routine screening with dual energy X-ray absorptiometry should be undertaken in combination with annual fasting and checking vitamin levels from around the age of 8–10 years, and repeated every 1–5 years, according to the BMD Z-score. In addition, annual bone densitometry should be considered in patients who are prescribed continuous systemic glucocorticoids [14].

Treatment should be guided by published guidelines, which are likely to change over time. It is presently suggested that bisphosphonate should be considered in adults with a lumbar spine or total hip or femoral neck Z-score ≤ -2 and significant bone loss on serial DXA measurements. Bisphosphonates have been associated with osteonecrosis of the jaw, and it is important to discuss this with the patient and ensure dental review.

Contraception

Women with CF should be given advice about safe and effective contraception, and pregnancy should always be planned. The high-dose combined oral contraceptive pill is often used.

Haemoptysis

Patients with mild haemoptysis are often treated with a short course of tranexamic acid. Large bleeds or recurrent medium volume bleeds may require embolization.

Lung Transplantation

Lung transplantation should be considered when patients enter the end stages of the disease and there is less than 50% predicted 2-year survival. In patients with CF, no single clinical parameter can accurately predict survival, but FEV_1 is the most frequently used variable. Increased hospitalisations, reducing exercise capacity, pulmonary hypertension, and progressive hypoxia/hypercapnia are all signs of end-stage disease. There are many contraindications for transplant, including severe osteoporosis, poor nutrition, renal impairment, and chronic infection with highly virulent organisms. At present, *B. cenocepacia* and *M. abscessus complex* are absolute contraindications. Following lung transplantation there is around 50% survival at 10 years.

New Therapies

The past decade has delivered scientific breakthroughs which have resulted in new effective therapies for correcting CFTR dysfunction [15]. These discoveries are the result of investment in high-throughput screening of hundreds of thousands of chemical compounds for activity against CFTR. Several small molecules have now been discovered, two of which have entered clinical practice. The first compound to get FDA approval was ivacaftor (Kalydeco®) which is a potentiator of class III (gating) mutations. Treatment is associated with a dramatic reduction in sweat chloride and pulmonary exacerbations, a greater than 10% improvement in lung function, and improved quality of life and nutritional status.

More recently, combination therapy of ivacaftor (corrector) plus lumacaftor (potentiator) (Orkambi®) was approved by the FDA in the U.S. for the treatment of patients homozygous for p.Phe508del. The p.Phe508del mutation has a class II and III defect and required a corrector so that it can be expressed in the membrane and a potentiator to stimulate function. Treatment with Orkambi® is associated with a modest improvement in lung function and reduction in pulmonary exacerbations [16]. Phase 2 trials using triple-combination therapy (tezacaftor, ivacaftor with VX-659 or VX-445) have recently been completed in patients heterozygous for one copy of the p.Phe508del and a second mutation with minimal CFTR function. Treatment was associated with a significant fall in sweat test and an increase in mean absolute change in percent predicted FEV1 of >13%. Multiple new trials are ongoing using CFTR correctors and potentiators. Placebo-controlled trials using cationic liposomes to transfer plasmid DNA encoding the CFTR gene into the lungs of patients with CF showed a modest improvement in lung function. This proof of concept study is the start of a series of trials to deliver more effective gene therapy.

Learning Points

- Treatment of CF is aimed at protecting the lung, reducing complications, and treating infections and inflammation before significant lung damage has occurred.
- A multidisciplinary approach is essential, and includes regular monitoring in combination with conventional therapy including pancreatic replacement, nutritional support, regular aerobic exercise, physiotherapy, mucolytics, antibiotics, and psychosocial support.
- DNase remains a safe, well-established, and effective treatment for patients with CF and should be considered first-line in patients with mild, moderate, or severe respiratory disease.
- Early and appropriate intervention with intravenous antibiotics is key, as neglecting early signs and symptoms may result in permanent damage to the respiratory tract and the onset of a slowly progressive deterioration in respiratory function.
- Low-dose macrolides are widely used in the treatment of CF for their anti-inflammatory properties. Long-term outcome data are needed.
- Good nutrition and early treatment of CF-related diabetes can have profound impact on morbidity and mortality.
- The introduction of CFTR potentiator drugs for class 3 gating mutations heralds a new era of transformational medicine. Phase 3 trials for class 2 mutations are ongoing.

References

1. Elborn JS, Bell SC, Madge SL, Burgel PR, Castellani C, Conway S, et al. Report of the European Respiratory Society/European Cystic Fibrosis Society task force on the care of adults with cystic fibrosis. Eur Respir J. 2015;47(2):420–8. https://doi.org/10.1183/13993003.00592-2015. PubMed PMID: 264536.

2. Kerem B, Rommens JM, Buchanan JA, Markiewicz D, Cox TK, Chakravarti A, et al. Identification of the cystic fibrosis gene: genetic analysis. Science. 1989;245(4922):1073–80. PubMed PMID: 2570460.

3. Green A, Isherwood D, Pollitt R. A laboratory guide to newborn screening in the UK for cystic fibrosis. 4th ed. London: UK National Screening Committee; 2014.

4. Farrell PM, Rosenstein BJ, White TB, Accurso FJ, Castellani C, Cutting GR, et al. Guidelines for diagnosis of cystic fibrosis in newborns through older adults: Cystic Fibrosis Foundation consensus report. J Pediatr. 2008;153(2):S4–S14. PubMed PMID: 18639722. Pubmed Central PMCID: PMC2810958.

5. Mayell SJ, Munck A, Craig JV, Sermet I, Brownlee KG, Schwarz MJ, et al. A European consensus for the evaluation and management of infants with an equivocal diagnosis following newborn screening for cystic fibrosis. J Cyst Fibros. 2009;8(1):71–8. PubMed PMID: 18957277.

6. De Boeck K, Derichs N, Fajac I, de Jonge HR, Bronsveld I, Sermet I, et al. New clinical diagnostic procedures for cystic fibrosis in Europe. J Cyst Fibros. 2011;10(Suppl 2):S53–66. PubMed PMID: 21658643.

7. Flight WG, Bright-Thomas RJ, Tilston P, Mutton KJ, Guiver M, Morris J, et al. Incidence and clinical impact of respiratory viruses in adults with cystic fibrosis. Thorax. 2014;69(3):247–53. PubMed PMID: 24127019.

8. Courtney JM, Bradley J, McCaughan J, O'Connor TM, Shortt C, Bredin CP, et al. Predictors of mortality in adults with cystic fibrosis. Pediatr Pulmonol. 2007;42(6):525–32. PubMed PMID: 17469153.

9. Jones AM, Dodd ME, Govan JR, Barcus V, Doherty CJ, Morris J, et al. Burkholderia cenocepacia and Burkholderia multivorans: influence on survival in cystic fibrosis. Thorax. 2004;59(11):948–51. PubMed PMID: 15516469. Pubmed Central PMCID: 1746874.

10. Yang C, Chilvers M, Montgomery M, Nolan SJ. Dornase alfa for cystic fibrosis. Cochrane Database Syst Rev. 2016;4:CD001127. PubMed PMID:27043279.

11. Nolan SJ, Thornton J, Murray CS, Dwyer T. Inhaled mannitol for cystic fibrosis. Cochrane Database Syst Rev. 2015;10:CD008649. PubMed PMID: 26451533.

12. Principi N, Blasi F, Esposito S. Azithromycin use in patients with cystic fibrosis. Eur J Clin Microbiol Infect Dis. 2015;34(6):1071–9. PubMed PMID: 25686729.

13. Koloušková S, Zemková D, Bartošová J, Skalická V, Šumník Z, Vávrová V, et al. Low-dose insulin therapy in patients with cystic fibrosis and early-stage insulinopenia prevents deterioration of lung function: a 3-year prospective study. J Pediatr Endocrinol Metab. 2011;24(7–8):449–54. PubMed PMID: 21932580. English.

14. Sermet-Gaudelus I, Bianchi ML, Garabedian M, Aris RM, Morton A, Hardin DS, et al. European cystic fibrosis bone mineralisation guidelines. J Cyst Fibros. 2011;10(Suppl 2):S16–23. PubMed PMID: 21658635.

15. Ramsey BW, Davies J, McElvaney NG, Tullis E, Bell SC, Dřevínek P, et al. A CFTR potentiator in patients with cystic fibrosis and the G551D mutation. N Engl J Med. 2011;365(18):1663–72. PubMed PMID: 22047557. Pubmed Central PMCID: PMC3230303.

16. Wainwright CE, Elborn JS, Ramsey BW, Marigowda G, Huang X, Cipolli M, et al. Lumacaftor-Ivacaftor in patients with cystic fibrosis homozygous for Phe508del CFTR. N Engl J Med. 2015;373(3):220–31. PubMed PMID: 25981758.

Mycobacterial Disease

13

Anda Samson and Hiten Thaker

Introduction

Tuberculosis (TB) has been affecting humans for thousands of years. Mankind is the only known reservoir for the disease, although animals can get infected. The disease may affect any dense community, will smolder amongst people living in poorly ventilated circumstances, and will flourish in the malnourished and weak.

TB infections decreased in the developed world as a consequence of better hygiene and nutrition; even before the discovery of *Mycobacterium tuberculosis* (MTB) infection in 1882, infection rates dropped. The discovery of streptomycin in the 1940s led to the world's first known randomised controlled trial. The development of para-amino salicylic acid (PAS) and combination therapy shortly after caused a paradigm shift in the treatment of tuberculosis; sanatoria and healthy food were replaced largely by antibiotic treatment. This subsequently caused a further reduction in tuberculosis cases in the UK and other developed countries.

However, despite being greatly reduced in wealthier nations, TB is far from eradicated. In developing countries, active TB is a major cause of death, especially since the global HIV epidemic. Recent estimates state about one in four people in the world have latent TB, [1] just under the 20-year-old WHO estimate of 1 in 3 [2]. In the UK there are around 6500 new TB cases per year, which is still one of the highest rates in Western Europe. The current TB case load in the UK is a reflection of global patterns; more than two-thirds of people diagnosed with active TB originate in high-prevalence countries, and another 10% of cases are people who have risk factors that might make them more vulnerable to falling ill with TB such as malnutrition, homelessness, or imprisonment [3]. The rest may be part of localized epidemics, or people with decreased immunity.

Since the late 1990s treatment-resistant TB strains have become a worldwide problem. Multi-drug-resistant TB (MDR-TB) and extensively-drug-resistant TB (XDR-TB) are major public health threats. This chapter intends to give practical guidance on the treatment of TB in adults; for the treatment of MDR-TB it is recommended to seek expert advice.

A. Samson (✉) · H. Thaker
Department of Infection, Hull and East Yorkshire Hospitals, Castle Hill Hospital, Cottingham, East Yorkshire, UK
e-mail: annette.samson@hey.nhs.uk

© Springer International Publishing AG, part of Springer Nature 2018
S. Hart, M. Greenstone (eds.), *Foundations of Respiratory Medicine*,
https://doi.org/10.1007/978-3-319-94127-1_13

Current Thinking on TB Immunology

Immunity to *M. tuberculosis* has largely been thought to be related to the activity of macrophages and cells of the adaptive immune system (CD4+ and CD8+ T lymphocytes) in the control of mycobacteria. Failure of this causes dissemination in the primary stage of disease. In addition to these adaptive mechanisms, innate immune responses are also involved in both the early and late responses to MTB. The concept that granuloma formation is a host-protective structure has changed, and granulomas are now actually seen as dynamic structures that may allow the mycobacteria to replicate and spread to other locations.

There appear to be two phases of immunological activity in the granuloma. The early stages of mycobacterial infection are dominated by the innate immune system, with increased macrophage accumulation (via TNF) as a consequence of mycobacterial replication. The subsequent adaptive phase involves IFN-γ-producing or polyfunctional (IL-2, IFN-γ and TNFα) CD4+ and CD8+ T lymphocytes and leads to the control of MTB replication. This process is also influenced by a number of other cells, including NK (natural killer) cells, regulatory CD4+ T cells (Tregs), and Th1 (T helper 1) CD4+ T cells. The CD4+ and CD8+ T cells produce high levels of TNF, and NK cells produce IFN-γ. Interaction of mycobacteria with TLR2 (toll-like receptor 2) on NK cells may directly affect entry of mycobacteria in the lung tissue.

The transition from latency to post-primary tuberculosis is a poorly understood process, with multiple non-mutually exclusive mechanisms contributing to exit from latency in infected individuals. Among any cohort of latently infected subjects, it is impossible to predict who will fall in the 10% that eventually will experience reactivation, but two clinical scenarios are well known. The first is when there is a depletion of CD4+T cells (e.g. during HIV infection), and the second is represented by impairment of TNF signaling (e.g. biological agents for rheumatoid arthritis). TLR-2 and TLR-9 polymorphisms are also asso-

ciated with an increased risk of TB in different populations, possibly due to attenuation of NK cell activation.

Diagnostic Testing

Tuberculin Skin Test and Interferon-γ Release Assays

The tuberculin skin test (TST) and Interferon-γ Release Assay (IGRA) tests rely on IFN-γ release from antigen-specific T-lymphocytes when re-exposed to MTB antigens. These tests do not distinguish between active and latent TB infection, and a positive result does not accurately predict progression to active tuberculosis. Moreover, in severely immunocompromised patients, patients with overwhelming tuberculosis infection or smear negative tuberculosis, IGRAs as well as TST may fail in the diagnosis of TB infection. Their use is therefore not recommended as the sole investigation for the diagnosis of active tuberculosis. Diagnosis, if clinically suspected, should be pursued by aggressive sampling, cultures, biopsies, and imaging.

Tuberculin Skin Test

During tuberculin skin testing a small amount of antigenic components of MTB (tuberculin) is injected intradermally. In patients previously exposed to TB, a T-cell mediated delayed-type hypersensitivity reaction will occur at the injection site. Ideally, the size of the resulting skin induration is measured 72 h after injection [4]. A positive TST will also occur in patients who have received BCG vaccination (a live attenuated mycobacterial strain derived from *M. bovis*) in childhood, but TST positivity tends to wane over time. Current UK guidelines thus consider any cutaneous response of 5 mm or more to be positive, regardless of BCG vaccination status [5]. It had been presumed that larger TST results correlated with active disease, but recent data challenge this presumption [6].

False positive results may occur due to prior vaccination with BCG, or due to cross-reaction with non-tuberculous mycobacteria. Because the TST it is cheap and does not require laboratory facilities, it is still used widely in low- and middle-income settings. Efforts are underway to produce a new TST unaffected by prior BCG vaccination.

Anergy can occur in a number of cases where immunity is compromised, including overwhelming active TB infection [7]. It is estimated that in up to 25% of microbiologically confirmed TB cases, the TST is negative. Those patients appear to be the more severe cases and have a higher likelihood of succumbing to their TB infection.

IGRA Testing

IGRAs measure the amount of interferon released from blood leukocytes when mixed with mycobacterial antigens. IGRAs require a single blood sample and produce a standardized, non-operator dependent result. They appear to be more sensitive than TST in detecting latent TB in most settings [8].

There are currently two types of commercially available IGRA test; Quantiferon-Gold™ and T-SPOT®.*TB*™. Quantiferon-Gold uses a standardized amount of blood and is less labour-intensive. T-SPOT®.*TB* uses a standardized number of peripheral blood mononuclear cells, giving this test a theoretical advantage in immunocompromised patients.

Lateral Flow Lipoarabinomannan Assay

The lateral flow lipoarabinomannan assay (LF-LAM) is a urine test for the presence of lipoarabinomannan, a glycolipid antigen from the MTB cell wall. Urine LAM testing may be a valuable and rapid adjunct to available tuberculosis testing tools in HIV-positive individuals with low CD4 counts who are seriously ill [9]. In other patients, LF-LAM sensitivity and specificity are too low to be used in daily practice; this includes ambulatory patients established in HIV care [10].

Acid-Fast Stains and Cultures

Sputum cultures are the cornerstone of TB diagnostics, but any material can be sent for TB culture. The first step in identifying MTB is conventional microscopy

using Ziehl-Nielsen or dark field electron microscopy using Auramine stains. Sensitivity of stains for detecting MTB in sputum in pulmonary TB infection is around 50–65%. Severely ill patients with TB are often unable to self-expectorate sputum, and may need sputum induction, or alternative invasive sampling such as bronchoscopy, to acquire material for diagnostic testing. Sensitivity of staining in other samples, such as CSF, tissue, or ascitic fluid can be much lower, ranging from 10% to 80% depending on sample site.

Definite diagnosis occurs after a positive mycobacterial culture. Because of the relatively slow growth of mycobacteria, it will take at least a week for colonies to form, but it is not unusual for a positive sample to emerge after 4–6 weeks of incubation.

Clear instructions for patients for sputum sample collection procedures are important for accurate TB diagnosis [11]. If not instructed well, saliva rather than sputum may be sampled, leading to false-negative results. In TB high-endemic settings the number of patients needed to screen in an in-patient population to find one case of active TB is less than ten, regardless of a patient's HIV status [12]. In reality, even in high-endemic settings, many more samples are needed to identify a case of TB [11]. Many simple and visual instruction cards are available readily and freely online.

Nucleic Acid Amplification Tests (NAAT)

Molecular methods can detect mycobacteria with high specificity by amplifying target DNA using methods based on polymerase chain reaction (PCR). The most commonly used assay is genXpert™ but there are several others available. The assays detect dead as well as live bacteria. Less than 200 bacilli per mL of sputum are needed for the NAAT to detect acid fast bacilli compared to 10,000 in microscopic examination.

The sensitivity for detecting mycobacterial DNA in smear-positive sputum samples is 95–98% which is close to that of culture, and can yield a result in about 90 min. Smear-negative but culture-positive sputum samples show a lower sensitivity of 68%. The sensitivity of NAAT in sputum samples from patients who are co-infected with TB and HIV is close to that in sputum samples from HIV-negative patients.

For the detection of spinal TB, NAAT showed a sensitivity of 70–96% and specificity of 96% in CSF samples. The World Health Organization recommends NAAT over conventional stain tests for diagnosis of TB in lymph nodes and other tissues, and as the preferred initial test for diagnosis of TB meningitis [13]. In specimens with a lower bacterial load, such as pleural or pericardial fluid, NAAT sensitivity drops to below 40%.

Chest Imaging

Standard chest-X ray is still a mainstay of TB diagnosis, and computed-tomography (CT) scanning provides additional detail. Upper lobe infiltrates and pulmonary cavities are the classic signs of pulmonary tuberculosis (Fig. 13.1a–d). Although previously deemed to be a sign of reactivation disease, these upper lobe infiltrates can also occur in primary disease. Some patients show a parenchymal infiltrate, making it difficult to distinguish from conven-

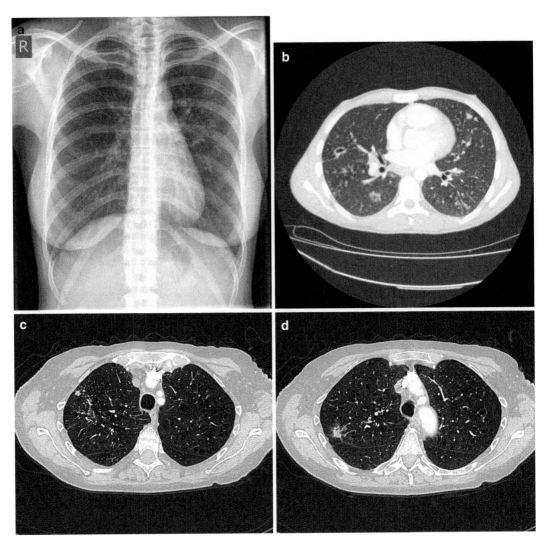

Fig. 13.1 (a–d) Reactivated TB. Examples of secondary (reactivated) pulmonary TB. (a) Focal left upper lobe infiltrate on chest-ray with patchy consolidation without visible cavitation. (b) Cavities and endobronchial disease on CT. Cavitation is a characteristic feature of reactivated TB and should immediately arouse suspicion of that diagnosis. A branching tree-in-bud pattern results from bron-chiolar inflammation and dilatation, is common in many infections including TB (as in this case). In larger airways, tuberculous granulomatous inflammation may progress to bronchial stricture and distal atelectasis. (c, d) Multifocal right upper lobe infiltrate on CT with a wide differential diagnosis including lung cancer, and which was confirmed as TB

tional bacterial pneumonia [14]. In patients with impaired immunity for any reason, adenopathy, effusion, or mid lower lung zone infiltrates or a miliary pattern (Fig. 13.2a, b) are more common. Around one-third of patients will develop a radiological scar after primary infection (Fig. 13.3) [14].

In patients with cavitation but without clear infiltrate on the chest X-ray, differentiation between active and old disease can be challenging. CT scan may be helpful in differentiating between the two, since it may detect early bronchogenic spread in active disease. Typical findings include a centrilobular branching linear structure, defined

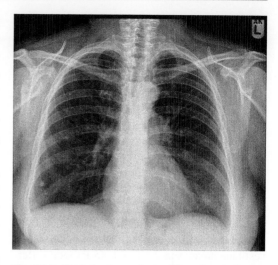

Fig. 13.3 Healed primary focus (Ghon focus). Healed primary tuberculosis, appearing as multifocal calcified scars in the right lung. The focus of primary tuberculosis is often unifocal, and may heal without trace, but calcified nodules or scars occur in about one-fifth of patients. Hilar (and sometimes mediastinal) lymphadenopathy is a very common radiological feature at the time of primary infection, and may resolve or leave hilar node calcification

small centrilobular peribronchiolar nodules, acinar shadows, and lobar consolidation. Patients with thoracic lymphadenopathy may be diagnosed by endobronchial ultrasound examination (EBUS) sampling. Preliminary data suggest that sonographic evidence of central necrosis in the lymph nodes favours tuberculosis over sarcoidosis [15].

In patients presenting with lymphadenopathy, PET-CT may be an additional aid in distinguishing between active disease and latent disease; metabolically active lymph nodes in a TB patient indicate active disease. The limitation of PET in this patient group is the inability to distinguish between infection and malignancy. Because PET-CT is very sensitive in detecting active TB, it may be used as a monitoring tool to assess treatment response, particularly during the treatment of MDR-TB or XDR-TB patients.

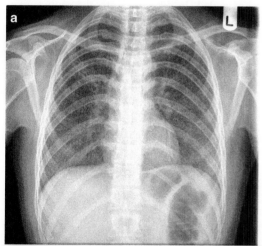

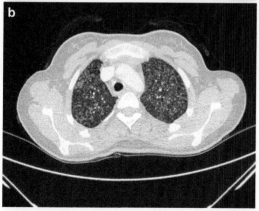

Fig. 13.2 (**a, b**) Miliary TB. Miliary pulmonary tuberculosis, appearing on a chest X-ray (panel **a**) and CT scan (**b**) as widespread multiple small (2–3 mm) granulomas. The millet seed radiological pattern only becomes apparent when the granulomas reach a certain size, and some patients with miliary TB will have a normal chest X-ray. Miliary TB may complicate either primary or reactivated disease. Whilst there are other causes of miliary nodulation on X-ray, TB should be the primary concern

Transmission of TB

Transmission of TB has resulted from airborne droplets not only from respiratory infections, but also droplets from drainage of abscesses, from third-space fluids (pleural and peritoneal), and organisms colonising the mouth. Even solid clinical waste can potentially produce an airborne risk. There is clear evidence that expectorated pathogens from a patient's room can contaminate susceptible individuals outside. Therefore, directional airflow control by negative pressure is recommended (particularly for MDR-TB) so that the airflow is directed from clean zones outwards through 'dirty' zones. This airflow from clean to dirty areas should be sufficient to overcome the escape of air, particularly when enhanced by the presence of ante-rooms. Most negative-pressure clinical areas are designed to provide around 2–15 Pa of negative pressure between neutral and vestibule areas, and 2.5 to 40–45 Pa total difference between neutral areas and patient rooms. Air control of the isolation area is also assisted by adequately engineered ventilation that allows 12–25 air changes per hour in the room.

Pulmonary Tuberculosis

The route of transmission of tuberculosis is in almost all cases through inhalation of aerosols. This can result in primary pulmonary tuberculosis, or in latent infection. Primary pulmonary TB typically presents with upper zone infiltrates on chest X-ray, as seen in Fig. 13.1, but can present as a common bacterial pneumonia, or with a miliary (disseminated) pattern, shown in Fig. 13.2.

Infections that do not cause primary TB often lead to a so-called Ghon complex—a small area of granulomatous inflammation with an associated lymph node that may be detected on a chest X-ray if calcified or large enough (see Fig. 13.3). Typically, these complexes appear in the upper zones of the lungs. They may contain dead or still-viable mycobacteria, and can thus be a source of reactivation later in life, which happens in around 10% of cases.

The presenting symptoms of pulmonary TB, primary or secondary, include cough, weight loss, night sweats, chest pain, increased sputum production, and hemoptysis. Occasionally, patients may present with severe hemoptysis when the infection erodes into a large pulmonary vessel. However, some patients have very few symptoms. Treatment usually improves symptoms rapidly, but may take a few months in those with a very heavy burden of disease.

In general, patients with pulmonary TB are infectious. Current UK guidelines recommend 2 weeks of isolation for those who are producing sputum that is positive for acid–fast bacilli (smear positive). It is generally recommended to repeat sputum testing until two negative samples have been produced, as a measure of treatment success. However, smears may not become negative in some patients with very large cavities, and this does not necessarily mean that treatment needs to be extended. In other patients, the sputum may convert to smear-negative after a few weeks of treatment, but the culture may remain positive. This is usually a sign of early treatment success.

Some patients may present with a large TB pleural effusion only, and this is considered to be a form of extrapulmonary TB. Immunocompromised patients or patients with advanced TB infection may present atypically, or with a miliary pattern on their chest X-ray. This is considered a sign of disseminated TB.

Extra-Pulmonary TB

Around one-fifth to one-half of TB in developed countries is extra-pulmonary. Although the overall incidence of tuberculosis in high-income countries is declining, the annual incidence of extra pulmonary TB is remarkably stable, with a notification level rate around 4/100,000 in Europe [16]. Since most cases originate from haematogeneous spread, tuberculosis can reactivate in any organ. The most common sites of extra-pulmonary disease are pleural (36%), lymph nodes (20%), bone, central nervous system, and gastro-intestinal tract. Although occasional transmission through aerosolisation of pus or needle stick incidents have been described, in general, patients with extra-pulmonary TB are not contagious. However, pulmonary involvement always needs to be ruled out, and each TB patient needs a full workup including a chest-X-ray and sputum cultures.

Lymph Node TB

Virtually all lymph nodes can be affected in TB infection. When biopsying a lymph node, enough tissue should be taken to provide a histological as well as a microbiological sample, and if lymphoma is in the differential diagnosis, a whole lymph node should be removed for diagnostic purposes. If this is not the case, fine-needle aspirates are a less-invasive and effective alternative.

Lymph nodes biopsies or aspirates may show a granulomatous pattern or acute inflammation. Stains for acid fast bacilli are not very sensitive in lymph node samples (perhaps only 30%). Diagnosis of TB lymphadenitis is often made on a combination of a positive screening test, histological pattern, and either culture or NAAT. The sensitivity of NAAT is around 70% in FNA aspirates and 43% in histological biopsies. NAAT can be performed on paraffinised tissue using special techniques; sensitivity is around 90% in tissue that is smear positive; it is much lower in smear-negative samples.

TB Meningitis/Tuberculoma

Lumbar puncture in the case of tuberculous meningitis will typically show a clear CSF with a raised protein count, with a normal to raised white cell count and a normal or decreased glucose concentration. Typically there is a predominance of lymphocytes, however, neutrophils can predominate, especially early in the course of CNS infection, and the CSF/serum glucose ratio can be normal. NAAT of CSF has a high sensitivity and is now recommended by WHO over the use of stains for the diagnosis of tuberculous meningitis [17]. However, despite a higher sensitivity, it is not 100%, and negative NAAT does not exclude tuberculous meningitis. MRI of the brain can aid in diagnosing TB meningitis; visibility of the meninges pre-contrast is highly suggestive of TB. Parenchymal lesions may appear as plaques—homogeneous, uniformly enhancing, dural-based masses.

Non-tuberculous Mycobacteria

Non-tuberculosis mycobacteria (NTM) is a term reserved for mycobacterial species other than *Mycobacterium tuberculosis* complex and *Mycobacterium leprae*. NTM are ubiquitous organisms found in water and soil, and can cause infections in lung, sinus, lymph node, joint, CNS, and disseminated infection. NTM, when infecting the lung, can cause lung disease or sometimes be asymptomatic. Pulmonary disease (NTM-PD) may be fibro-cavitary or nodular. NTM are divided into slow-growing and rapid-growing species. The most common species causing lung infection are the slow-growing *M. avium* complex (MAC; consisting of *M. avium*, *M. intracellulare*, and *M. chimaera*), *M. kansasii*, *M. malmoense*, and *M. xenopi*, and the rapid-growing *M. abscessus*, *M. chelonae*, and *M. fortuitum*. Currently there is an increasing incidence of NTM infections worldwide, but more so in the resource-rich settings. This may be due to a number of reasons including reduced incidence of MTB, more contact with shower aerosols, and increased use of antibiotics and immunosuppressive treatments. Host susceptibility factors seem to be primarily associated, including impaired mucociliary clearance in patients with chronic lung diseases. Other risk factors include co-morbidities such as gastro-oesophageal reflux, rheumatoid arthritis, and immunodeficiency states.

The mechanism of transmission remains unclear, but there is growing evidence through whole genome sequencing that although person-to-person spread is unlikely, spread may be possible through fomites and long-lived infected aerosols.

The diagnosis is based on ATS/IDSA criteria for NTM-PD. A patient must have characteristic symptoms, compatible radiology, and two or more positive sputum samples of the same NTM species, or one positive bronchial wash/lavage, or compatible histopathological findings with one positive culture. Other potential causes of pulmonary disease must also be excluded. Although culture remains the gold standard of diagnosis, direct molecular detection by PCR is now available, though less sensitive. Culture itself can be difficult, but a combination of liquid

Table 13.1 Treatment of *M. avium* complex pulmonary disease

M. avium complex pulmonary disease	Antibiotic regimen
Non-severe	Rifampicin 600 mg 3× per week Plus ethambutol 25 mg/kg 3× per week Plus azithromycin 500 mg 3× per week Or clarithromycin 500 mg BD 3× per week Continue for at least 12 months after culture conversion
Severe	Rifampicin 600 mg daily Plus ethambutol 15 mg/kg daily Plus azithromycin 250 mg daily or clarithromycin 500 mg twice daily Consider intravenous or nebulized amikacin Continue for at least 12 months after culture conversion
Clarithromycin-resistant	Rifampicin 600 mg daily Plus ethambutol 15 mg/kg daily Plus isoniazid 300 mg daily (+pyridoxine) Or moxifloxacin 400 mg daily Continue for at least 12 months after culture conversion

systems (mycobacteria growth indicator tube) and solid systems tend to give the best positive yields. Currently many laboratories have Matrix-assisted laser desorption ionisation-time of flight (MALDI-TOF) mass spectrometry which provides early speciation of the NTM.

Treatment and the clinical value of *in vitro* drug susceptibility testing remains uncertain. Currently the best approach may be to determine the exact MICs to determine susceptibility. There are no RCTs to help guide when treatment should be commenced. Current NICE guidelines suggest that treatment should be started after taking into consideration both the patient's characteristics and the severity of the clinical syndrome (rate of progression, severity, radiological change, underlying lung disease) and mycobacterial factors (bacterial load, time to positivity of culture, smear positivity). The patient's views should also be taken into consideration, as their disease can remain stable without antibiotic treatment and "no treatment" may be a reasonable option. Antibiotic treatments are summarized in Table 13.1.

Treatment

Latent Tuberculosis

Treating latent tuberculosis decreases the risk of developing active TB by 60–80%. Commonly used treatment strategies for latent tuberculosis include a 3-month course of a combination of rifampicin and isoniazid, or a 6–9 month course of isoniazid monotherapy. However, other strategies such as rifampicin monotherapy for 3–4 months, or weekly rifapentin plus daily isoniazid for 3 months, may offer similar efficacy and lower toxicity. The optimum strategy for targeting patients for latent TB screening and offering chemoprophylaxis is controversial, and depends on the balance between perceived risks of active TB versus therapy-induced toxicity. Recent NICE guidance advises offering treatment to all patients up to 65 years of age who have a positive screening test. However, the risk of therapy-related toxicity increases significantly with age, and a careful judgement on a case-by-case basis is warranted. A pragmatic approach to offering therapy for latent TB is shown below.

Patients Who should Be Offered Therapy for Latent TB (Once Active TB Has Been Excluded)
- Significant past TB exposure
- TST >5 mm in patients regardless of prior BCG vaccination
- Positive IGRA

Latent TB in Immunocompromised Patients

Patients with latent TB undergoing treatment with TNF-blocking biologic agents have an approximately fivefold increased risk of progression to active TB. This risk can be substantially reduced by treatment for latent TB prior to starting anti-TNF therapy. The risk of progressing to active TB for patients with latent TB taking other immunosuppressive agents is not exactly known, but in general the risk increases with the degree of immunosuppression. Patients in this severely immunocompromised category could be (but are not limited to) those with HIV and CD4 counts of fewer than 200 cells/mm³, or after solid organ or allogeneic stem cell transplant, those on dual or more immunosuppressive agents, or those after severely immunosuppressive chemotherapy for cancer.

In severely immunocompromised patients, TST as well as IGRA may not be sensitive enough to detect latent TB. It would be pragmatic in those patients to offer both IGRA and TST *alongside* the clinical risk-assessment. In case of extensive exposure to TB, chemoprophylaxis can still be offered despite negative screening tests. If active TB develops during anti-TNF therapy, therapy should be stopped until TB treatment is well established. In other cases, a risk-benefit assessment of stopping immunosuppressive medication against treating TB should be made.

In the case of exposure to MDR-TB, there currently are no clear guidelines regarding chemoprophylaxis. Although a few case series suggest efficacy of pyrazinamide and a quinolone, randomised trials are needed to confirm this effect. Since the highest risk of converting to active disease is during the first 2 years after inoculation, a practical approach may be to regularly assess the patient clinically, and to repeat chest X-rays on a serial basis during the first 24 months.

First Line-TB Treatment

Before the widespread availability of anti-mycobacterial chemotherapy in the 1950s, the mainstays of treatment of pulmonary TB were collapse therapy and bed rest. Cavitatory disease was likely to become widespread with aspiration to previously unaffected lung, and carried a poor prognosis. Strict and prolonged bed rest in a dependent position was sometimes able to close cavities, but to prevent them from reopening when the patient became ambulant required some other procedure, such as a phrenic crush combined with a pneumoperitoneum, regular artificial pneumothoraces, two-stage thoracoplasty, or extra periosteal plombage with foreign material such as lucite balls.

Anti-mycobacterial therapy should be used as follows:

- For people with active TB without central nervous system involvement, offer:
  1. Isoniazid (with pyridoxine), rifampicin, pyrazinamide, and ethambutol for 2 months, then
  2. Isoniazid (with pyridoxine) and rifampicin for a further 4 months.
  3. Modify the treatment regime according to drug susceptibility testing.

Rifampicin and Isoniazid are dependent on gastric acid for absorption, so they should thus be taken at least 30 min before a meal or 2 h after a meal.

- For people with active TB of the central nervous system, offer:
  1. Isoniazid (with pyridoxine), rifampicin, pyrazinamide and ethambutol for 2 months, then
  2. Isoniazid (with pyridoxine) and rifampicin for a further 10 months.
  3. Modify the treatment regimen according to drug susceptibility testing.

Therapy Duration

Therapy should be given for 6 months for fully sensitive pulmonary tuberculosis and most cases of extra-pulmonary tuberculosis, including abdominal. In tuberculous meningitis, treatment duration should be extended to 12 months. In a small review, spinal TB treatment for 6 months was non-inferior to a treatment of longer than 6 months However, if there is CNS involvement of spinal TB, treatment duration has to be extended to 12 months. Fluoroquinolones add anti-tuberculosis activity to the standard treatment regimen, but to improve outcomes of TB meningitis, they must be started early, before the onset of coma.

There can be other factors that favour longer treatment duration, such as a very long duration of sputum to become culture-negative, patients receiving chemotherapy for malignancy as well as antituberculous drugs, and a very high burden of disease.

Despite a faster sputum culture conversion time by the addition of moxifloxacin to the standard four-drug combination, attempts to shorten the total duration of treatment to 4 months by adding moxifloxacin have not been successful [18].

Side Effect Profiles of Antituberculous Drugs

> **Main Drugs**
> *Rifampicin*: Hepatitis, skin reactions, gastrointestinal, thrombocytopenia, flu-like symptoms. Rarely haemolytic anaemia, acute renal failure, shock.
> *Isoniazid*: Hepatitis, skin reactions, peripheral neuropathy. Neurological symptoms including seizure, optic neuritis, giddiness, mental symptoms. Pyridoxine now routinely co-prescribed.
> *Ethambutol*: Retrobulbar neuritis, arthralgia. Rarely hepatitis, skin reactions, neuropathy, renal failure.
> *Pyrazinamide*: Anorexia, nausea, photosensitivity, hepatitis, arthralgia. Rarely gout, vomiting.

> **Reserve Drugs**
> *Streptomycin*: Skin reactions, numbness, giddiness, tinnitus. Rarely vertigo, deafness, renal damage, ataxia.
> *Thiacetazone*: Gastrointestinal, skin reactions, vertigo, conjunctivitis. Rarely hepatitis.

> **Significant Drug Interactions Requiring Dose Adjustment or Alternatives**
> *Rifampicin*: potent inducer of cytochrome P450 and so may reduce the levels of many drugs including: antiretrovirals[1], oral anticoagulants, oral contraceptive, ciclosporin, digoxin, glucocorticoids, itraconazole, methadone, midazolam, phenytoin, quinidine, theophylline, verapamil.
> *Isoniazid*: inhibits cytochrome P450 and may increase levels of some drugs including: benzodiazepines, anticonvulsants.

Treatment in Special Circumstances and Management of Complications

Rifampicin, isoniazid, ethambutol, and pyrazinamide are safe in pregnancy, but streptomycin should be avoided because of foetal ototoxicity. Only small subtherapeutic amounts of first-line antituberculous drugs are secreted in breast milk, so breastfeeding is regarded as safe. Pregnant patients with MDR-TB will need a specialist-selected regime where toxicity for the foetus and survival of the mother are carefully weighed.

In patients co-infected with hepatitis B or C, usually treatment can be commenced without any problem; however it is advised to seek hepatology

---

[1] Depending on drug. Rifabutin may be preferred. Advise to seek HIV specialist opinion.

specialist advice if there is liver cirrhosis or severe fibrosis. There is no dose adjustment in this patient group.

In renal failure, isoniazid and rifampicin are used in normal doses. Ethambutol and aminoglycosides require monitoring of drug levels. For stage four or five CKD, or patients on haemodialysis, dosing intervals should be increased to three times weekly for ethambutol, pyrazinamide, and aminoglycosides, and the medication given after haemodialysis.

Mild gastrointestinal symptoms are common, lessen with time, and can be managed symptomatically. Hepatitis with enzymes 5× normal or jaundice occurs in 3%. Pyrazinamide, rifampicin, and isoniazid, in descending order, are the most likely culprits. If it is possible to interrupt treatment, then one approach is to wait until ALT has fallen to <2× normal then reintroduce two drugs (ethambutol and rifampicin or isoniazid) over 10 days. If the patient is too ill or infectious to stop treatment, continue two low risk drugs (ethambutol, streptomycin, quinolone). A similar strategy can be used for severe cutaneous hypersensitivity.

Ethambutol oculotoxicity in patients with normal renal function is rare when using a dosing regimen of 15 mg/kg. Any eye symptoms should be reported and referred to ophthalmology urgently. Formal visual assessment prior to starting treatment is not usually required in patients with no visual impairment, although an informal check is advisable. Ethambutol should be stopped if there is likely to be a delay and, if appropriate, substituted with another drug.

Compliance and Directly Observed Therapy (DOT)

If there are no concerns about compliance and the treatment response is satisfactory, then regular medication checks and opportunistic urine screening for orange (rifampicin-induced) discolouration is usually sufficient. Rifampicin levels can confirm the drug is being taken and may help tailor dose adjustments when the response to treatment is suboptimal or the pharmacokinetics might have altered (e.g. in pregnancy).

DOT is considered when assessment suggests adherence is likely to be poor (see box below). Treatment (isoniazid 15 mg/kg, rifampicin 600–900 mg, pyrazinamide 2.0–2.5 g, ethambutol 30 mg/kg) is given thrice weekly under direct observation. This regime is for 2 months, then rifampicin and isoniazid thrice weekly for a further 4 months. The toxicity profile includes flu-like symptoms, dyspnoea, abdominal symptoms, renal failure, haemolytic anaemia, thrombocytopenic purpura, and anaphylactic shock.

> **Indications for Directly Observed Therapy (DOT) for TB**
> - Current or previous non-adherence to treatment
> - Previous treatment for TB
> - Homeless or drug/alcohol misuse
> - Prison within the previous 5 years
> - Major psychiatric, memory or cognitive disorder
> - In denial of diagnosis
> - Multidrug-resistant TB
> - Requests directly observed therapy
> - Too ill to self-administer treatment

Use of Steroids and Paradoxical Reactions

The occurrence of paradoxical reactions in HIV-negative patients is well recognized. In up to 20% of patients with tuberculous lymphadenitis, a worsening of symptoms can occur paradoxically during the first 2–3 months of treatment, or even after completion of treatment. Predictive factors seem to be a swelling >3 cm and simultaneous extra-lymph node TB [19]. If the lymph node swelling occurs after completion of treatment, paradoxical (sterile) reaction is much more likely than recurrence of infection. Hence follow-up rather than re-treatment is routinely recommended. Other sites of paradoxical reactions in HIV-negative patients can be the pericardium, pleura, bone, muscle, and brain.

Despite a more frequent occurrence of immune reconstitution syndrome (IRIS) after initiating antiretroviral therapy in TB co-infected HIV patients, starting antiretroviral therapy as soon as 2 weeks after initiation of TB treatment rather than later has shown to improve survival in this group.

In some patients, the addition of corticosteroids can be beneficial; in HIV patients with IRIS and in patients with TB meningitis, steroids can reduce mortality [20]. In patients with tuberculous pericarditis there is conflicting evidence, but in clinical practice the use of steroids is usually recommended [5].

Drug-Resistant TB

The classification of drug resistant TB includes four major types:

- Isoniazid-resistant
- Rifampicin-resistant (RR-TB)
- Multidrug-resistant (MDR-TB)
- Extensively drug-resistant (XDR-TB)

The drugs used in the management of resistant TB are also now regrouped based on the current evidence of their effectiveness and safety (Table 13.2). Combination treatment with these drugs depends on the groups. Clofazimine and linezolid are now recommended as core second-line medicines in the MDR-TB regimen, while para-aminosalicylic acid is an add-on agent. Clarithromycin and other macrolides are no longer included among the medicines to be used for the treatment of MDR/RR-TB. MDR-TB treatment is recommended for all patients with RR-TB.

The current WHO recommendations are that shorter MDR-TB treatment is now preferred. These shorter MDR-TB treatment regimens

Table 13.2 Grouping to guide longer treatment regimens for rifampicin-resistant TB and MDR-TB[a]

Group A Fluoroquinolones	Levofloxacin Moxifloxacin Gatifloxacin
Group B Second line injectable agents	Amikacin Capreomycin Kanamycin (streptomycin)
Group C Other core second line agents	Ethionamide/prothionamide Cycloserine/terizidone Linezolid Clofazimine
Group D Add-on agents	Pyrazinamide Ethambutol Isoniazid (high dose)
D2	Bedaquiline Delamanid
D3	Para-aminosalicylic acid Imipenem-cilastatin Meropenem Amoxicillin-clavulinic acid Carriage return - (thioacetazone)

[a]Medicines in Groups A and C are shown by decreasing order of usual preference for use (subject to other considerations). In patients with RR-TB or MDR-TB, a regimen with at least five effective TB medicines during the intensive phase is recommended, including pyrazinamide and four core second line TB medicines—one chosen from Group A, one from Group B, and at least two from Group C. If the minimum number of effective TB medicines cannot be composed as given above, an agent from Group D2 and other agents from Group D3 may be added to bring the total to five. In patients with RR-TB or MDR-TB, it is recommended that the regimen be further strengthened with high-dose isoniazid and/or ethambutol. (Adapted from WHO treatment guidelines for drug-resistant TB, 2016 update)

are standardized in content and duration and split into two distinct parts. First, an intensive phase of 4 months (extended up to a maximum of 6 months in case of lack of sputum smear conversion) includes the following drugs: gatifloxacin (or moxifloxacin), kanamycin, prothionamide, clofazimine, high-dose isoniazid, pyrazinamide, and ethambutol. This is followed by a continuation phase of 5 months with the following drugs: gatifloxacin (or moxifloxacin), clofazimine, pyrazinamide, and ethambutol. These guidelines also recommend partial lung resection as the surgical procedure of choice in appropriate situations.

Vaccination

The only currently registered vaccine against TB is the BCG vaccination. The BCG is derived from a live attenuated strain of *M. bovis* and contains a mix of over 4000 antigens [21]. Despite variability over the years, it has been shown to be effective in preventing the most severe cases of TB in children, such as TB meningitis and disseminated TB. Little is known about its efficacy in those over age 16. The vaccine does not prevent primary infection or pulmonary tuberculosis, which is the main route of infection in adults, and it does not prevent reactivation of latent tuberculosis. The effect on the spread of tuberculosis in endemic settings is thus dubious.

Caution is warranted when using the vaccine in immunocompromised patients; cases of reactivation of *M. bovis* after vaccination have been described.

Health care workers who are frequently exposed to TB (laboratory workers, employees in a chest clinic) should be given the opportunity to be vaccinated against TB; however they should be aware that there is little evidence for the effectiveness of the vaccine in persons aged 35 and over.

Several trials are currently running with the aim to induce a more sustained immune response in adults by using adjuvant vaccines targeting various antigens, modifying the current BCG vaccine, or by using attenuated MTB strains. These are phase 1, 2, and 3 trials, some of which are promising in HIV-infected as well as HIV-uninfected patients. Alternative routes of vaccination such as inhalation are being explored, but are in a very preliminary phase of development.

References

1. Houben RM, Dodd PJ. The global burden of latent tuberculosis infection: a re-estimation using mathematical modelling. PLoS Med. 2016;13(10):e1002152.
2. Dye C, Scheele S, Dolin P, Pathania V, Raviglione MC. Consensus statement. Global burden of tuberculosis: estimated incidence, prevalence, and mortality by country. WHO Global Surveillance and Monitoring Project. JAMA. 1999;282(7):677–86.
3. TB alert UK. 2016. Available at: https://www.tbalert.org.
4. Singh D, Sutton C, Woodcock A. Tuberculin test measurement: variability due to the time of reading. Chest. 2002;122(4):1299–301.
5. National Institute for Health and Care Excellence. Tuberculosis NG33. NICE guideline published January 2016. Last updated May 2016. Available at: https://www.nice.org.uk/Tuberculosis.
6. Al Zahrani K, Al Jahdali H, Menzies D. Does size matter? Utility of size of tuberculin reactions for the diagnosis of mycobacterial disease. Am J Respir Crit Care Med. 2000;162(4 Pt 1):1419–22.
7. Redelman-Sidi G, Sepkowitz KA. IFN-gamma release assays in the diagnosis of latent tuberculosis infection among immunocompromised adults. Am J Respir Crit Care Med. 2013;188(4):422–31.
8. Diel R, Loddenkemper R, Meywald-Walter K, Gottschalk R, Nienhaus A. Comparative performance of tuberculin skin test, QuantiFERON-TB-gold in tube assay, and T-spot.TB test in contact investigations for tuberculosis. Chest. 2009;135(4):1010–8.
9. Zijenah LS, Kadzirange G, Bandason T, Chipiti MM, Gwambiwa B, Makoga F, et al. Comparative performance characteristics of the urine lipoarabinomannan strip test and sputum smear microscopy in hospitalized HIV-infected patients with suspected tuberculosis in Harare, Zimbabwe. BMC Infect Dis. 2016;16:20.
10. Hanifa Y, Fielding KL, Chihota VN, Adonis L, Charalambous S, Karstaedt A, et al. Diagnostic accuracy of lateral flow urine LAM assay for TB screening of adults with advanced immunosuppression attending routine HIV care in South Africa. PLoS One. 2016;11(6):e0156866.
11. Bos JC, Smalbraak L, Macome AC, Gomes E, van Leth F, Prins JM. TB diagnostic process management of patients in a referral hospital in Mozambique in comparison with the 2007 WHO recommendations for the diagnosis of smear-negative pulmonary TB and extrapulmonary TB. Int Health. 2013;5(4):302–8.
12. Shapiro AE, Chakravorty R, Akande T, Lonnroth K, Golub JE. A systematic review of the number needed to screen to detect a case of active tuberculosis in different risk groups. Geneva: WHO; 2013.
13. World Health Organization. Updated WHO recommendations Xpert MTB/RIF test. Geneva: WHO; 2014.
14. Skoura E, Zumla A, Bomanji J. Imaging in tuberculosis. Int J Infect Dis. 2015;32:87–93.
15. Dhooria S, Agarwal R, Aggarwal AN, Bal A, Gupta N, Gupta D. Differentiating tuberculosis from sarcoidosis by sonographic characteristics of lymph nodes on endobronchial ultrasonography: a study of 165 patients. J Thorac Cardiovasc Surg. 2014;148(2):662–7.
16. Sandgren A, Hollo V, van der Werf MJ. Extrapulmonary tuberculosis in the European Union and European Economic Area, 2002 to 2011. Euro Surveill. 2013;18(12):20431.
17. World Health Organization. WHO Xpert MTB/RIF implementation manual. Technical and operational

'how-to': practical considerations. Geneva: WHO; 2014.

18. Gillespie SH, Crook AM, McHugh TD, Mendel CM, Meredith SK, Murray SR, et al. Four-month moxifloxacin-based regimens for drug-sensitive tuberculosis. N Engl J Med. 2014;371(17):1577–87.

19. Chahed H, Hachicha H, Berriche A, Abdelmalek R, Mediouni A, Kilani B, et al. Paradoxical reaction associated with cervical lymph node tuberculosis: predictive factors and therapeutic management. Int J Infect Dis. 2016;54:4–7.

20. Prasad K, Singh MB, Ryan H. Corticosteroids for managing tuberculous meningitis. Cochrane Database Syst Rev. 2016;4:CD002244.

21. Husain AA, Daginawala HF, Singh L, Kashyap RS. Current perspective in tuberculosis vaccine development for high TB endemic regions. Tuberculosis (Edinb). 2016;98:149–58.

Lung Diseases Caused by Aspergillus and Pulmonary Eosinophilia

Simon P. Hart

Lung Diseases Caused by Aspergillus

Introduction

Aspergillus fumigatus is the most frequent cause of fungal lung disease in humans, but occasionally other Aspergillus species (e.g. *A. flavus, A. niger*) may cause human disease. Colonies of Aspergillus fungus live on dead or decaying matter in the environment and release abundant tiny (2–3 μM) conidia (spores) into the atmosphere, which are readily respired. Highest conidia levels occur in late summer and early autumn, and climatic events such as thunderstorms can increase the number and allergenic potency of airborne fungal spores. In healthy individuals, respired spores are cleared from the airways by the mucociliary escalator and from the alveoli by the innate immune system. Thermotolerant fungi such as Aspergillus species are able to grow both in the environment and at body temperature, and are thus able to colonise the airways under certain conditions if inhaled conidia are not cleared. In immunocompromised individuals or patients with chronic lung disease in whom lung defence

Table 14.1 Aspergillus lung diseases

Allergic fungal airways disease
• Fungal asthma/severe asthma with fungal sensitisation (SAFS)
• Allergic bronchopulmonary aspergillosis (ABPA)
Invasive aspergillosis (IA)
Chronic pulmonary aspergillosis (CPA) [1]
• Aspergillus nodule
• Simple aspergilloma
• Chronic cavitary pulmonary aspergillosis (CCPA; complex aspergilloma)
• Chronic fibrosing pulmonary aspergillosis (CFPA)
• Subacute invasive (chronic necrotising) pulmonary aspergillosis

is impaired, germination of spores in the airways leads to growth of a mass of branching filamentous hyphae (mycelium), which can infiltrate the surrounding lung tissue.

The Table 14.1 below shows a classification of Aspergillus lung diseases. There is often overlap between the various presentations such that patients may exhibit features of more than one form of aspergillosis.

Allergic Fungal Airways Disease

Fungal Asthma

Fungal asthma (also called severe asthma with fungal sensitisation, SAFS) is caused by IgE-mediated immune reactions against inhaled fungal spores. There is no mycelial colonisation.

S. P. Hart
Respiratory Research Group,
Hull York Medical School, Castle Hill Hospital,
Cottingham, East Yorkshire, UK
e-mail: s.hart@hull.ac.uk

Sensitisation occurs commonly to *Aspergillus fumigatus*, but also to other fungi including Cladosporium, Penicillium, Alternaria, and Saccharomyces species. Fungal sensitisation is related to asthma severity, with up to 75% of patients with severe asthma showing a positive skin test or serum IgE reactivity against Aspergillus or other fungi. Higher environmental fungal spore counts (typically in summer/autumn) are associated with more severe asthma hospitalisations.

Asthma treatment follows the usual stepwise algorithm. Episodes of acute severe asthma are relatively unusual in fungal asthma, and the clinical picture is one where periods of poorly controlled chronic disease predominate. Allergen avoidance is not feasible for most fungi causing sensitisation due to their ubiquitous presence in the environment. There is no evidence to support use of antifungal drugs in patients with asthma and fungal sensitisation.

Fungal Rhinosinusitis

In allergic fungal rhinosinusitis (AFRS), mycelial colonisation of a sinus occurs in a sinus with impaired drainage, similar to ABPA in the lower airways although the two conditions rarely co-exist. Surgery is usually required in AFRS to clear the affected sinuses and allow access of nasally-delivered corticosteroids. Antifungal drug therapy is usually ineffective.

Allergic Bronchopulmonary Aspergillosis (ABPA)

The term ABPA was first used in the 1950s to describe a series of patients with lung damage and fungal sensitisation. Occasionally, a fungus other than *A. fumigatus* may be implicated, in which case the term allergic bronchopulmonary mycosis is applied. ABPA occurs most commonly in people with asthma or cystic fibrosis, and it occurs when the airways become colonised with growing fungal hyphae, combined with immune responses characterised by increased

levels of Aspergillus-specific IgE and IgG. It typically presents as asthma complicated by flitting eosinophilic lung infiltrates, and may progress to bronchiectasis and fibrosis. Typically, the blood eosinophil count is markedly elevated ($>1.0 \times 10^9$/L). Antibody-mediated immune responses to *A. fumigatus* are the hallmark of ABPA, with raised serum total IgE (often >1000 IU/L) and strongly positive Aspergillus-specific IgE RAST tests. Serum aspergillus precipitins (IgG antibodies) may also be present. Patients may report coughing up bronchial casts, which are laden with eosinophils, and Aspergillus can often be cultured from sputum. Haemoptysis may occur. In late disease, bronchiectasis supervenes, and is typically but not invariably in a proximal (central) distribution as demonstrated on CT.

Numerous radiologic features have been described in ABPA. Fleeting or persistent lung opacities, tramline shadows due to bronchial wall thickening, and finger-in-glove opacities may be seen on chest X-ray. CT features include central bronchiectasis with peripheral tapering, mucoid impaction or bronchocoele (classically high attenuation, shown in Fig. 14.1a), mosaic attenuation, centrilobular nodules, and tree-in-bud opacities. Whilst central bronchiectasis (Fig. 14.1b) distinguishes ABPA from fungal asthma, not all patients with ABPA have bronchiectasis. Precise diagnostic criteria for ABPA have not been agreed, and often a period of monitoring and retesting is required for confirmation once the diagnosis is suspected.

Susceptibility to germination and colonisation of Aspergillus in the airways leading to ABPA is not well understood. A number of genetic variations have been described that are over-represented in ABPA, including HLA class I, surfactant proteins, cytokines, and innate immune defence proteins.

Treatment is aimed at controlling asthma using the standard algorithm. Oral corticosteroids may be required, and in the past were regarded as the mainstay of treatment of ABPA to prevent bronchiectasis and reduce the risk of permanent lung damage. However, the natural history of ABPA is poorly understood, and the effect of steroids on

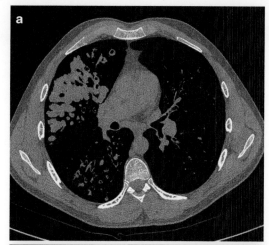

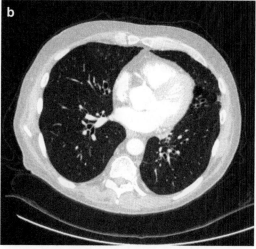

Fig. 14.1 (a) ABPA in a patient with cystic fibrosis. CT demonstrates mucoid impaction in multiple dilated airways. (b) Proximal bronchiectasis demonstrated on CT in a patient with asthma and ABPA

disease progression is uncertain. Typically, oral corticosteroid therapy is used for at least several months, with treatment response determined by reduction in symptoms and lung infiltrates. Typically, a fall in serum total IgE by 35–50% is associated with treatment response. Anti-IgE therapy with omalizumab has been reported to be beneficial, but has not subjected to randomised controlled trials. Coexisting bronchiectasis and bacterial colonisation and infection are managed accordingly (see Bronchiectasis chapter). Pulmonary rehabilitation is recommended for patients with fixed airflow obstruction.

Antifungal treatment for ABPA is often disappointing in clinical practice. Some of the clinical trial benefits reported with itraconazole could be attributed to its steroid-enhancing effect (itraconazole is a potent inhibitor or CYP3A4, which breaks down prednisolone in the liver). Triazoles do not penetrate the bronchial lumen particularly effectively, and are poor at eradicating airway fungi, so are likely to be most effective when there is heavy colonisation with active infection or invasion (i.e. co-existing subacute invasive aspergillosis, see below). In ABPA, trial data supporting antifungal treatment with triazoles are weak, and the decision to treat has to be balanced against the risk of adverse effects. Typically, a trial of oral corticosteroid therapy will be given first, with antifungal triazole treatment reserved for steroid-resistant cases.

Invasive Aspergillosis (IA)

Invasive aspergillosis occurs as a complication of severe immunodeficiency, seen in transplant recipients, patients with acute leukaemia, advanced HIV (infection with human immunodeficiency virus), patients in critical care, and those taking immunosuppressive drugs, particularly high-dose corticosteroids. Patients with severe neutropenia ($<0.5 \times 10^9$/L, and particularly $<0.1 \times 10^9$/L) are at highest risk, particularly if prolonged. The incidence is rising because of the growing number of iatrogenically immunosuppressed patients, and mortality remains high (50% during neutropenia, 90% with bone marrow grafts). It can occur in the lungs or sinuses, reflecting the common mode of entry of Aspergillus into the body, or in a disseminated form with fungaemia and multi-organ involvement including the brain.

Clinical features reflect the affected organs. In the lungs IA may mimic bronchopneumonia, but pleuritic chest pain (due to vascular invasion causing pulmonary infarction) and haemoptysis are common. A fever unresponsive to antibacterial treatment should raise the suspicion of fungal disease. CT appearances in the lungs include multifocal infiltrates, nodules, and cavities.

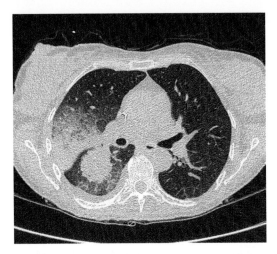

Fig. 14.2 Invasive pulmonary aspergillosis in a neutropenic patient with acute leukaemia. CT demonstrates rounded consolidation with surrounding ground glass opacification

Rounded areas of consolidation are characteristic, often with a surrounding halo of ground glass opacity (Fig. 14.2). Cavitation occurs later.

Aspergillus tracheobronchitis represents a more limited form of IA, and is seen particularly in lung transplant recipients. Diagnosis is made at bronchoscopy and microscopy and fungal cultures from the affected tissue. There is an ulcerative tracheobronchitis with abundant fibrin in the immediate vicinity of the airway anastomosis. One-third of patients may progress to IA, so early aggressive treatment is critical.

Diagnosis

Microscopy and Cultures

Diagnosis of IA requires a high index of suspicion. Cultures are the mainstay of diagnosis, but interpretation can be complicated in samples from non-sterile sources (including the respiratory tract) since respired Aspergillus spores are commonly present in sputum from normal individuals. Positive sputum cultures for aspergillus are unlikely to be of clinical significance in the immunocompetent patient. Conversely, in an immunocompromised host, a positive culture may be regarded as a marker of invasive infection and should raise a high level of suspicion. Fungal blood cultures are rarely positive in IA.

The presence of branching fungal hyphae on microscopy or histopathological analysis of a biopsy specimen is characteristic. Fungal cultures should always be performed to determine whether the fungus is Aspergillus, and if so which species since some may be resistant to amphotericin.

Testing for Aspergillus DNA by PCR has been evaluated and shows some promise, but like cultures, it is unable to distinguish between colonisation and infection. However, a high DNA load measured by quantitative methods may be more indicative of infection, and in the context of antifungal drug therapy, could indicate likely drug resistance.

Antigen Testing

Galactomannan (GM) is a polysaccharide released from the fungal cell wall that can be measured in serum or bronchoalveolar lavage (BAL). Sensitivity and specificity of serum GM for IA are approximately 70% and 90% respectively. The test is most useful in patients with acute leukaemia or haematopoietic stem cell transplant (HSCT) recipients. False positives may occur due to GM absorption from food in the gut, especially in the presence of mucositis, or from administration of β-lactam antibiotics. GM is not species-specific and is produced by many moulds, so careful microbiological testing is also required to make a precise diagnosis.

Beta (1,3)-D-glucan is also present in the fungal cell wall, and measurement in serum shows similar accuracy to GM testing. Combining the two tests may improve diagnostic accuracy.

Serology

Serological testing for Aspergillus antibodies is frequently unhelpful in the immunocompromised patient.

Treatment

Because of the severity and high mortality of IA, treatment is commonly initiated based on clinical suspicion. Intravenous Amphotericin B has been used for the treatment of fungal infections for decades, and was hitherto regarded as the gold standard for treatment of IA. Lipid formulations are generally better tolerated than conventional amphotericin, although the efficacy is similar. Drawbacks include poor solubility in water and side effects, including nephrotoxicity, electrolyte disturbance, local infusion reactions, and vomiting.

The newer broad-spectrum triazoles voriconazole and posaconazole seem to be better tolerated, and the former is now regarded as first-line treatment for IA, whereas posaconazole has a more established role as prophylaxis. Triazoles block production of ergosterols in fungal cell membranes, causing toxic methylsterols to accumulate in the fungal cell wall leading to inhibition of fungal growth and replication. Common side effects include visual disturbance and hepatotoxicity. Drawbacks include variable absorption following oral administration, and cytochrome P450 CYP3A4 inhibition leading to numerous drug interactions, including sirolimus, ciclosporin, carbamazepime and anti-HIV treatments. There is considerable variation in plasma levels between individuals, so in refractory aspergillosis measurement of blood drug levels is advised. Addition of caspofungin can be considered as salvage therapy in resistant cases.

A long duration of treatment is often required and depends on patient response and the nature of the underlying immunodeficiency. Correction of underlying neutropenia with recombinant human granulocyte colony stimulating factors such as filgastim may help speed recovery.

Chronic Pulmonary Aspergillosis

Subacute invasive (previously chronic necrotising) aspergillosis

Subacute invasive (previously chronic necrotising) aspergillosis is more indolent than invasive aspergillosis, with slower onset (several months) and locally invasive infection affecting the lung, particularly in patients with mild immunocompromise (e.g. long-term corticosteroid therapy) or debilitation due to chronic lung disease including COPD, cystic fibrosis, and chronic sarcoid-

Table 14.2 Diagnosis of chronic pulmonary aspergillosis

• Consistent imaging (usually CT)
• Direct evidence of Aspergillus infection (microscopy, culture, histology)[a]
• And/or Serological response (Aspergillus IgG)
• Exclusion of alternative diagnoses

[a]If a fungal ball is observed on CT, then direct evidence of Aspergillus infection is not required if serum IgG tests are positive [1]

osis. Local invasion of lung tissue by growing fungal hyphae is associated with an acute inflammatory response and tissue necrosis, which is recognisable on histological examination of a tissue biopsy. The differential diagnosis often includes lung cancer, mycobacterial infection, bacterial infection, and vasculitis. It is important to recognise that these conditions may co-exist with aspergillosis.

Diagnosis is made according to the Table 14.2 above. Serological testing for aspergillus infection (serum IgG (precipitins)) is usually positive. GM antigen testing in BAL has superior accuracy compared to serum antigen testing. The principles of management are the same as for invasive aspergillosis. Drug treatment with a triazole (itraconazole, voriconazole) should be given first-line, usually for 3–6 months.

Aspergilloma

An aspergilloma (mycetoma) may be found in all forms of CPA. It typically occurs when Aspergillus colonises a pre-existing cavity in one or both lungs. Most commonly aspergillomas occur in old TB cavities, but sometimes they can be found in a cavitating squamous cell lung cancer, a cavitating pulmonary infarct, sarcoidosis, or ankylosing spondylitis. Radiologically, the aspergilloma appears as a fungal ball partially filling the cavity, with a crescent (meniscus) of air separating it from the cavity wall. The fungal ball is usually attached to the cavity wall at one or more points. The cavity wall is often thick, especially in longstanding aspergillomas, and there may be adjacent pleural thickening. The fungal ball is well seen on CT, appearing as a sponge-like mass with the air crescent sign (Fig. 14.3).

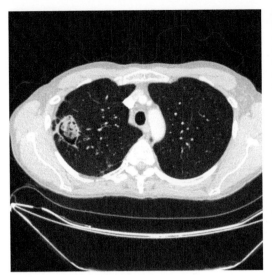

Fig. 14.3 Simple aspergilloma. CT demonstrates a sponge-like fungal ball with a surrounding air crescent within a lung cavity

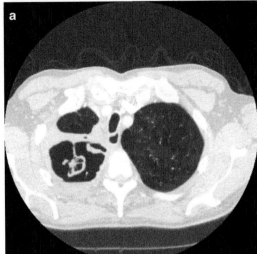

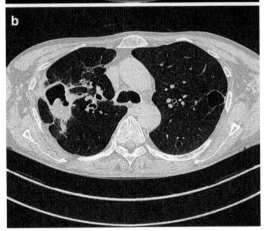

The mobility of the fungal ball within the cavity can be demonstrated with decubitus or lateral views. Invasion into the surrounding lung (semi-invasive disease) sometimes occurs, with adjacent consolidation and lung destruction seen on CT (Fig. 14.4a, b). An early aspergilloma may appear as strands or a membrane within a pre-existing cavity before the fungal ball is visible on plain CXR. Haemoptysis is the usual presenting symptom, arising from the inflamed cavity wall with a systemic vascular supply from the bronchial arterial circulation. Investigations typically reveal strongly positive serum IgG antibodies (precipitins) against aspergillus, and fungi may be identified in sputum or bronchial washings.

Surgical resection of a simple aspergilloma is often recommended and may be curative, but if the patient is asymptomatic and given the unclear natural history of the condition, there is an argument for an expectant observational approach. In symptomatic patients the disease may be more complex—with thick walled cavities, parenchymal scarring, and pleural thickening—and surgery is more complicated and with higher morbidity, particularly as lung function is almost always severely compromised. Tranexamic acid may be effective for treating episodes of haemoptysis. Bronchial artery embolization may be required

Fig. 14.4 Chronic cavitary aspergillosis is a patient with COPD. (**a**) An upper lobe cavity contains a fungal ball (aspergilloma). (**b**) Lower CT slice demonstrating the aspergilloma with neighbouring bronchiectasis and local invasion with an inflammatory response in surrounding lung tissue

to relieve recurrent or severe haemoptysis. Antifungal drug therapy with a triazole (itraconazole, voriconazole) may be attempted, and there is some evidence from trials that up to 6 months of therapy leads to superior response rates (measured using composite endpoints) compared with placebo. Drug tolerability may be a problem for some patients, and the effects of triazole therapy in the long term are unclear. Intra-cavity instillation of antifungal drugs has been tried in selected cases, but not subjected to rigorous trials. Some patients have an indolent systemic illness with fever, weight loss, and excessive sputum production, and systemic steroids are sometimes dramatically effective. In chronic cavitary pulmonary aspergillosis, complex aspergilloma may progress to end-stage lung destruction and dense fibrosis, referred to as chronic fibrosing pulmonary aspergillosis (CFPA).

Aspergillus Nodule

Single or multiple pulmonary nodules due to aspergillus are uncommon. Cavitation may or may not occur. An aspergillus nodule may mimic lung cancer, tuberculoma, or other fungal infections. The value of testing for Aspergillus serum IgG antibodies is unknown. Diagnosis is usually made by histology, and surgical resection leads to cure.

Pulmonary Eosinophilia

Pulmonary eosinophilia describes a heterogeneous group of lung diseases characterised by infiltration of the alveolar spaces and interstitium with eosinophils [2], as listed in the Table 14.3 below. Healthy lung tissue does not normally contain eosinophils. These conditions typically present with pulmonary infiltrates, combined usually with blood eosinophilia ($>0.45 \times 10^9$/L). Pulmonary eosinophilia may be demonstrated by bronchoscopy and bronchoalveolar lavage (BAL). The normal BAL eosinophil count is <5%, but in pulmonary eosinophilia syndromes it may be markedly raised (e.g. to more than 40%). Investigation of pulmonary eosinophilia should look for a cause, particularly helminthic infec-

Table 14.3 Classification of pulmonary eosinophilia

• Eosinophilic granulomatosis with polyangiitis (EGPA, Churg-Strauss syndrome)
• Allergic bronchopulmonary aspergillosis
• Simple pulmonary eosinophilia (Löffler's syndrome)
• Acute eosinophilic pneumonia (AEP)
• Chronic eosinophilic pneumonia (CEP)
• Hypereosinophilic syndrome

tions, drug reactions to prescribed and recreational drugs, or systemic vasculitis. Sometimes, no cause can be found. Eosinophils readily undergo apoptosis (programmed cell death) upon exposure to corticosteroids, and the pulmonary eosinophilia syndromes tend to respond rapidly to steroid treatment. However, because these conditions are rare, there is no consensus on dose or duration of steroid therapy, which should be guided by patient response.

Some of the causes of pulmonary eosinophilia have been described elsewhere (see above for ABPA and see the chapter on Vasculitis for EGPA). The various forms of eosinophilic pneumonia are described below.

Simple Pulmonary Eosinophilia (Löffler's Syndrome)

This is a self-limiting condition that presents with cough and mild fever, and blood eosinophilia up to 2.0×10^9/L. Eosinophilic lung infiltrates on chest X-ray often appear to radiate from the hila and may appear migratory. It resolves spontaneously within 1 month. Hypersensitivity to drugs is a common cause, particularly antibiotics and nonsteroidal analgesics (see Table 14.4 below).

Löffler's syndrome was originally described as hypersensitivity to larval forms of filarial nematodes during their life cycle in human hosts. Ingestion of eggs of roundworms such as *Ascaris lumbricoides* is followed by larvae hatching in the gut, penetration into the mesenteric lymphatics, and entering the venous circulation, where they become lodged in the pulmonary capillaries. The larvae then penetrate the alveolar walls and ascend the bronchial tree and are swallowed. However, since its original description, it has been recognised that Löffler's syndrome can also occur in association with parasites whose life cycle does not involve the lungs, such as *Wuchereria bancrofti* and *Brugia malayi*, causes of lymphatic filariasis. It is seen in indigenous residents where filariasis is endemic, and is only rarely seen in visitors. Fine linear infiltrates may be seen on CXR. Treatment is with an antihelminthic drug such as diethylcarbamazine.

Acute Eosinophilic Pneumonia (AEP)

AEP is a more recently described entity that presents as an acute illness with fever and fulminant respiratory failure. It is a rare disease, being reported in only a small number of case series. The cause is unknown, but there appears to be an association with recent onset of cigarette smoking. Alveolar opacification on chest X-ray or CT is often bilateral, and associated with interstitial lines/reticulation and pleural effusions in the absence of left heart failure. The differential diagnosis includes infection. Other causes of eosinophilic pneumonia need to be ruled out, including parasitic infection, drug reaction, EGPA (Churg-Strauss syndrome), and hypereo-

Table 14.4 Commoner causes of drug- or treatment-related pulmonary eosinophilia

• Amiodarone
• Antibiotics (nitrofurantoin, penicillins, sulphonamides, tetracyclines)
• Cocaine
• Gemcitabine
• Heroin
• Ibuprofen (and other NSAIDs)
• Imatinib
• Infliximab
• Marijuana
• Mesalazine (and sulphasalazine)
• Nivolumab
• Phenytoin
• Propylthiouracil
• Radiotherapy
• Simvastatin
• Tryptophan
• Venlafaxine

sinophilic syndrome. There is marked eosinophilia (>25%) on bronchoscopy/BAL. The blood eosinophil count may be normal, particularly in the early phase of the disease. There is prompt response to steroid therapy and, unlike chronic eosinophilic pneumonia, it does not recur.

Chronic Eosinophilic Pneumonia (CEP)

The presentation and imaging findings of CEP are similar to cryptogenic organising pneumonia (COP), with fever, cough and sputum, weight loss, crackles on auscultation, and raised blood inflammatory markers. In CEP there is marked eosinophilic infiltration of the lung parenchyma. The cause is unknown, but there is an association with atopy, and a history of asthma can be elicited in up to two-thirds of patients. The characteristic homogeneous peripheral consolidation on CXR, described in its classical form as "a photographic negative of pulmonary oedema," is seen in a minority of cases. Blood eosinophilia is usual but not invariable, and marked eosinophilia (>40%) on BAL or tissue infiltration with eosinophils on biopsy confirms the diagnosis. Rapid resolution with prednisolone is the norm. Some cases recur and require longer tapering courses of corticosteroids, and some patients may go on to fulfill diagnostic criteria for EGPA (Churg-Strauss syndrome).

Hypereosinophilic Syndrome

Hypereosinophilic syndrome describes a group of haematological disorders (Table 14.5) characterized by high blood eosinophil counts and

Table 14.5 Causes of hypereosinophilic syndrome

Myeloproliferative variant	Chromosome 4 deletion leading to FIP1L1/PDGFRA fusion gene Anaemia, high serum vitamin B12, endomyocardial fibrosis, myelofibrosis, splenomegaly
Lymphoproliferative variant	Abnormal T cells Angioedema, immune complex disease, high serum IgE, rash, dermatographism
Eosinophilic leukaemia	Very high blood eosinophil counts
Gleich syndrome (episodic eosinophilia and angioedema)	Rare. High serum IgM. Associated with eosinophil degranulation but without organ damage.
Familial hypereosinophilic syndrome	Linked to 5q 31-33

eosinophilic infiltration of many tissues, which may include the lungs, and therefore needs to be discriminated from other forms of eosinophilic pneumonia. The presence of extrapulmonary manifestations should prompt further investigation for a hypereosinophilic syndrome. Diagnosis requires bone marrow biopsy with cytogenetic and mutation testing to identify the associated genetic abnormalities.

References

1. Denning DW, Cadranel J, Beigelman-Aubry C, Ader F, Chakrabarti A, Blot S, et al. Chronic pulmonary aspergillosis: rationale and clinical guidelines for diagnosis and management. Eur Respir J. 2016;47(1):45–68.
2. Jeong YJ, Kim KI, Seo IJ, Lee CH, Lee KN, Kim KN, et al. Eosinophilic lung diseases: a clinical, radiologic, and pathologic overview. Radiographics. 2007;27(3):617–37. discussion 637–9.

Interstitial Lung Disease

15

Simon P. Hart

Introduction

Interstitial lung disease (ILD), also known as diffuse parenchymal lung disease, describes a group of disorders that affect the gas-exchanging alveolar interstitium of the lungs. In health, efficient gas exchange requires a short path comprising thin type I alveolar epithelial cells (AEC), a basement membrane, and capillary endothelial cells to facilitate gaseous diffusion between the airspaces and the pulmonary capillaries. Extracellular matrix in the normal alveolar interstitium comprises principally elastin, which gives the lungs their characteristic stretchiness and elastic recoil.

In ILD the alveolar walls become thickened due to a combination of a cellular infiltrate and deposition of excessive extracellular matrix. The cellular infiltrate may comprise inflammatory cells such as lymphocytes, monocytes, or neutrophils, or more commonly fibroblasts and their active forms called myofibroblasts, which express smooth muscle actin and secrete collagen. Deposition of collagen types I and III within the alveolar interstitium is the key pathological feature of pulmonary fibrosis and is a prominent feature of many ILDs. Thickening of the alveolar

walls leads to longer paths for gas exchange, and loss of elasticity results in lung restriction manifested by reduction in lung volumes, particularly forced vital capacity (FVC) and total lung capacity (TLC).

Classification of ILD

Interstitial lung diseases can be classified as shown in Table 15.1 [1–3]. Much of the terminology used nowadays was originally proposed by Liebow and Carrington in 1969, and descriptive terms such as usual interstitial pneumonia (UIP) have persisted into common usage. To accurately classify ILD, careful history taking and physical examination should focus on known causes or associations. These include the connective-tissue diseases, particularly rheumatoid arthritis, scleroderma, polymyositis/dermatomyositis, and the recently recognized anti-synthetase syndromes. Many drugs have been linked with increased risk of ILD, but for only a few is there convincing evidence of a causative link. Bleomycin, a cytotoxic anti-cancer drug are used for the treatment of head and neck cancers, lymphoma, and testicular cancer, is an accepted cause of pulmonary fibrosis. The risk of bleomycin-induced pulmonary fibrosis can be minimised by careful attention to dosing because toxicity is dose-related. Nitrofurantoin, an antibiotic which is used for long-term prevention of urinary tract infections,

S. P. Hart
Respiratory Research Group,
Hull York Medical School, Castle Hill Hospital,
Cottingham, East Yorkshire, UK
e-mail: s.hart@hull.ac.uk

© Springer International Publishing AG, part of Springer Nature 2018
S. Hart, M. Greenstone (eds.), *Foundations of Respiratory Medicine*,
https://doi.org/10.1007/978-3-319-94127-1_15

Table 15.1 Classification of ILD

ILD with known cause or association	Idiopathic interstitial pneumonias (IIP)	Granulomatous ILD	Rare ILD
Connective tissue diseases	*Chronic fibrosing* Idiopathic pulmonary fibrosis (IPF)	Sarcoidosis	Langerhans cell histiocytosis
Scleroderma	Non-specific interstitial pneumonia (NSIP)	Hypersensitivity pneumonitis (extrinsic allergic alveolitis)	Lymphangio-leiomyomatosis
Rheumatoid arthritis		Lymphocyic granulomatous ILD associated with common variable immunodeficiency	Alveolar proteinosis
Polymyositis/dermatomyositis	*Smoking-related* Desquamative interstitial pneumonia (DIP)		Idiopathic lymphoid interstitial pneumonia
Anti-synthetase syndromes	Respiratory bronchiolitis-ILD		Pleuroparenchymal fibroelastosis
Drugs	*Acute/subacute* Acute interstitial pneumonia (AIP)		
Bleomycin			
Nitrofurantoin	Cryptogenic organising pneumonia (COP)/ bronchiolitis obliterans organizing pneumonia (BOOP)		
Amiodarone			
Inorganic dusts/fibres			
Asbestos			
Coal dust			
Silica			

can also cause ILD with prolonged usage. ILD associated with the class 3 anti-arrhythmic drug amiodarone was particularly common when high-maintenance doses (up to 800 mg/d) were routinely used, but it is rarely seen nowadays. Methotrexate may induce an acute pneumonitis, but reports of pulmonary fibrosis caused by methotrexate are confounded by its frequent usage for treatment of rheumatoid arthritis, itself commonly associated with ILD. Recent evidence suggests that the risk of ILD is not increased in patients treated with methotrexate for conditions other than CTDs, such as psoriasis or inflammatory bowel disease [4]. Inhalation of fibrogenic dusts or fibres, particularly asbestos, silica, and coal dust, are well recognized causes of pulmonary fibrosis, and where careful history taking can establish exposures to occupational and environmental dusts and fibres.

The most commonly encountered group of ILD is the idiopathic interstitial pneumonias.

Here the term pneumonia is using its broadest term, meaning inflammation of the lungs. Idiopathic pulmonary fibrosis (IPF) is the commonest condition in this group and the commonest ILD overall. A number of other idiopathic interstitial pneumonias, some of which resemble IPF, are encountered less commonly.

Granulomatous ILD refers to the characteristic histopathological finding of non-caseating granulomata, similar to those seen in tuberculosis, but usually without accompanying central necrosis. Sarcoidosis is a multisystem inflammatory granulomatous disease that commonly affects the lungs (see Chap. 16). Hypersensitivity pneumonitis (HP), also known as extrinsic allergic alveolitis, is an immune-mediated hypersensitivity reaction to inhaled organic dusts, particularly bird dander and fungi. The rare (orphan) interstitial lung diseases are described in the chapter on *Vasculitis and Rare Lung Diseases*.

Patterns of ILD on High-Resolution CT Scanning

The key investigation in patients with suspected ILD is high-resolution computed tomography (HRCT) of the lungs, and a number of distinct patterns may be seen (Table 15.2 and Fig. 15.1a–f). In patients with suspected IPF, HRCT is used to answer the key question of whether the pattern of fibrosis is consistent with UIP.

Lung Function Testing

Typical lung function abnormalities in ILD are reduction in FVC and lung volumes (restriction) and reduced gas transfer (diffusing capacity for carbon monoxide, TLco and Kco). However, patients with mild disease may have a normal FVC at presentation. A mixed obstructive/restrictive pattern may be seen in sarcoidosis or HP, or in patients with combined ILD and emphysema. In fibrotic ILD, change in lung function at 1 year is the single best indicator of prognosis regardless of HRCT pattern or histology. FVC decline is the most reproducible measure of prognosis in IPF and has been adopted as the standard primary endpoint in clinical trials.

Bronchoalveolar Lavage

When a patient undergoes bronchoscopy and bronchoalveolar lavage (BAL), cells from the alveolar spaces and terminal bronchioles are sampled by instillation and aspiration of sequential aliquots of lavage fluid (total volume 100–300 ml for adults) in an affected area of the lung. BAL may be useful investigation in patient with ILD in whom the clinical and radiological picture is not suggestive of UIP. A differential cell count is performed on the BAL fluid to look for evidence of an inflammatory alveolitis, characterised by increased proportions of lymphocytes, neutrophils, or eosinophils compared with normal BAL (Table 15.3) [5]. BAL is rarely diagnostic in ILD, but sometimes a diagnosis of pulmonary eosinophilia or alveolar proteinosis may be made fairly confidently. In patients with unclassified ILD, the presence of BAL lymphocytosis is inconsistent with UIP, and high lymphocyte counts (>25%) may be seen in chronic HP, non-specific interstitial pneumonia (NSIP), or organising pneumonia (OP). The presence of a BAL eosinophilia (>20%) suggests eosinophilic lung disease, which may or may not be accompanied by eosinophilia in peripheral blood. A predominance of pigment-laden macrophages is

Table 15.2 Patterns of ILD seen on high-resolution CT scanning

Pattern	Disease associations	CT features
Usual interstitial pneumonia (UIP)	Idiopathic pulmonary fibrosis Rheumatoid arthritis Other connective tissue disease, e.g. scleroderma Asbestosis	Peripheral and basal reticulation Honeycomb cysts Traction bronchiectasis Little ground glass change
Non-specific interstitial pneumonia (NSIP)	Scleroderma Other connective tissue disease, e.g. anti-synthetase syndromes Idiopathic NSIP	Ground glass change Traction bronchiectasis
Organising pneumonia (OP)	Post-infective Post-chest radiotherapy Drug reactions Polymyositis Anti-synthetase syndromes Idiopathic—COP	Patchy consolidation Air bronchograms
Diffuse alveolar damage (DAD)	Adult respiratory distress syndrome Exacerbation of IPF Acute interstitial pneumonia	Diffuse ground glass change

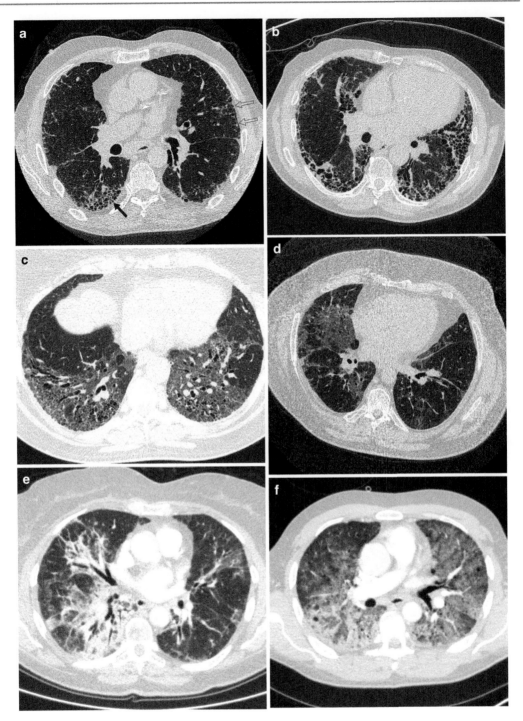

Fig. 15.1 Patterns of interstitial lung disease on chest CT scans. (**a**) Usual interstitial pneumonia (UIP). The characteristic features of UIP on CT scan are shown. Reticulation (lines) is present in a predominantly peripheral and basal distribution (open arrows), and there is honeycomb change (subpleural clusters of small cysts, closed arrow). Traction bronchiectasis may be present, but is not demonstrated on this image. Features regarded as inconsistent with UIP (profuse ground glass change, nodules, bronchocentric distribution, discrete cysts, consolidation, air trap-ping) are absent. (**b**) Advanced UIP, showing extensive honeycomb change. (**c**) Non-specific interstitial pneumonia (NSIP), showing patchy ground glass change with traction bronchiectasis. (**d**) Ground glass change in this patient was due to desquamative interstitial pneumonia (DIP). (**e**) Organising pneumonia, with bilateral consolidation including air bronchograms. (**f**) Diffuse alveolar damage (DAD) appearing as widespread ground glass change in a patient with acute interstitial pneumonia (AIP)

Table 15.3 Normal BAL differential cell counts in non-smoking adults

Cell type	Differential cell count (%)
Macrophages	>85
Lymphocytes	5–15
Neutrophils	≤3
Eosinophils	≤1
Epithelial cells	≤5

compatible with smoking-related ILD, such as respiratory bronchiolitis-ILD (RB-ILD) or desquamative interstitial pneumonia (DIP). If performing a surgical lung biopsy is not feasible, BAL lymphocytosis may be regarded as a non-specific marker of likely response to anti-inflammatory drug therapy, although the utility of BAL cell count as a therapeutic biomarker remains to be studied prospectively.

Lung Biopsy

The value of transbronchial biopsy (TBB) in ILD is limited to patients in whom a diagnosis can be made in a targeted manner on a small piece of tissue. Typically, TBB is most informative in sarcoidosis, malignancy (lymphangitis carcinomatosa), or pulmonary eosinophilia. TBB may sometimes provide helpful information in HP or cryptogenic organising pneumonia (COP), but in IPF and other IIPs an accurate picture of the spatial distribution of the disease is important for the pathologist, so larger samples of lung tissue obtained by surgical lung biopsy are required. Transbronchial biopsy using a freezing cryoprobe (cryobiopsy) has the potential to achieve larger biopsies without crush artefact less invasively than surgical biopsy, but the risk of complications, including bleeding and pneumothorax, is higher than conventional forceps TBB.

Video-assisted thoracic surgical (VATS) lung biopsy provides large tissue samples and is less invasive than open surgical biopsy. VATS biopsy is the investigation of choice in IIPs when clinical and HRCT information does not show a typical pattern of IPF/UIP, provided the patient is fit enough and willing to accept the risk of biopsy. Mortality following VATS biopsy is less than 2%

for elective cases, but 16% if the procedure is performed urgently, [6] for example in patients admitted because of new or worsening symptoms in respiratory failure. In IPF, there is a risk of acute exacerbation following surgical lung biopsy. In IIPs, VATS biopsy aims to demonstrate features of UIP, if present, and biopsies from multiple lobes are recommended because of the heterogeneity of the disease. Areas of established honeycombing, or areas of entirely normal lung on HRCT, should be avoided. Discordance may occur between biopsy findings in different lobes, for example NSIP in one lobe and UIP in another. If discordance occurs, prognosis is determined by the least favourable biopsy pattern (typically UIP). Biopsy is not required if a confident diagnosis of IPF can be made based on clinical-radiological correlation.

Idiopathic Pulmonary Fibrosis

IPF (previously called cryptogenic fibrosing alveolitis (CFA) in the UK) has an incidence of about 10 per hundred thousand people per year, and in the UK it is estimated there are about 5000 new cases diagnosed each year and about 15,000 people living with the disease. It is a disease of older people, with a mean age at presentation around 70 years. IPF is unusual in patients aged younger than 50. There is a slight male predominance, but the disease occurs worldwide and across ethnicities. Median survival is 3–4 years from diagnosis, and 5-year survival figures for IPF are worse than most common cancers.

Pathogenesis

The cause of IPF is unknown. Prevailing views about IPF pathogenesis have shifted away from the idea that fibrosis results from chronic inflammation (alveolitis), largely because of the ineffectiveness of anti-inflammatory therapies. A currently favoured hypothesis is that pulmonary fibrosis ensues from an aberrant healing response following injury to the alveolar epithelium in susceptible individuals. Proposed injurious stimuli include viruses, cigarette smoke, micro-aspiration of gastric refluxate, inhaled metal or wood dusts, or autoimmunity. Multiple injuries may occur together or sequentially. The abnormal healing response is characterised by alveolar epithelial cell damage, apoptosis, and proliferation. Fibroblasts accumulate in the alveolar interstitium and differentiate into collagen-producing myofibroblasts, best seen histologically within fibroblastic foci. Transforming growth factor-beta (TGF-β) is a key cytokine produced by alveolar epithelial cells that drives differentiation of myofibroblasts.

Epidemiological studies have identified associations between IPF and vascular risk, including arterial disease and venous thromboembolism, and systemic hypercoagulability. There is also evidence of local activation of coagulation factors in fibrotic lung, which may directly activate fibroblasts through protease-activated receptors (PARs).

Genetics and Familial IPF

Genetic factors can increase a person's risk of developing IPF, and it has been estimated that 5–20% of patients with IPF have an affected first-degree relative. Genes encoding several proteins, including surfactant proteins, telomerase, and mucins, have been associated with familial and sporadic IPF (Table 15.4). The prevalence of genetic mutations is highest in patients with familial IPF. TERT and TERC genes encode components of telomerase, an enzyme responsible for maintaining the length of telomeres (structures at the ends of chromosomes) that otherwise shorten with each cell division. Variations in surfactant protein C (encoded by the gene SFTPC) and surfactant protein A2 (SFTPA2), which are expressed exclusively by type II alveolar epithelial cells, have been identified in some families with IPF. A naturally occurring variation (polymorphism) in the promoter region of MUC5B accounts for the highest genetic risk for IPF that has been identified so far. MUC5B encodes a gel-forming mucin expressed by bronchial epithelial cells, implying a role for mucociliary dysfunction in IPF aetiology. Pulmonary

Table 15.4 Prevalance of genetic mutations and risk of developing IPF

Gene	Familial IPF (%)	Sporadic IPF (%)	Controls (%)
SFTPC Surfactant protein C	1–25	<1	
SFTPA2 Surfactant protein A	<1	0	
TERT Telomerase reverse transcriptase	8–18	3	
TERC Telomerase RNA component	1	0	
MUC5B Mucin 5B rs35705950	34	38	9

fibrosis also occurs in rare multisystem inherited diseases, including dyskeratosis congenita and Hermansky-Pudlak syndrome.

Clinical Features

The typical patient with IPF is older than 50 years and presents with progressive exertional breathlessness for a year or more, sometimes associated with a dry cough. No cause or association is found on history taking or physical examination. Characteristic physical examination findings are bibasal fine late inspiratory crackles ("velcro® crackles") on chest auscultation. Finger clubbing may be present.

The natural progression of IPF (and hence prognosis) is notoriously difficult to predict for an individual patient at the time of diagnosis. Slow progression is the norm, with average FVC decline about 200 ml per year in patients treated with placebo in IPF clinical trials. However, prior disease behaviour is not always a good predictor of future behaviour. Patients are prone to periods of rapid, often catastrophic deterioration—termed acute exacerbations of IPF once alternative diagnoses have been excluded (see section below on diffuse alveolar damage syndromes). Exacerbations presenting as acute respiratory failure are often fatal despite supportive treatment, and patients who survive are left with significantly impaired lung function.

In patients with IPF, worsening symptoms are commonly due to progressive fibrosis, but important potential co-morbidities should be carefully looked for, including ischaemic heart disease, pneumothorax, pulmonary hypertension, and lung cancer. Pulmonary hypertension is common in IPF, particularly in advanced disease, being present in 50% of patients referred for lung transplantation. Whilst the presence of pulmonary hypertension is associated with shorter survival, treatment with pulmonary vasodilator drugs has not been shown to improve outcomes, and risks worsening hypoxaemia by increasing blood flow to regions of fibrotic lung with poor gas exchange. The risk of developing lung cancer is increased sevenfold in patients with IPF compared with controls even after adjusting for tobacco smoking, with squamous cell and adenocarcinomas being the predominant histological subtypes.

Investigations

Spirometry in established disease will show restriction, with reduced forced vital capacity and a normal FEV_1/FVC ratio. However, in mild disease, FVC may be well preserved, i.e. without evidence of restriction. Baseline abnormalities on lung function testing and 6-min walk test (6MWT) are prognostic indicators in IPF, and serial measurements every 3–12 months are used to assess disease progression. Baseline TLco <40% predicted or desaturation on a 6-min walk test to $SaO_2 \leq 88\%$ indicate severe disease and a worse outcome. Serial measurements are informative, since decline in FVC $\geq 10\%$ or TLco $\geq 15\%$ over 1 year indicate progressive disease and worse prognosis.

The chest X-ray in IPF typically shows bilateral reticular opacities consisting of multiple fine lines. HRCT typically demonstrates a UIP pattern, consisting of reticular opacities in a predominantly basal and peripheral (subpleural) distribution. Reticulation may extend caudally where it is characteristically becomes more prominent anteriorly, whereas the distribution is mainly posterior at the lung bases. Honeycombing refers to clusters of small cysts (3–10 mm) in a subpleural location, and is regarded as pathognomic of UIP. A "definite UIP" HRCT scan with all these features is sufficient to make a diagnosis of IPF in a patient with consistent clinical findings. Sometimes peripheral and basal reticulation may not be associated with honeycombing (a so-called "possible UIP" pattern), in which case the presence of traction bronchiectasis is highly predictive of UIP pathology. In the absence of honeycombing or traction bronchiectasis, or in the presence of significant ground glass change, VATS lung biopsy should be considered to exclude non-UIP pathologies such as NSIP or chronic HP. However, in the absence of histology, the extent of reticulation and increasing age of the patient (>70 years) are good predictors of underlying UIP.

Characteristic blood test findings in IPF include a polyclonal increase in serum immunoglobulins, raised lactate dehydrogenase, and mild elevations of inflammatory parameters (erythrocyte sedimentation rate, plasma viscosity, C-reactive protein). Positive antinuclear antibodies may be found, and the term interstitial pneumonia with autoimmune features (IPAF) has been proposed to describe patients without clinical evidence of connective tissue disease who have positive autoantibodies. However, it is unclear whether disease course, prognosis, or treatment response are influenced by positive autoantibodies.

In the majority of cases of IPF, a diagnosis can be made with careful clinical-radiological correlation, but sometimes further information in the form of a surgical lung biopsy is required to make an accurate diagnosis by multidisciplinary consensus. The histopathological features of UIP are patchy fibrosis with architectural distortion and the presence of fibroblastic foci (Fig. 15.2a, b).

Treatment of IPF

Lung transplantation should be considered for suitable people (see Chap. 20), since there is no treatment that can cure IPF or halt its progression. There have been many randomised controlled trials of different interventions in IPF

Fig. 15.2 Histology of usual interstitial pneumonia (UIP) on a VATS lung biopsy stained with H&E. (**a**) Low-power photomicrograph demonstrating the patchy nature of disease in UIP. Beneath the pleural surface (left) are areas of normal lung (open arrows) adjacent to grossly abnormal areas containing pink-staining fibrosis (black arrows) and a patchy chronic inflammatory cell infiltrate (white arrow). (**b**) High-power photomicrograph of UIP showing a characteristic fibroblastic focus (black arrow) lying beneath metaplastic bronchiolised epithelium (open arrow) in an airspace containing alveolar macrophages (white arrow). Photomicrographs provided by Dr. Anne Campbell

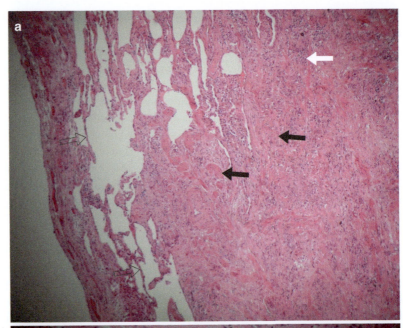

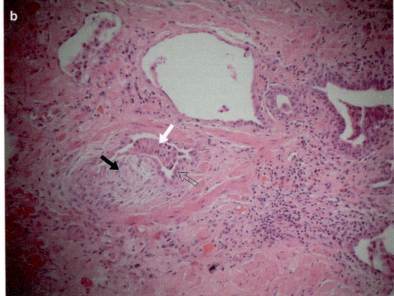

which have been summarised in international guidelines (Table 15.5) [7, 8]. Most of the interventions that are given a positive recommendation are based on only weak evidence, whereas stronger evidence exists for interventions which are not recommended, reflecting the fact that most clinical trials of novel interventions in IPF have proved negative. Two disease-modifying drugs, nintedanib and pirfenidone, are recom-

mended for use in some patients, whereas treatment regimes containing corticosteroids (e.g. prednisolone) should not be used for people with IPF.

Corticosteroids

A placebo-controlled trial (PANTHER-IPF) of a previously widely prescribed treatment regime comprising prednisone, azathioprine, and the

Table 15.5 Recommendations for treatment of IPF

Strong Yes Most people would want the intervention	Weak Yes The majority of people would want the intervention, but many would not	Weak No The majority of people would not want the intervention, but some would	Strong No Most people would not want the intervention
Lung transplantation + Long term oxygen therapy in patients with significant resting hypoxaemia +	Nintedanib +++ Pirfenidone +++ Pulmonary rehabilitation + Treatment of asymptomatic acid reflux + Corticosteroids for exacerbations +	Sildenafil +++ Macitentan or bosentan ++ N-acetylcysteine monotherapy ++ Treatment of pulmonary hypertension ++ Mechanical ventilation for exacerbations ++	Prednisolone, azathioprine, and N-acetylcysteine ++ Warfarin ++ Imatinib +++ Ambrisentan ++

Quality of evidence: + very low; ++ low, +++ moderate, ++++ high

Table 15.6 Comparison of nintedanib and pirfenidone for treatment of IPF

	Nintedanib	Pirfenidone
Mechanism of action	Tyrosine kinase inhibitor	Unknown
Licence	EU marketing authorisation FDA approved	EU marketing authorisation FDA approved
UK regulatory approvals	NICE: FVC 50–80% predicted SMC: FVC≤80%	NICE: FVC 50–80% SMC: FVC≤80%
Adverse effects	Diarrhoea, nausea, vomiting, anorexia, weight loss	Nausea, dyspepsia, anorexia, vomiting, weight loss, photosensitive rash (requires sun-avoidance measures)
Contraindications	Anticoagulant therapy (warfarin, direct oral anticoagulants)	
Pill burden	2 pills per day	up to 9 pills per day

EU European Union, *FDA* Food and drug administration, *FVC* forced vital capacity, *NICE* National Institute for Health and Care Excellence, *SMC* Scottish Medicines Consortium

antioxidant N-acetylcysteine (NAC) was stopped early after an interim analysis showed significantly more deaths and hospitalisations in the steroid-containing triple therapy arm compared with placebo [9]. The worse outcomes were mainly due to progressive pulmonary fibrosis rather than specific side effects of the drugs. Based on this evidence, patients with IPF should not be treated with steroids or other anti-inflammatory drugs.

Disease-Modifying Drug Therapy

Nintedanib and pirfenidone are approved in Europe and the U.S. for treatment of IPF. These drugs were studied in separate placebo-controlled randomised trials of similar designs. The primary endpoint of the trials was rate of decline of FVC. Although the two drugs are different struc-turally and pharmacologically, their efficacy compared with placebo was similar. Both slowed the rate of decline in forced vital capacity over 1 year by about half. Neither improved lung function or halted the progression of IPF. There were no demonstrable effects of either drug on patient-reported outcomes such as breathlessness or quality of life. There were trends to improved survival with both drugs, but the trials were not statistically powered to detect changes in patient-reported outcomes or mortality.

Whilst drug treatment can slow progression of disease, this has to be balanced against potential adverse effects. The most frequently occurring adverse events are listed in Table 15.6. Both drugs caused significantly more upper gastrointestinal side effects than placebo. Nintedanib caused more diarrhoea, whereas pirfenidone caused more rashes, typically due to photosensitivity affecting light-exposed skin.

Although the two drugs have not been directly compared, their efficacy against placebo is similar, and so choice should be determined by appropriately informed patient preference. Whilst the development of nintedanib and pirfenidone represents progress in drug treatment for IPF, significant issues remain. Treatment does not halt disease progression, and the drugs are expensive. Patients with chronic fibrosing ILDs other than IPF, whether idiopathic or CTD-related, are disenfranchised with no approved treatments. With two drugs showing disease-modifying effects in IPF, future placebo-controlled trials will be more challenging, since new experimental treatments will have to show an effect in addition to existing therapy.

Non-pharmacological Treatment for IPF

There should be a focus on palliation of symptoms, and it is important to consider referral to multidisciplinary palliative care services when advancing IPF is identified as disease progression can be unpredictable. Conveying appropriate disease-related information is important, and input from a specialist ILD nurse in this setting is valuable. Lung disease charities provide useful information for patients and carers in print and electronic form. Addressing chronic refractory breathlessness may involve simple measures such as using a handheld fan, which has been shown to result in a significant reduction in breathlessness after only 5 min of use when directed across the nose and mouth. Drug therapy with opioids (e.g. slow-release morphine 10 mg once daily) or benzodiazepines may be helpful. The evidence for pulmonary rehabilitation in IPF is predominantly extrapolated from its use in the context of COPD, where it has been found to be of benefit. Long-term oxygen therapy is recommended if a patient is breathless and hypoxaemic at rest, again extrapolating evidence from COPD studies. Patients with severe ILD are often tachypnoeic at rest and desaturate markedly on ambulation, and may require high oxygen flow rates to maintain oxygenation (SaO_2 around 90%). Systems are available to deliver up to 15 L/min of heated humidified supplemental oxygen in a patient's home to support them in the advanced stages of their disease. Patients can be offered ambulatory oxygen for use during exercise in a pulmonary rehabilitation programme if they have demonstrated an improvement in exercise endurance.

Cough is often a difficult symptom for patients with IPF. Studies have shown that patients with IPF have a high incidence of acid and non-acid reflux when compared to controls, and it has been suggested that reflux may contribute to the pathogenesis and progression of IPF. It is often informative to look for symptoms suggestive of a reflux cough in patients with IPF, and to offer trials of anti-reflux treatment if appropriate (see Chap. 5).

For many patients with IPF, recruitment to an ongoing randomised controlled trial of an experimental treatment is a good option.

ILD Associated with Connective Tissue Disease

Patients with connective tissue disease (CTD) make up 10–20% of all patients with ILD, with the most common associations being rheumatoid arthritis, scleroderma, polymyositis/dermatomyositis, and anti-synthetase syndromes. Antinuclear antibody testing should be performed in patients presenting with ILD, including Jo-1 (anti-histidyl transfer RNA synthetase), Scl70 (anti-topoisomerase), and rheumatoid factor. Anti-CCP antibodies and serum creatine kinase may be helpful in identifying patients with rheumatoid arthritis and and occult myositis respectively. The increasing recognition of polymyositis-related anti-synthetase syndromes, characterised by non-Jo-1 antibodies against other tRNA synthetases, means that extended antibody testing may be valuable. Characteristic clinical features of anti-synthetase syndromes include ILD, oesophageal dysmotility, "mechanics hands" (thickening and fissuring of skin on the fingertips and thenar aspects of the fingers), Raynaud's phenomenon, and muscle pain or weakness with raised serum creatine kinase. Some patients with an IIP and positive antinuclear antibodies have no clinical features of a CTD, and the term IPAF (interstitial pneumonia with autoimmune features) has been coined to describe these patients. Generally the prognosis for patients with CTD-ILD is better than those with IPF. In ILD associated with myositis or anti-synthestase syndrome, where the predominant pattern of ILD on HRCT is a combination of OP and NSIP, a good initial response to steroid therapy can be expected. In scleroderma-ILD, typically associated with NSIP pattern but sometimes UIP, the response to anti-inflammatory therapy is less predictable. The Scleroderma Lung Trial demonstrated that oral cyclophoshamide conferred a very small benefit over placebo in terms of slowing decline in lung function at 1 year. Oral mycophenolate may be a less toxic and more acceptable alternative to cyclophosphamide. In RA-ILD the typical UIP pattern of ILD often mimics IPF and is resistant to anti-inflammatory therapy, but there are no good-quality clinical trials to guide management. Aggressive therapy with intravenous methylprednisolone and cyclophosphamide may be tried in patients with rapidly progressive RA-ILD, provided the patient is willing to accept the risk of therapy balanced against the small chance of disease response.

Idiopathic Non-specific Interstitial Pneumonia

Some patients present in a similar manner to IPF but with a "NSIP pattern" on HRCT, comprising bilateral patchy ground glass changes most pronounced at the lung bases. The presence of accompanying reticular shadowing or traction bronchiectasis indicates that the ground glass change represents fine diffuse fibrosis histologically, rather than inflammation. Patients are usually younger, with a female preponderance. A careful search for underlying CTD should be performed and may reveal suggestive features such as arthritis, muscle pain or weakness, skin

changes, periungual erythema with dilated capillary loops on nailfold capillaroscopy, telangiectasia, Raynaud's, or swallowing problems. Antinuclear antibody testing should be supplemented with an extended myositis antibody screen to look for an occult anti-synthetase syndrome. If no CTD can be found, VATS lung biopsy is recommended, which may show features of fibrotic NSIP, principally comprising varying degrees of interstitial inflammation and fibrosis which appear uniform, without the temporally and geographically patchy appearance seen in UIP. Fibroblastic foci may be seen, but are fewer in number than in UIP. Such patients often present a dilemma because it is unclear whether the focus of treatment should be anti-inflammatory or anti-fibrotic. Typically, anti-inflammatory/immunosuppressant treatment is tried with monitoring of response over 3–6 months, and if improvement is demonstrated, then maintenance treatment is continued in the same as for CTD. In contrast, progressive disease often indicates behaviour similar to IPF. NSIP and UIP frequently occur together in the same patient if biopsies from multiple lobes are taken, in which case UIP is dominant in determining prognosis.

Pneumoconiosis

Pneumoconiosis refers to the accumulation of solid inorganic dust in the lungs and the ensuing fibrotic tissue reaction. In coal workers' pneumoconiosis (CWP), deposition in the alveoli will occur when fine particles of dust 0.5–5 μm in diameter are inhaled. Particles not cleared by the mucociliary escalator are ingested by alveolar macrophages, seen pathologically as black focal centrilobular nodules. Coal dust may be transported within macrophages via the lymphatics to draining lymph nodes.

Simple CWP typically occurs in coal workers after at least 10 years of coal dust exposure. It appears on a chest X-ray as multiple pulmonary nodules 1–4 mm in diameter. Simple CWP alone does not lead to significant symptoms, physical signs, or lung function impairment, and prognosis is good. However, significant disability may result from co-existing coal dust-related chronic bronchitis and emphysema.

Progressive massive fibrosis (PMF) occurs when simple CWP is complicated by multiple larger (>1 cm) nodules, typically occurring peripherally in the upper lobes. PMF may progress even after removal from dust exposure, leading to breathlessness and respiratory failure. Features of chronic bronchitis and emphysema commonly coexist and contribute to functional and physiological impairment. Other complications include chest pain, pneumothorax, haemoptysis, and melanoptysis (coughing black sputum).

Caplan's Syndrome

Caplan's syndrome occurs in coal workers with rheumatoid factor-positive rheumatoid arthritis, and is characterized by multiple larger (0.5–5 cm) nodules lying in a subpleural location with background changes of simple CWP. The pulmonary nodules in Caplan's syndrome demonstrate histological features of rheumatoid nodules, with an outer fibrous layer, an inner cellular palisade of radially-arranged macrophages and fibroblasts, and central fibrinoid necrosis. Caplan's nodules may calcify or cavitate due to central necrosis.

Silicosis

Silicosis occurs due to inhalation of respirable crystalline silica (silicon dioxide, quartz). Silica is widely occurring in stone, rocks, sand, glass, and clay. At-risk occupations include tunneling, quarrying, mining coal and metals, sand blasting, potteries, foundry work, and stone masonry. Even though silica often contributes to other forms of pneumoconiosis, silicosis should be used to describe disease caused primarily by inhalation of free silica. Silica particles are highly fibrogenic in the lung, with dense, glassy, fibrotic nodules occurring following particle ingestion by macrophages. Multiple small pulmonary nodules throughout the lung fields, but more pronounced in the upper and mid zones, are characteristic, along with hilar lymph node enlargement and calcification ("eggshell calcification") which can be confused with sarcoidosis if the occupational history is unclear. In complicated silicosis, PMF may occur due to conglomeration of nodules. Acute silicosis occurs following a short (6 months) but intense exposure to inhaled silica, but is extremely rare. There is no specific treatment for silicosis other than removal from exposure to silica dust. Inhalation of silica also increases the risk of tuberculosis and lung cancer.

Asbestosis

Asbestosis is pulmonary fibrosis secondary to inhalation of asbestos fibres. The diagnosis of asbestosis requires a history of sufficiently heavy occupational exposure to asbestos, along with establishing the presence of pulmonary fibrosis. Often there will be evidence of co-existing asbestos-related pleural disease, but this is not required for a firm diagnosis. Clinically, radiologically, physiologically, and pathologically asbestosis is similar to IPF, and distinction is important in terms of prognosis, eligibility for financial compensation, and access to disease-modifying anti-fibrotic drugs. A detailed occupational exposure history is vital. At-risk occupations include those involving asbestos mining, milling, or transport (dock workers); manufacture of asbestos products; or handling asbestos, including laggers, electricians, joiners, pipe fitters, sheet metal workers, or boiler makers.

Asbestosis typically occurs after a latent period of 15–30 years following prolonged occupational exposure (e.g. 10–20 years) to asbestos, but it may occur following short, intense exposures equating to at least daily exposure for 1 year. It is thought that clinical asbestosis is unlikely if cumulative exposure is much below 25[f/ml]y (i.e. exposure equivalent to 1 fibre/ml for 25 years, 2.5 fibres/ml for 10 years, etc.) but this view has been challenged, and it is likely that lower exposures may cause fibrosis in some individuals.

Tobacco smoking increases the risk of asbestosis in asbestos-exposed workers and makes progression more likely. Inhaled asbestos fibres deposited in small airways migrate through the lung tissue, causing local injury, inflammation (alveolitis), and fibrosis. Peri-bronchiolar fibrosis might cause pathological changes in the small airways, but there is no physiological evidence of airflow obstruction in non-smokers with asbestosis. The characteristic physiological findings are those of restriction with reduced gas transfer caused by the interstitial fibrosis. Asbestos fibres phagocytosed by lung macrophages may be cleared from the lungs through draining lymphatics, or may dissolve slowly over time. Some fibres within macrophages become coated with an iron-rich proteinaceous material and can be visualised with special stains on light microscopy as asbestos bodies. The presence of fibrosis and asbestos bodies in lung tissue or BAL is sufficient to diagnose asbestosis, but lung biopsy purely to support a medico-legal claim is not justifiable. Chrysotile asbestos is cleared relatively quickly from the lung, whereas amphiboles are retained, perhaps explaining their greater propensity to cause fibrosis. Most asbestos fibres remain uncoated and invisible on light microscopy, but may be identified and quantified by methods including electron microscopy, which may be helpful in assessing the degree of asbestos exposure.

In distinguishing asbestosis from IPF or other chronic fibrosing ILD, the presence of pleural plaques or thickening support a history of asbestos exposure, but do not confirm that heavy exposure has taken place. The prognosis of asbestosis is better than IPF, with most patients demonstrating stability or very slow progression. There is no intervention that will prevent development of asbestosis once exposure has occurred, or slow disease progression once fibrosis has developed. The risk of lung cancer is increased by smoking and asbestosis in a multiplicative manner and is one of the commonest causes of death. Individuals with heavy asbestos exposure are at greater risk for lung cancer even in the absence of asbestosis.

In the UK, patients with pneumoconiosis or asbestosis may be eligible to claim financial compensation in the form of industrial injuries disablement benefit if it can be demonstrated that their occupation contributed to the disease. The amount of compensation received is based on the degree of disability suffered.

Hypersensitivity Pneumonitis (Extrinsic Allergic Alveolitis)

Hypersensitivity pneumonitis (HP), also known as extrinsic allergic alveolitis (EAA), is caused by immunological responses to inhaled antigens of organic origin, derived from bacteria, fungi, plants, or animals. History taking should focus on possible occupational or environmental exposures, some of which are listed in Table 15.7. Inhaled particles are small enough to be deposited in the small airways, or alveoli, where a susceptible individual responds with a combination of hypersensitivity reactions type III (mediated

Table 15.7 Examples of exposures to inhaled allergens that cause hypersensitivity pneumonitis

Allergen	Exposure	Disease
Micropolyspora faeni	Mouldy hay	Farmer's lung
Avian proteins	Feathers and droppings	Bird fancier's lung
Microbial contamination	Metalworking fluid mists	Metal worker's lung
Thermophilic actinomycetes	Humidifier mist	Humidifier lung
Mycobacterium avium complex	Hot tub mist	Hot tub lung
Thermophilic actinomycetes	Sugar cane	Bagassosis
Aspergillus clavatus	Mouldy barley	Malt worker's lung
Thermophilic actinomycetes	Compost	Mushroom worker's lung
Aquatic animal proteins	Shellfish	Prawn/mollusk worker's lung
Penicillium glabrum	Mouldy cork dust	Suberosis

by IgG antibody production and immune complex formation) and type IV (delayed type, mediated by activated T lymphocytes). The hallmark of the disease has been regarded as the formation of IgG antibodies ("precipitins") which can be measured in blood, although many exposed individuals will have measurable antibodies without disease, and some individuals with HP have negative antibody tests if their disease is driven by a predominantly cellular (type IV hypersensitivity) immune response. Pathologically, lymphocytic inflammation is centred on the small airways and alveoli, with loosely-formed non-caseating granulomata.

In acute and subacute disease, the patient presents with breathlessness and cough, often with constitutional symptoms that may be misdiagnosed as infection. On chest auscultation, characteristic inspiratory squeaks or squawks may be heard, reflecting small airways disease.

The chest X-ray is abnormal, with diffuse bilateral opacification of the lung fields (Fig. 15.3a, b). Typically there is upper/mid lung predominance, but this is not universal. Lung function tests are usually abnormal, showing evidence of restriction with reduced FVC, often with co-existing obstruction due to small airways

inflammation. Gas transfer (TLco) is often markedly reduced and desaturation occurs on a 6-min walk test.

The key investigation is a high-resolution CT scan of the chest which demonstrates widespread centrilobular nodules most marked in the upper and mid-zones, with sparing adjacent to the pleural surface, and which is particularly apparent around the oblique fissures (Fig. 15.3). This pattern indicates disease centered on small airways. The upper parts of the lungs are worst affected. Toward the bases of the lungs there are more spared areas of normal lung leading to a mosaic pattern, which is accentuated on an expiratory scan because of small airways disease and gas trapping.

In clear-cut cases with a history of exposure, positive serum precipitins, and a compatible HRCT scan, pursuing tissue histology may be unnecessary, and the patient should be advised to completely avoid exposure to the causative antigen. In cases of uncertainty, BAL or a transbronchial or VATS lung biopsy will demonstrate lymphocytic interstitial information and loosely formed granulomata. Recovery following removal of exposure to antigen may take many months, with lung function improvements often lagging behind resolution of symptoms.

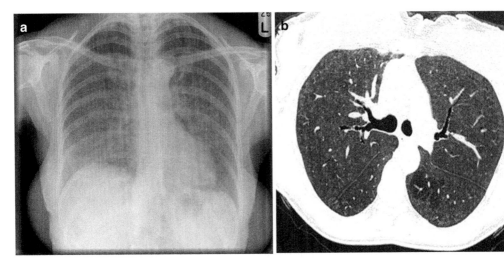

Fig. 15.3 Hypersenstivity pneumonitis (extrinsic allergic alveolitis). (**a**) Chest X-ray showing diffuse bilateral opacification. (**b**) High-resolution CT scan showing widespread soft centrilobular nodularity with sparing of the subpleural and peri-fissural regions

Chronic Hypersensitivity Pneumonitis

A chronic fibrosing ILD may occur in patients with persistent low-grade allergen exposure, which may be difficult to distinguish from IPF or other IIPs. In contrast to acute and subacute forms of the disease, the pathogenesis of chronic HP is poorly understood. The disease may mimic IPF with chronic breathlessness, crackles on chest auscultation, reticulation and honeycombing on HRCT, and interstitial fibrosis with fibroblastic foci on biopsy. Additional clues to the aetiology include evidence of small airways disease with squeaks or squawks on auscultation, mosaic pattern with air trapping, upper lobe reticulation or nodules with sparing of the lung bases, peribronchial fibrosis on HRCT, BAL lymphocytosis, or granulomata on biopsy. Removal from antigen exposure often does not lead to clinical improvement, and the disease is likely to progress. Even more challenging are cases of chronic fibrosing ILD suggestive of chronic HP where no inciting antigen exposure can be identified. In up to a third of cases with a histological appearance suggesting chronic HP, no causative environmental exposure can be identified. It is unknown whether "idiopathic chronic HP" genuinely results from a chronic hypersensitivity reaction to an unidentified inhaled allergen, or whether a similar histological pattern results from an alternative pathogenesis. Response to anti-inflammatory therapy is often disappointing.

Acute/Subacute ILD

Organising Pneumonia

Organising pneumonia (OP) describes a pattern seen on CT scanning or lung biopsy which should not be regarded as a disease, but rather an aberrant healing response following lung injury. OP can occur in a variety of conditions including infection, CTD, malignancy, following radiother-

apy, in some drug reactions, and immunodeficiency. If no cause can be found it is known as cryptogenic organising pneumonia (COP) (previously known as bronchiolitis obliterans organising pneumonia (BOOP)). Surgical lung biopsy is generally required to make a confident diagnosis of COP, although TBB may be sufficient in radiologically typical cases.

CT scan of the chest in OP the shows patchy consolidation with air bronchograms, typically in subpleural locations, which may appear to be migratory on serial imaging (Fig. 15.1). There may be patchy ground glass change, and sometimes reticulation or nodules. A similar pattern may be seen in classical pneumonia due to a community-acquired infection with *Streptococcus pneumoniae* or other organisms, so this has to be put in the context of the clinical presentation. COP tends to present with progressive breathlessness and cough over several weeks or months, and may be accompanied by fever, myalgia, and elevated blood inflammatory markers. Lung function tests will typically show restriction with impaired gas transfer.

On lung biopsy, the features of OP include granulation and fibroblastic tissue within the small airways and the alveoli. There is often patchy fibrosis involving alveoli and distal bronchioles. Fibroblasts and inflammatory cells are seen embedded in extracellular matrix, forming polypoid masses within the airspaces known as Masson bodies.

The prognosis of COP is good, with at least half of cases regressing spontaneously. In nonremitting or progressive COP, corticosteroids are often used on the basis that there may be an autoimmune aetiology, although there have been no good-quality clinical trials. In steroid-responsive cases, relapse may occur after stopping therapy.

COP may sometimes present as fulminant acute respiratory failure, in which case the prognosis is poor. In other cases it behaves more like a fibrotic IIP, with progressive breathlessness unresponsive to steroid therapy. Biopsy in these cases will often show a mixed picture of OP and interstitial fibrosis.

Diffuse Alveolar Damage Syndromes

Diffuse alveolar damage (DAD) is a pathological pattern seen in acute respiratory distress syndrome (ARDS), which typically ensues several days following major trauma or sepsis. DAD is also a feature of exacerbations of IPF in people with pre-existing pulmonary fibrosis. Rarely, DAD may occur in patients without an inciting cause, when it is referred to as acute interstitial pneumonia (AIP, also known as Hamman Rich syndrome). DAD syndromes tend to present acutely and CT scan shows widespread ground glass change (Fig. 15.1). The prognosis of DAD is poor.

Acute exacerbations of IPF (AE-IPF) are characterised by rapidly increasing breathlessness, typically over several days or weeks, associated with new ground glass opacities on chest X-ray and CT scan on a background of pre-existing reticulation and honeycomb change. The differential diagnosis includes infection, heart failure, and pulmonary embolism. Investigations should be performed to rule out these alternative diagnoses as much as possible, and if no clear evidence can be found, then a diagnosis of AE-IPF can be made. Recognised triggers include viral infections, trauma, and surgery (including VATS lung biopsy). The risk of AE-IPF seems to be higher in patients with more severe IPF. Mortality is high, up to 85% for patients admitted to hospital with respiratory failure. There is no specific treatment for AE-IPF, and management should be focussed on supportive care. Corticosteroids are frequently administered despite a lack of evidence supporting their use. Because of the poor prognosis, mechanical ventilation should be avoided.

Smoking-Related ILD

RB-ILD and DIP can be regarded as forms of smoking-related macrophage pneumonia, in which exposure to an inhaled irritant leads to pronounced accumulation of macrophages in small airways and alveolar air spaces. Most smokers will display some evidence of respiratory bronchiolitis up to 3 years after quitting. RB-ILD is more extensive than simple respiratory bronchiolitis and is characterised on HRCT scanning by centrilobular nodules and ground glass change. Histologically, pigmented macrophages are seen in airspaces centred on bronchioles, and there may be mild peri-bronchiolar fibrosis. Smoking cessation will usually lead to remission. In DIP the changes are more extensive still. The CT scan in DIP typically shows widespread or patchy ground glass change, worse in the lower lobes (Fig. 15.1), and biopsy shows extensive accumulation of pigmented macrophages in the alveolar airspaces, with accompanying interstitial inflammation and fibrosis. Smoking cessation is the mainstay of treatment. Thirty percent of DIP cases occur in non-smokers, making diagnosis and management difficult. Progressive or non-remitting disease is often treated with steroid-containing immunosuppressive regimes, although this practice is not supported by robust clinical trial evidence.

References

1. American Thoracic Society/American Thoracic Society/European Respiratory Society International Multidisciplinary Consensus Classification of the Idiopathic Interstitial Pneumonias. This joint statement of the American Thoracic Society (ATS), and the European Respiratory Society (ERS) was adopted by the ATS board of directors, June 2001 and by the ERS Executive Committee, June 2001. Am J Respir Crit Care Med. 2002;165(2):277–304.
2. Travis WD, Costabel U, Hansell DM, King TE Jr, Lynch DA, Nicholson AG, et al. An official American Thoracic Society/European Respiratory Society statement: update of the international multidisciplinary classification of the idiopathic interstitial pneumonias. Am J Respir Crit Care Med. 2013;188(6):733–48.
3. Bradley B, Branley HM, Egan JJ, Greaves MS, Hansell DM, Harrison NK, et al. Interstitial lung disease guideline: the British Thoracic Society in collaboration with the Thoracic Society of Australia and New Zealand and the Irish Thoracic Society. Thorax. 2008;63(Suppl 5):v1–58.
4. Conway R, Low C, Coughlan RJ, O'Donnell MJ, Carey JJ. Methotrexate use and risk of lung disease in psoriasis, psoriatic arthritis, and inflammatory bowel disease: systematic literature review and

meta-analysis of randomised controlled trials. BMJ. 2015;350:h1269.

5. Meyer KC, Raghu G, Baughman RP, Brown KK, Costabel U, du Bois RM, et al. An official American Thoracic Society clinical practice guideline: the clinical utility of bronchoalveolar lavage cellular analysis in interstitial lung disease. Am J Respir Crit Care Med. 2012;185(9):1004–14.

6. Hutchinson JP, Fogarty AW, McKeever TM, Hubbard RB. In-hospital mortality after surgical lung biopsy for interstitial lung disease in the United States. 2000 to 2011. Am J Respir Crit Care Med. 2016;193(10):1161–7.

7. Raghu G, Collard HR, Egan JJ, Martinez FJ, Behr J, Brown KK, et al. An official ATS/ERS/ JRS/ALAT statement: idiopathic pulmonary fibrosis: evidence-based guidelines for diagnosis and management. Am J Respir Crit Care Med. 2011;183(6):788–824.

8. Raghu G, Rochwerg B, Zhang Y, Garcia CA, Azuma A, Behr J, et al. An official ATS/ERS/JRS/ALAT clinical practice guideline: treatment of idiopathic pulmonary fibrosis. an update of the 2011 clinical practice guideline. Am J Respir Crit Care Med. 2015;192(2):e3–19.

9. Idiopathic Pulmonary Fibrosis Clinical Research Network, Raghu G, Anstrom KJ, King TE Jr, Lasky JA, Martinez FJ. Prednisone, azathioprine, and N-acetylcysteine for pulmonary fibrosis. N Engl J Med. 2012;366(21):1968–77.

Sarcoidosis

16

Robina K. Coker

Introduction

The cutaneous lesions of sarcoidosis were first recognised and described by Jonathan Hutchinson in London in 1869 and by Caesar Boeck in Norway in 1899. It is now clear that sarcoidosis affects the lungs in over 90% of cases, and accounts for around a third of the patients with interstitial lung disease (ILD) seen in specialist respiratory clinics. Although the twenty-first century has given us a better appreciation of potential predisposing environmental and genetic factors, the pathogenesis and optimal management of this multisystem condition remain poorly understood.

A significant proportion of patients with active disease are limited in their daytime activities by breathlessness, fatigue, or arthralgia. The course of sarcoidosis varies considerably. While there is a high rate of spontaneous remission, the disease may persist in up to one-third. It is currently not possible to predict with certainty which patients will develop chronic or progressive disease, or how best to manage them.

Treatment is indicated for vital organ involvement and usually consists of systemic corticosteroids with or without other immunosuppressive agents. Biologic drugs such as infliximab may be of value in some patients. Supplemental oxygen may be required. Lung transplantation is reserved for those with respiratory failure who fail to respond to maximal therapy, and is limited by organ availability. Other potential serious complications include pulmonary hypertension, lung cavitation with mycetoma formation, and opportunistic infections resulting from immunosuppression.

Epidemiology

Sarcoidosis is recognised worldwide and affects all racial and ethnic groups. It can present at any age, with a peak incidence between the ages of 20 and 50 years. Variations in incidence around the world probably reflect different environmental exposures, reporting methods, predisposing HLA alleles, and genetic factors. The highest annual incidence of 5–40 cases per 100,000 is reported in northern Europe, while annual incidence in Japan is just 1–2 per 100,000. The condition is much more prevalent in Afro-Caribbean and black populations. Annual incidence among black Americans is approximately three times that in white Americans, with around 35 cases per 100,000 compared with 11 per 100,000. Afro-Caribbean and black patients are also more likely to develop chronic and potentially fatal disease. The condition is more common in

R. K. Coker
Respiratory Medicine, Hammersmith Hospital,
Imperial College Healthcare NHS Trust, London, UK
e-mail: r.coker@nhs.net

© Springer International Publishing AG, part of Springer Nature 2018
S. Hart, M. Greenstone (eds.), *Foundations of Respiratory Medicine*,
https://doi.org/10.1007/978-3-319-94127-1_16

females across all racial and ethnic groups. It has been estimated that around 3000 cases are diagnosed each year in the UK.

Pathogenesis

Seasonal clustering of sarcoidosis, with new cases presenting more frequently in the spring and early summer, is well described. This observation, and the fact that the commonest organs involved are the skin, lungs, and eyes, has led to extensive investigation into possible environmental triggers. A number have been reported, including exposure to tree pollen, wood-burning stoves, insecticides, and moulds. Occupational associations have been noted with naval service, metalworking, and handling of building materials. An increased incidence of sarcoidosis was reported in New York City Fire Department rescue workers involved in the aftermath of the 2001 World Trade Center terrorist attack. Berylliosis may be clinically indistinguishable from sarcoidosis; those at risk include workers in aerospace, electronics, and nuclear industries. A careful occupational history is therefore essential. Studies have reported finding T cells and serum antibodies that recognise mycobacterial antigens in patients with sarcoidosis.

Familial sarcoidosis is well documented, with concordance in monozygotic twins apparently higher than in dizygotic twins. In the North American A Case Control Etiological Sarcoidosis Study (ACCESS), patients with sarcoidosis reported siblings or parents with the disease five times as often as control subjects [1]. Phenotypic features and outcomes do not appear to be concordant in siblings, with the exception of eye and liver involvement.

A number of HLA associations are reported with sarcoidosis, including with class I HLA-B8 antigens, and class II antigens encoded by HLA-DRB1 and DQB1 alleles. Associations with non-HLA candidate genes, such as tumour necrosis factor α (TNF-α), interferon-γ, and chemokine receptors, have not been confirmed. The outcomes of genome-wide scans for loci associated with sarcoidosis appear to vary with the population being studied.

Taking into consideration the above, it is presumed that sarcoidosis results from immune responses to various environmental triggers in genetically susceptible individuals. Epigenetic studies to identify interactions between genetic and environmental factors, for instance specific genetic loci and environmental modifiers, would appear to be essential to define the aetiology more precisely.

Pathology

Although not specific for sarcoidosis, the histological hallmark of the condition is the presence of non-caseating granulomas in affected tissues. The process whereby granulomas are generated is incompletely understood, but exposure to unknown antigen(s) appears to result in acquired cellular immunity, with granuloma formation dependent on interaction between antigen-presenting cells and antigen-specific CD4+ T lymphocytes. Triggering antigen(s) appear to favour accumulation and activation of selective T cell clones. Activated CD4+ cells differentiate into type 1 helper T (Th1) cells, predominantly secreting interleukin-2 (IL-2) and interferon-γ (IFN-γ). They thereby augment TNF-α production by macrophages and amplify the local cellular immune response. Despite extensive local inflammation, peripheral anergy may also develop, manifest as a depressed immune response to the tuberculin skin test (TST).

Granulomas may resolve without adverse sequelae, but pulmonary fibrosis is a complication in up to 25% of patients. The precise causes are unclear, but may reflect a shift to a Th2 cell phenotype with increased production of interleukins 4, 10, and 13. Alveolar macrophages activated in the presence of a Th2 cytokine profile produce increased levels of fibronectin and the CC motif ligand 18 (CCL18) chemokine. CCL18 increases lung fibroblast collagen production, which in turn increases macrophage release of CCL18, perpetuating the development of fibrosis which can result in irreversible damage.

Clinical Presentations

Patients may present in a variety of ways (Fig. 16.1a–j). Good education for healthcare practitioners who may not previously have encountered the condition is thus vital to help prevent delays in referral and diagnosis. Patients may be asymptomatic, and physical examination may be normal. Abnormalities on chest radiograph (CXR) or computed tomography (CT) scanning may be noted as an incidental finding during pre-employment screening or while undergoing investigations for an unrelated condition. Patients may present acutely with the classic Löfgren's syndrome, comprising erythema nodosum, arthritis, and bilateral hilar lymphadenopathy (BHL) on CXR. Alternatively, they may present with a more insidious onset of non-specific symptoms including fatigue, sweats, weight loss, and arthralgia. Cough (usually dry) and breathlessness are frequently reported. Less common but well described is Heerfordt's syndrome, consisting of fever, parotid enlargement, anterior uveitis, and facial nerve palsy.

Other extra-pulmonary symptoms and signs depend on the affected organ(s). Acute uveitis is a potential cause of irreversible blindness, which mandates urgent ophthalmology review and treatment. Patients with cutaneous lesions including erythema nodosum, nodules, and plaques may present to the dermatology clinic; those with arthralgia or dactylitis may be referred to the rheumatology service. Neurosarcoidosis can present acutely with the effects of a space-occupying lesion causing hemiplegia or seizures, or with encephalitis, aseptic meningitis, or isolated nerve palsies. Hypercalcaemia in sarcoidosis results from conversion of 25-hydroxyvitamin D3 to the active 1,25 di-hydroxy-vitamin D3 metabolite by macrophages in sarcoid granulomas. Patients with hypercalcaemia and/or hypercalcuria may present to the emergency unit, endocrinology, or renal clinics. Patients may present to infectious diseases or fever clinics with lymphadenopathy and/or pyrexia of unknown origin, or to the haematology service with anaemia and/or hepatosplenomegaly. Although rare, intrahepatic cholestasis and portal hypertension may prompt initial referral to gastroenterology or hepatology. Ventricular tachycardia is an increasingly recognised presentation of cardiac sarcoidosis; other complications include conduction abnormalities and heart failure.

Patients may thus present not only to respiratory specialists, but to a wide variety of clinicians in other disciplines. The range of organ involvement has important implications for diagnosis and management in individual cases. Optimal management of sarcoidosis therefore frequently requires close working across different specialities. How this is best delivered in any particular unit will depend on local referral patterns, available resources, and service configuration.

As there is no single, specific diagnostic test for sarcoidosis, making the diagnosis requires the clinician to establish a compatible clinical picture, where possible with histology, after excluding other conditions capable of producing a similar clinical or histological picture. A thorough and detailed history is an essential pre-requisite. In suspected sarcoidosis, investigations should be aimed at providing histological confirmation, evaluating the extent and severity of organ involvement, assessing whether the disease is likely to progress, and whether treatment is indicated.

Investigations (see Table 16.1)

Laboratory Evaluation

Initial laboratory investigations include full blood count to look for anaemia and/or lymphopenia; and renal, liver, and bone profile. Liver function tests are abnormal in around 10% of cases, most commonly in Afro-Caribbean and black patients. Liver ultrasound and biopsy may be required subsequently to help confirm the diagnosis. Hypercalcaemia resulting from sarcoidosis is an indication for systemic treatment, but other causes need to be excluded. Urine dipstick is part of the necessary work-up in ILD patients to help exclude vasculitis or nephritis. Twenty-four-hour urinary excretion of calcium should be measured in all patients; intrarenal calcium deposition can lead to renal failure, although renal failure due to granulomatous nephritis is rare.

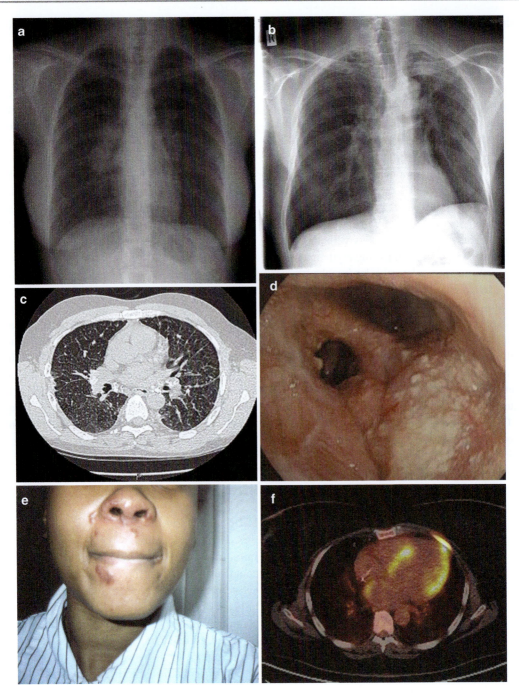

Fig. 16.1 (**a**) Chest X-ray showing bilateral hilar lymph-adenopathy. (**b**) Chest X-ray showing bilateral upper lobe fibrosis with left apical mycetoma. (**c**) High-resolution CT scan showing parenchymal nodularity and characteristic beading of the fissures. (**d**) Endobronchial nodularity seen at bronchoscopy (image courtesy of Prof. Martin Walshaw). (**e**) Cutaneous sarcoidosis. (**f**) [18]FDG-PET CT axial image showing avid patchy activity in the myocardium. (**g**) [18]FDG-PET scan from a patient with sarcoidosis showing extensive lymphadenopathy. Arrows indicate FDG uptake in lymph nodes, spleen and liver. (**h**) Gallium scan showing panda (periorbital and parotid glands) and lambda (medi-astinal and hilar nodes) pattern of uptake (image courtesy of Mike Hughes). (**i**) brain MRI (T2-weighted spin echo image) showing signal abnormality in left temporopari-etal white matter in a patient with neurosarcoidosis. (**j**) brain MRI (post-gadolinium contrast T1-weighted image) showing focal nodular leptomeningeal contrast enhance-ment (blue arrowheads) in a patient with neurosarcoidosis (image courtesy of Dr. Chris Rowland-Hill)

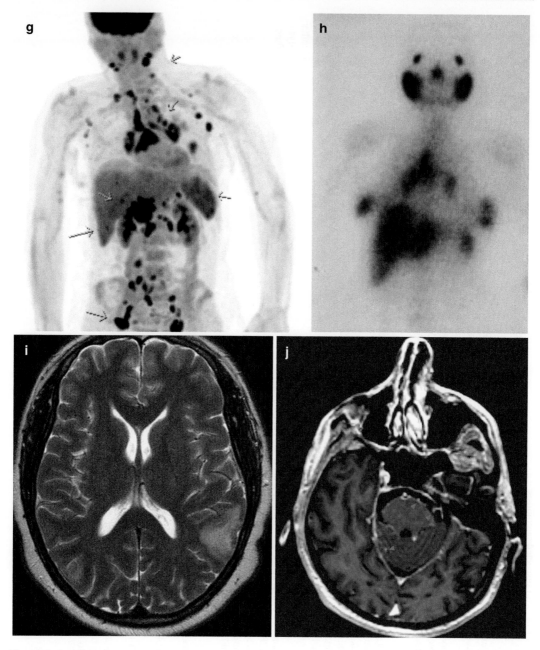

Fig. 16.1 (continued)

Serum angiotensin converting enzyme (ACE) activity levels are raised in up to two-thirds of patients because of excess ACE production by sarcoid granulomas. Although the test lacks sensitivity and specificity, it does reflect granuloma burden. Elevated ACE activity usually falls with treatment and may be a guide to compliance as well as disease activity. A polyclonal increase in immunoglobulins may help to distinguish sarcoidosis from other less frequently encountered granulomatous conditions such as common variable immunodeficiency. Measurements of serum levels of soluble IL-2 receptor have been reported to correlate with disease activity, but are not routinely available in clinical practice.

Table 16.1 Clinical evaluation of patients with suspected sarcoidosis

Initial assessment	Laboratory evaluation	Radiology	Physiology	Biopsy	Further investigations as required for extra-pulmonary disease
History, including occupational or environmental exposures and family history	Full blood count	PA chest X-ray	Pulmonary function tests (before bronchoscopy): Spirometry, total lung capacity and diffusion (TLCO/KCO)	Bronchial, transbronchial biopsy and/or EBUS-TBNA, or biopsy of an affected extra-pulmonary organ	Fundoscopy and slit-lamp examination
	Inflammatory markers: C reactive protein (CRP) and erythrocyte sedimentation rate (ESR)	High-resolution computed tomography is usually indicated to evaluate the lung parenchyma, except in clear-cut cases of Löfgren's syndrome. It is essential in the following circumstances: • atypical clinical and/or chest X-ray findings, including massive or suspicious lymphadenopathy • suspected bronchiectasis, mycetoma, pulmonary fibrosis or malignancy • normal chest X-ray but clinical suspicion of sarcoidosis	12 lead electrocardiogram (ECG)		Echocardiography
Examination	Biochemical profile: Renal function; liver enzymes including alkaline phosphatase, aspartate aminotransferase and alanine aminotransferase; bone profile including serum calcium				Holter monitoring
	Serum angiotensin converting enzyme (ACE)* *ACE levels are suppressed and therefore unreliable if the patient is taking an ACE inhibitor				Cardiac PET and/or MRI
	Immunoglobulins				Right heart catheterisation
	Urine dipstick				Brain MRI and lumbar puncture with analysis of cerebrospinal fluid
	24-h urinary calcium				
	T cell-based blood test and/or skin testing for tuberculosis according to local guidelines				

An important differential diagnosis is tuberculosis (TB). Because of peripheral anergy, the tuberculin skin test (TST) in sarcoidosis patients has a high specificity but poor sensitivity for TB. Thus, although a negative TST in the general population is a feature of sarcoidosis, a positive TST in a patient suspected to have sarcoidosis mandates thorough investigation for TB. Interferon gamma release assays have a higher specificity and sensitivity for detecting TB infection because they employ antigens specific for *Mycobacterium tuberculosis* complex. Current data suggest that their predictive value for TB is good, even in patients with sarcoidosis. They remain positive in many patients and may detect latent TB infection more accurately. Local guidelines should be followed when deciding which investigation(s) to employ to help exclude TB.

Radiology

CXR is essential, and in all but the mildest of cases, such as acute and self-limiting Löfgren's syndrome, high-resolution computed tomography (HRCT) scanning is advisable to examine the lung parenchyma for abnormalities. Scadding's original staging of CXR changes (see below) underestimates the extent of pulmonary involvement when compared with HRCT, but still has prognostic value, with stage 0 conferring the best prognosis and stage IV the least favourable outcome.

Scadding's Chest Radiograph (CXR) Staging in Sarcoidosis [2]

Stage 0   Normal CXR
Stage I   Bilateral hilar lymphadenopathy (BHL) with clear lung fields
Stage II   Hilar lymphadenopathy with interstitial infiltrates[1]
Stage III Interstitial infiltrates
Stage IV   Pulmonary fibrosis

---

[1]Typically predominant in the upper zones.

Physiology

Lung function tests (spirometry, lung volumes and diffusion capacity) should be performed to exclude or confirm physiological defects. Normal lung function tests, despite widespread radiographic abnormalities, is a characteristic feature of sarcoidosis. Conversely, there may be significant physiological dysfunction with clear lung fields, for example in endobronchial sarcoidosis. Classically there is restriction with reduced gas transfer, but airflow obstruction is not uncommon, resulting from endobronchial involvement. Routine electrocardiography (ECG) is recommended to exclude obvious conduction defects which may be asymptomatic.

Biopsy

Aside from TB, the other important differential for BHL in younger patients is lymphoma. Bronchoscopy and/or endobronchial ultrasound-guided transbronchial needle aspiration (EBUS-TBNA) should be considered if the radiology is abnormal. Bronchoscopy should include bronchial washings to exclude infection, and bronchoalveolar lavage (BAL) for differential cell count. This typically shows a lymphocytic picture, with neutrophilia in patients with pulmonary fibrosis. Endobronchial biopsies (EBB) yield a diagnosis in around 40% of cases, especially if the mucosa is visibly abnormal. Transbronchial biopsy (TBLB) has an estimated 60% sensitivity for finding granulomas in patients with sarcoidosis, but confers a 2–6% risk of significant haemorrhage and pneumothorax. Studies of a combined transbronchial and endobronchial approach report a positive diagnosis up to 86% of cases. Biopsies should also be sent in saline for culture in order to exclude TB.

Both endoscopic ultrasound (EUS) and EBUS-TBNA have a higher sensitivity for obtaining non-caseating granulomas from affected lymph nodes. EBUS-TBNA is safer than TBLB, conferring only a 1% risk of significant haemorrhage, pneumothorax or other complications. Current data suggest that EBUS-TBNA provides the highest diagnostic yield, especially when combined with TBLB, but many clinicians prefer to avoid TBLB because of the associated risks. EBUS-TBNA is generally safe and well-tolerated, but procedure time for EBUS-TBNA is significantly longer than for conventional bronchoscopy alone.

Where there is evidence of disease involving other tissues, for instance peripheral lymphadenopathy or skin lesions, these should be considered as less invasive targets for biopsy. Biopsy of erythema nodosum reveals non-specific panniculitis and is not diagnostic.

Further Investigations in Extra-Pulmonary Disease

Echocardiography should be performed if there is concern about possible myocardial sarcoidosis, or in suspected pulmonary hypertension. Symptomatic cardiac sarcoidosis is estimated to occur in around 5% of patients; autopsy studies in North America suggest a prevalence of around 25%. The prevalence of pulmonary hypertension ranges between 5% and 15%. Although more common in stage IV disease, it can also occur with relatively normal lung parenchyma and function. Referral for consideration of right heart catheterisation is important if there is evidence of pulmonary hypertension on echo.

Further investigations in suspected cardiac sarcoidosis include gadolinium-enhanced cardiovascular magnetic resonance (CMR), and referral to cardiology for consideration of myocardial biopsy. However, myocardial biopsy is not highly sensitive because of the patchy nature of the disease, and may not be required if there is positive histology from a non-cardiac site in the presence of a compatible clinical picture [3]. There are no pathognomonic features for sarcoidosis on CMR, but sub-epicardial lesions in the free ventricular wall or interventricular septum that demonstrate late enhancement with gadolinium are suggestive. Correct interpretation requires a cardiologist or radiologist with specific expertise in the condition. Ambulatory electrocardiography (Holter monitoring) may be required for investigation of arrhythmias.

In patients with suspected neurosarcoidosis, gadolinium-enhanced MRI is indicated to look for brain lesions; MRI can also help monitor response to treatment. Lumbar puncture and analysis of cerebrospinal fluid (CSF) should be considered in collaboration with neurology. Lymphocytic inflammation is characteristic; ACE level estimation can be of value as a pointer to the diagnosis despite its limitations. Oligoclonal immunoglobulin bands may be elevated in CSF, and the condition may be difficult to differentiate from multiple sclerosis.

Further investigations which may be helpful in some patients include ^{67}Ga gallium scanning and ^{18}F fluoro-deoxyglucose positron emission tomography (^{18}FDG PET). The basis of gallium scanning is the ability of the active, freely dissolved gallium ion Ga^{3+} to bind to bacterial products, leucocyte lactoferrin, and inflammatory proteins. It is therefore non-specific, highlighting tumours, inflammation, and areas of acute or chronic infection. However, ^{67}Ga scanning in sarcoidosis may reveal classic "lambda" or "panda" patterns of radiotracer uptake, which help support the diagnosis in atypical cases. The technique entails significant radiation exposure and cannot be used sequentially to monitor response to treatment. Gallium scanning has largely been replaced with FDG-PET scanning.

FDG is taken up by metabolically active cells, so that ^{18}FDG PET may also yield false positives in malignancy or other inflammatory conditions. However, it can help to identify potential diagnostic biopsy sites in patients with possible sarcoidosis, and confers a lower radiation dose than gallium scanning. It may also be a valuable alternative to CMR in patients with suspected or proven cardiac sarcoidosis and a non-MRI compatible pacemaker or defibrillator, and may be used to monitor response to treatment. Interpretation of the findings of these nuclear imaging techniques requires a specialist with specific expertise.

The eye is involved in up to 80% of patients with sarcoidosis. All patients with symptomatic, biopsy-proven, or a firm clinical diagnosis of sarcoidosis should have ophthalmology review including slit-lamp examination and fundoscopy.

Treatment

General Strategies

Clear communication to patients regarding diagnosis and management is essential, given the uncertainty in the majority of cases as to the cause of the condition, treatment, and prognosis. Many North American, European, and British professional societies and charities provide high-quality patient information.

Erythema nodosum alone is not an indication for corticosteroid treatment, but can be painful. It is best managed with paracetamol and/or a non-steroidal anti-inflammatory drug.

Smoking cessation advice should be given to all patients. The outcomes of randomised controlled trials of pulmonary rehabilitation in sarcoidosis are awaited. However, patients with sarcoidosis and pulmonary disease causing deconditioning, disabling breathlessness, impaired quality of life, nutritional deficits, fatigue, and social isolation share many features in common with those suffering from chronic obstructive pulmonary disease (COPD), and should be considered for pulmonary rehabilitation.

Fatigue may be troublesome and impact severely on the patient's daily life and employment. Other causes, including depression and hypothyroidism, should be excluded. Corticosteroids are not usually indicated for sarcoidosis-associated fatigue; they may ultimately worsen matters by inducing weight gain, diabetes, and obstructive sleep apnoea. Lifestyle measures, including attention to diet, weight, sleep, and regular exercise, are important. Small case series have shown improvement with the neuro-stimulant methylphenidate, and two small, randomised controlled trials, one of dexmethylphenidate and one of armodafinil, have also reported benefit [4, 5]. These agents are not currently licensed for use in sarcoidosis in the UK.

Gastro-oesophageal reflux should be treated to help limit cough and possibly prevent potential exacerbation of pulmonary fibrosis. Patients with pulmonary disease and/or pulmonary hypertension who fulfil criteria for supplemental oxygen, whether ambulatory or long-term, should be assessed and managed according to national guidelines. Referral for lung transplantation may be appropriate in patients with respiratory failure. Palliative care referral may be necessary in a minority of patients in whom all other forms of treatment have been exhausted. Avoidance of excessive sun exposure is commonly advised, particularly for patients who have suffered from hypercalcaemic or who have hypercalciuria.

Wherever possible, patients with sarcoidosis should be consented for inclusion into appropriate national registries and/or high-quality clinical trials. Only by collecting relevant data can the epidemiology be better understood and service delivery improved; only by prosecuting high-quality research can therapeutic advances be made which will benefit patients with this intriguing condition.

Pharmacological Strategies

Systemic Corticosteroids

There are no clear criteria for initiating corticosteroid therapy for pulmonary disease. Spontaneous remission occurs in up to 90% of patients, and the natural history is variable. The long-term value of corticosteroid treatment remains unclear, and there are important potential adverse effects [6, 7]. Nevertheless, the effectiveness of oral corticosteroids in pulmonary sarcoidosis was first reported in the 1950s, and they have been widely used since the 1960s. An early study showed that a short course of adreno-corticotrophin hormone (ACTH) or cortisone attenuated infiltrates seen on CXR, and that prolonged cortisone treatment induced remission of granulomas in repeat biopsy samples. Subsequent studies have confirmed clinicians' observations of short- to medium-term (weeks to months) symptomatic, radiographic, and functional improvement. Even in patients with chronic disease previously untreated for several years, oral steroids can be of short-term clinical value.

In contrast, the long-term benefits of oral corticosteroids, and in particular whether they prevent pulmonary fibrosis and/or improve survival, are much less clear, with most studies showing no definite evidence of benefit. The numbers of patients in these studies ranges from under 20 to over 150. Interpretation is complex because of differences in disease phenotype, with some patients showing spontaneous regression and varying degrees of residual scarring, while others develop persistent disease. Significant long-term disability resulting from pulmonary fibrosis is estimated to arise in up to 20% of patients.

Many studies have included patients with stage I disease on CXR. This has cast doubt on the interpretation of the results, because in many of these patients the condition resolves spontaneously without treatment. In most series steroids were started at the time of presentation, whereas in everyday practice most respiratory specialists delay treatment in favour of careful monitoring. Many studies used a treatment protocol which did not include gradual tapering of the dose according to response, although this is also common clinical practice. Ethnic diversity is a further important consideration: most North American studies included a large proportion of black and Afro-Caribbean patients in whom sarcoidosis is often more severe. Their results may therefore not be applicable in white European populations.

The British Thoracic Society (BTS) open-label study attempted to model real-life practice more closely by including a 6 month observation period before starting oral corticosteroid treatment [7]. Patients with no evidence of spontaneous improvement after this time were started on treatment, and alternately allocated to one of two groups. The first group were treated with steroids for at least 18 months (prednisolone 30 mg daily for 1 month, reducing by 5 mg every month to a maintenance dose of 10 mg daily) with the goal of achieving and maintaining maximal radiographic improvement. In the second group, treatment was restricted to those who required symptom relief or who had deteriorating lung function. Patients were followed up for 5 years.

Patients in the prednisolone group showed greater improvements in symptoms, lung function, and radiographic appearances than those in the control group, with an average difference in vital capacity at final review of 9% predicted. Of the 149 subjects recruited, 39% showed spontaneous radiographic resolution after 6 months, and 22% needed steroids for symptoms. Most of the patients in this study were Caucasian. Side effects of treatment were frequent but mostly mild, and led to withdrawal in only two patients.

Symptom relapse on reducing or withdrawing steroids is well-recognised. One retrospective study suggested that relapse occurred more often in patients previously treated with steroids than in those who had experienced spontaneous resolution, raising concern that steroid treatment itself could contribute to disease prolongation. However, most of the patients included in this study were treated for extra-pulmonary disease, most were black or Afro-Caribbean, and those experiencing spontaneous remission had milder disease initially. Current BTS guidelines on pulmonary sarcoidosis conclude that it is unclear whether steroid treatment might have a negative effect on longer-term prognosis.

A systematic review of steroid treatment in pulmonary sarcoidosis endorsed data from just eight studies out of 150. Six studies examined oral steroids alone, one study treated patients with oral steroids followed by inhaled steroids, and the final study examined inhaled steroids alone. The authors concluded that oral corticosteroids improve CXR appearances after 6–24 months of treatment and result in small increases in vital capacity and diffusing capacity. It is not known whether these benefits are maintained after 2 years, and there are no data confirming that steroid treatment influences long-term disease progression. For these reasons, most clinicians agree that oral corticosteroids are not indicated in patients with Stage 0 or Stage I disease unless lung function parameters are declining.

The starting dose of prednisolone in controlled studies has varied from 30 to 60 mg daily, usually tapering each month according to response, to an average of 10 mg daily. This dose is generally maintained for between 6 and 12 months before attempting slow withdrawal. Anecdotal observations suggest that in some patients, treatment is best continued for at least 2 years to prevent relapses. Alternate-day dosing, with the dose kept equivalent to the average daily dose, may limit side effects and has been shown in at least one controlled study to be as effective as daily treatment. Such a regime should be discussed carefully with patients before deciding whether to implement it. Diabetic patients may prefer daily dosing to maintain consistent blood glucose readings, and others may have greater difficulty remembering to take their treatment if it not prescribed daily.

Patients with life-threatening or severe vital organ involvement, for instance cardiac disease, neurosarcoidosis, or other complicated extra-pulmonary disease, should be managed in collaboration with the appropriate specialist(s). They may be treated initially with pulsed-dose intravenous methylprednisolone. After 3 days, treatment is usually converted to oral prednisolone at a once-daily dose of at least 60 mg.

Steroid treatment guidelines are summarised in Table 16.2. There is agreement that oral corticosteroids should be considered in patients with severe, persistent, or progressively worsening respiratory symptoms, or declining lung function. Severe symptoms are those which interfere with essential aspects of the patient's daily life, such as work or caring for young children. Many physicians monitor lung function (VC and TLCO) for 6 months before deciding that there is progressive deterioration. There are no absolute cut-offs to determine when treatment is necessary,

Table 16.2 Guidelines on steroid therapy for sarcoidosis

	Steroid therapy	Prednisolone dose	Treatment failure
American Thoracic Society (ATS), European Respiratory Society (ERS), World Association of Sarcoidosis and Other Granulomatous Disorders (WASOG) joint statement 1999 [17]	Steroids are effective short-term but it is not known whether they alter the natural history of the disease, or for how long treatment should continue. Patients with progressive symptomatic disease, or asymptomatic patients with infiltrates on CXR and progressively worsening lung function, should probably be treated	Initial dose 20–40 mg/day for pulmonary sarcoidosis, or the equivalent taken alternate days Further evaluation of response after 2–3 months. In steroid responders, gradually tapering the dose to 5–10 mg/day (or an equivalent alternate day dose), and treat for at least 12 months	In patients who fail to respond to steroids after 3 months, consider reasons for failure such as the presence of irreversible fibrosis, non-compliance, or inadequate dosage
British Thoracic Society (BTS)	Steroid treatment is not indicated for asymptomatic stage I disease, nor in asymptomatic patients with stage II or III disease with mild lung function abnormalities and stable parameters. Oral corticosteroids are first-line therapy in patients with disease progression (as indicated by radiology or lung function) or significant symptoms	Initial dose 0.5 mg/kg/day for 4 weeks, tapering to a maintenance dose which controls symptoms and disease progression, for a period of 6–24 months	Consider other immunosuppressive agents when corticosteroids are not controlling the disease, or when side-effects are unacceptable. Methotrexate is the second-line agent of choice

but a fall in VC of 10% and/or TLCO of >15% is generally considered significant. There is agreement that neither oral nor inhaled corticosteroids are indicated in asymptomatic patients in the absence of other organ involvement.

Inhaled Corticosteroids

The value of inhaled budesonide was first reported in an open study of 20 patients with pulmonary sarcoidosis. Several subsequent studies have investigated the potential of inhaled steroids, either used first-line or as maintenance treatment, after a response is obtained with oral steroids. Only two studies, both using budesonide, have showed conclusive benefit.

Current evidence suggests that inhaled steroids are less consistently effective than oral steroids in pulmonary sarcoidosis. It is generally agreed that they should not be employed routinely. They may, however, have a role in maintenance treatment, or as steroid-sparing agents; they may also be of value in those patients whose main symptom is a troublesome cough and/or who have evidence of endobronchial involvement.

Alternative Immune-Suppressants

A number of patients with severe or persistent sarcoidosis require treatment with alternative agents, usually in combination with corticosteroids, but sometimes alone. Treatment with an alternative agent may be required for patients in whom corticosteroids are contra-indicated, for those unable to tolerate the side-effects of steroids, for those whose disease is refractory to corticosteroids, or for those who are continuing to require unacceptably high doses. In the absence of clear evidence, such decisions need to be made on a case-by-case basis. It seems reasonable to consider adding a second-line agent if the patient is continuing to require in excess of 10 mg prednisolone once daily after 6 months, and if there is no indication of likely improvement or potential to reduce the dose over the following 6 months.

The range of potential alternative immunosuppressive agents is wide. It includes methotrexate (MTX), azathioprine, hydroxychloroquine, cyclophosphamide, mycophenolate mofetil

(MMF), ciclosporin A, and chlorambucil; as well as anti-TNFα agents including pentoxifylline, thalidomide, infliximab, and etanercept. Most of the literature examining these agents consists of small case series, and many have focused on the effects of these agents on extra-pulmonary rather than pulmonary disease. The most commonly used are generally MTX, azathioprine, hydroxychloroquine, and MMF. Limited evidence supports MTX as the second-line drug of choice after corticosteroids. However, there is no clear evidence as to which immunosuppressant should be used thereafter, if prednisolone and/or MTX fail to control the disease.

Methotrexate

MTX has been employed as a steroid-sparing agent for many years in the treatment of rheumatoid arthritis. It is a folic acid analogue which inhibits dihydrofolate reductase and transmethylation reactions. At low doses it has anti-inflammatory properties, attributable largely to enhanced adenosine release. Adenosine suppresses TNFα release from monocytes, macrophages, and neutrophils; suppresses neutrophil reactive oxygen species release; and inhibits lymphocyte proliferation.

A randomised controlled trial of MTX (10 mg once weekly) or placebo plus oral prednisolone in 24 patients, conducted over 1 year, showed that patients taking MTX required significantly less prednisolone in the second 6-month period. However, the trial was limited by a high drop-out rate, with only 15 patients remaining in the study after 6 months. MTX did not differ from placebo on an intention-to-treat basis, and lung function, radiology, and symptoms did not differ between the two groups.

With the exception of teratogenicity, the most important side effects of MTX are hepatic fibrosis and leucopenia. Baseline liver function should be documented before starting treatment, but abnormal liver function resulting from sarcoidosis is not a contra-indication to MTX. Where appropriate, serology for HIV and hepatitis B and C should be sent before starting treatment. Significant renal disease, and acute or chronic infection, are contra-indications to treatment with MTX.

Continued regular monitoring of liver function and full blood count is vital. There is uncertainty around the value of surveillance liver biopsy in patients exposed to MTX for prolonged periods of time. In some centres, the advent of the Fibroscan (Transient Elastography) to measure liver fibrosis is increasingly obviating the need for biopsy. Its advantages are that it is non-invasive and cheaper, does not carry the risk of pain and bleeding, and avoids the sampling errors inherent in biopsy. Interpretation and subsequent recommendations require close collaboration with gastroenterology.

Co-treatment with folic acid is advised to limit toxicity. A typical protocol is folic acid 5–10 mg once weekly. Pregnancy should be excluded in females before starting treatment, and both men and women receiving MTX must employ effective contraception. British authorities advise continuing contraception for men and women for at least 3 months after stopping MTX. North American advice is that pregnancy should be avoided for at least 3 months after treatment in male patients, and for at least one ovulatory cycle in females. International guidelines on the use of MTX in sarcoidosis provide a resource for developing local management guidance and shared-care monitoring protocols for primary care physicians [8].

Azathioprine

Azathioprine is a purine analogue. Its precise mechanism of action in sarcoidosis is unclear. Its metabolite mercaptopurine affects RNA and DNA synthesis, thereby inhibiting lymphocyte proliferation. Cellular immunity is suppressed to a greater degree than humoral immunity. There are no randomised controlled trials of azathioprine in sarcoidosis. Case series have shown it can improve chest X-ray appearances and reduce breathlessness; however a retrospective review suggested benefit in only two out of ten patients. An open-label study examined the effect of azathioprine (2 mg/kg per day) combined with glucocorticoid treatment in 11 patients with chronic or relapsing pulmonary sarcoidosis [9]. All patients had significant symptomatic relief and showed improved radiographic and physiological parameters, without significant side-effects, despite reducing their prednisolone dose to 0.1 mg/kg/day within 2–3 months of starting the study. Cytokine release in BAL fluid was reduced. Eight patients remained in stable remission for between 4 months and 6 years after stopping treatment.

Regular blood counts to check for myelosuppression, and liver function monitoring, are essential. Azathioprine is metabolised by the enzyme thiopurine methyltransferase (TPMT), and the risk of myelosuppression is increased in the minority of the population who are homozygous for low TPMT activity. Consequently, many clinicians check TPMT levels before starting azathioprine, despite limited evidence to support this practice. Azathioprine should not be started in pregnancy, as there have been reports of premature birth and low birth weight following exposure; spontaneous abortion has been reported after both maternal and paternal exposure.

Hydroxychloroquine

Hydroxychloroquine (like chloroquine) is an anti-malarial agent, which has been used with some success in patients with hypercalcaemia, cutaneous disease, and neurosarcoidosis. Two randomised controlled trials have compared chloroquine and placebo in pulmonary sarcoidosis [10, 11]. In the early British study, 52 patients who had not received steroids but either had pulmonary infiltrates for 6 months and breathlessness, or progressive lung infiltrates for 6 months, or persistent infiltrates for 1 year, were randomised to receive chloroquine or placebo for 16 weeks. Chloroquine treatment conferred no benefit but resulted in a greater number of adverse events. In the subsequent Canadian study, 23 patients received chloroquine at a dose of 750 mg daily for 6 months, gradually tapering every 2 months to 250 mg daily. Eighteen patients were then randomised to a maintenance group or to an observation group. Patients randomised to the maintenance group had a slower decline in lung function and fewer relapses than those in the observation group. Side effects were mainly limited to the high-dose treatment phase. The authors conclude that chloroquine should be considered in chronic pulmonary sarcoidosis; in practice, hydroxychloroquine is preferred because it has lower ocular toxicity.

Hydroxychloroquine should be used with caution in liver or renal impairment, and regular blood count monitoring (to check for agranulocytosis and thrombocytopenia) and liver function is needed. The British Royal College of Ophthalmologists advises that patients should be asked about visual impairment before starting treatment, and that visual acuity should be recorded. If eye disease is present, an ophthalmologist should be consulted before starting treatment. Patients should be asked about visual symptoms during treatment, and visual acuity monitored annually. If treatment is required for over 5 years, individual arrangements should be made with the local ophthalmology service.

Hydroxychloroquine should be used in caution in glucose-6-phosphate (G6PD) deficiency, as it may precipitate acute haemolytic anaemia. As deficiency is highly prevalent in Africans, in whom persistent and severe sarcoidosis is more common, it appears prudent to check G6PD levels before starting hydroxychloroquine.

Mycophenolate

Like azathioprine, MMF is an anti-proliferative immunosuppressant. However, it is metabolised to mycophenolic acid, which has a more selective action than azathioprine. Several authors report employing MMF successfully as a steroid-sparing agent in extra-pulmonary sarcoidosis, but there are no controlled studies in pulmonary disease. In practice it may be used empirically when other options, including corticosteroids, MTX and azathioprine, have been exhausted.

Leflunomide

Leflunomide is an anti-metabolite similar to MTX, with reduced gastrointestinal toxicity. There are no randomised controlled trials in sarcoidosis, and evidence in favour of its use comes from small case series. Some authors report successful use in sarcoidosis, extrapolating from experience in rheumatoid arthritis.

Minocycline

Minocycline has been used in cutaneous sarcoidosis; one study of 12 patients showed effectiveness in treating skin lesions in 10 patients, and in treating pulmonary involvement in two patients. Possible modes of action of tetracyclines in sarcoidosis include inhibition of matrix metalloproteinases, angiogenesis, apoptosis, and granuloma formation.

Ciclosporin A

Ciclosporin A is a T cell suppressor which has been reported to improve neurosarcoidosis in retrospective studies. However, a randomized controlled trial in 37 patients with pulmonary sarcoidosis treated over 18 months showed no effect on breathlessness or lung function, and side-effects were significantly greater in the treatment group. It is not therefore currently recommended for pulmonary sarcoidosis.

Cyclophosphamide

Cyclophosphamide is an alkylating agent which has been used with apparent benefit in cardiac and neurosarcoidosis. There are no controlled studies in pulmonary disease, and routine use is therefore not currently recommended.

Anti-TNF agents

Agents which more specifically target TNF-α include thalidomide, pentoxifylline, infliximab, and etanercept. Individual case reports and small series support the use of thalidomide in cutaneous sarcoidosis, but there are no studies in pulmonary disease. Teratogenic concerns strictly limit its use in women of child-bearing age, and side-effects can be troublesome. Pentoxifylline in high doses has been shown to improve lung function in mild pulmonary sarcoidosis.

Infliximab is a chimeric humanised monoclonal antibody that neutralises TNF-α. Its effectiveness in sarcoid was first reported in refractory cutaneous and pulmonary disease in 2001. Since then a series of case reports and small series have noted the effectiveness of infliximab in skin, eye, brain, lung, sinus, and muscle disease. Two larger studies were published in 2006. The first, by Doty and colleagues, was a retrospective study of ten patients with sarcoidosis refractory to conventional agents [12]. Six patients had lung involvement, although the indication for using infliximab was extra-pulmonary disease. Nine patients reported symptomatic improvement with infliximab, and all had objective evidence of improvement. In five of six patients taking concomitant corticosteroids, the dose was reduced. The authors did not comment on lung function or radiology. They nevertheless concluded that infliximab appeared safe and effective in refractory sarcoidosis.

The second study, conducted by Baughman and colleagues [13] was a phase II, multi-centre, double-blind, placebo-controlled clinical trial in which patients were randomised in a 1:1:1 ratio to receive intravenous placebo, infliximab 3 mg/kg, or infliximab 5 mg/kg at weeks 0, 2, 6, 12, 18, and 24. Patients were followed up for 1 year. One hundred and thirty eight patients were randomised; 44 completed the placebo arm, 46 completed the lower dose infliximab arm, and 45 completed the higher dose infliximab arm. In all cases the indication for recruitment to the study was refractory pulmonary disease. Patients in the combined infliximab groups had an average increase in forced vital capacity (FVC) of 2.5% predicted at week 24. Post hoc exploratory analyses suggested that patients with more severe disease (longer disease duration, lower FVC or more symptoms) benefit the most.

Although these benefits appear modest, they are significant in patients with life-threatening fibrotic disease who would also potentially be candidates for transplantation. Even stability represents a significant treatment response, and improvement would be exceptional.

Etanercept is a soluble TNF-α receptor fusion protein that binds TNF-α and has a longer half-life than the native soluble receptor. It has not been shown to be effective in sarcoidosis, possibly because it is inferior to infliximab in achieving tissue penetration and cell-mediated lysis of TNF-α secreting cells.

Adalimumab is a fully human anti-TNF-α antibody. A few case reports and small series have reported benefit in extra-pulmonary sarcoidosis. Golimumab is a humanised anti-TNFα antibody, and ustekinumab is a monoclonal antibody which inhibits IL-12 and IL-23. A placebo-controlled trial of these agents in patients with chronic pulmonary and/or skin sarcoidosis failed to demonstrate effectiveness in lung disease, although there was a trend towards improvement in cutaneous disease with ustekinumab.

At present, therefore, infliximab may be considered in life-threatening pulmonary sarcoidosis when all other options have been exhausted. It remains expensive, and patients need careful assessment for evidence of TB before starting therapy.

Important Complications of Treatment

In patients with sarcoidosis requiring treatment, preventing, monitoring for, and managing potential side effects is an important component of clinical follow-up. Several studies have shown that weight gain, skin thinning, sleep disturbance, osteoporosis, and neuropsychiatric disorders occur not infrequently in patients taking corticosteroids, even at relatively low doses. There is limited guidance for clinicians on monitoring for adverse effects in sarcoidosis. Some may arise with little warning; others are potentially preventable by using the lowest steroid dose possible, careful monitoring, and appropriate prophylaxis. They appear to be dependent on dose and duration of treatment. More recent data reinforce previous observations suggesting that oral corticosteroids significantly increase the risk of infection. Diabetes is a notable potential complication, and appropriate monitoring is required.

There is increasing recognition that rapid decline in bone mineral density (BMD) begins in the first 3 months of glucocorticoid use, with a peak after 6 months and further slow decline with continued treatment. This has justifiably heightened concern about the impact on fracture risk. Although Afro-Americans may be at a lower risk of glucocorticoid-induced osteoporosis, a study of BMD in women with sarcoidosis has suggested that post-menopausal women with sarcoidosis may be at greater risk of bone mineral loss compared with controls.

The American College of Rheumatology (ACR) 2010 recommendations for prevention and treatment of glucocorticoid-induced osteoporosis adopt a risk-stratification approach [14]. After measurement of the T score with dualenergy X-ray absorptiometry (DEXA), and taking into account the patient's age, gender, and ethnic origin, the patient's 10-year fracture risk, using the WHO Fracture Risk Assessment Tool (FRAX), is categorised as low, medium, or high. Other risk factors for osteoporosis are low body mass index, parental history of hip fracture, current cigarette smoking, and alcohol intake in excess of three drinks a day. The daily dose and duration of glucocorticoid therapy are taken into consideration. Patients with any of these additional risk factors may be placed in a higher risk category at the clinician's discretion. Bisphosphonates and/or lifestyle measures are advised according to the patient's risk, age, and glucocorticoid exposure, and in women, their child-bearing potential.

British guidelines on prevention and management of glucocorticoid-induced osteoporosis were published in 2002 [15]. Evaluation of all patients taking corticosteroids for three or more months is recommended. General measures advised in all cases include minimising the corticosteroid dose, considering steroid-sparing agents, and switching to topical steroids where possible. Lifestyle measures recommended for all patients include ensuring adequate calcium and vitamin D intake, regular weight-bearing exercise, maintenance of a healthy body weight, smoking cessation, and avoidance of alcohol abuse. In patients with a T score above 0, repeat DEXA is not advised unless very high doses of corticosteroids are required. In patients with a T score between 0 and −1.5, repeat DEXA is advised after one to 3 years if steroids are continued. If the T score is −1.5 or lower, specific treatment is advised in addition to lifestyle measures. Specific treatments include alendronate, cyclical etidronate, hormone replacement therapy in women, pamidronate, and risedronate.

The National Institute for Health and Care Excellence (NICE) recommends DEXA scanning in patients taking prednisolone at doses of 7.5 mg or more daily for 3 months or more [16]. BTS guidelines advise using bisphosphonates as appropriate to minimize steroid-induced osteoporosis. Hypercalcaemia and hypercalcuria arising in sarcoidosis may be exacerbated by supplementary calcium and vitamin D. Some authors therefore advise measuring baseline serum and urine calcium and repeating measurements 4–8 weeks after starting calcium supplements, with continued subsequent monitoring.

A further consideration in sarcoidosis is that patients are relatively young, with females often of reproductive age. Since manufacturers caution against bisphosphonates in pregnancy, physicians must either not prescribe these agents in females of child-bearing age or else counsel them appropriately. Local guidelines should be followed when deciding whether to refer to an osteoporosis clinic.

Since the first report in 2003, hundreds of cases of bisphosphonate-associated mandibular osteonecrosis have been described. This complication has mostly been associated with intravenous pamridonate and zoledronic acid. It may arise spontaneously or follow an invasive procedure such as dental extraction. Length of treatment is a risk factor, especially if it exceeds 36 months. An initial dental examination with appropriate preventative dentistry should be considered before starting a bisphosphonate. Patients with risk factors should be advised to avoid invasive dental procedures while on treatment, if possible.

Opportunistic infections are a potential consequence of immunosuppression. Prophylaxis against pneumonia caused by *Pneumocystis jiroveci* should be given to all patients with a history of the infection, and should be considered for severely immunocompromised patients. North American guidelines for preventing opportunistic infection in HIV-infected individuals, endorsed by the British Infection Society, provide the basis for current recommendations. Oral co-trimoxazole is the drug of choice for prophylaxis, either 960 mg daily or three times a week. The dose can be reduced to 480 mg daily to improve tolerance. In patients unable to tolerate co-trimoxazole, nebulised pentamidine is effective, as is oral dapsone; atovaquone has also been employed. Co-trimoxazole and dapsone can cause bone marrow suppression and skin rashes, among other side-effects. Neither North American nor British sarcoidosis guidelines recommend Pneumocystis prophylaxis routinely in otherwise immuno-competent patients.

Lung Transplantation

A small number of patients with severe and progressive pulmonary sarcoidosis, despite medical therapy, may be candidates for transplantation. Patients should be assessed for common co-morbidities as well as bronchiectasis, right ventricular impairment, infection, and mycetomas. Close liaison with the transplant centre is required at an early stage.

Sarcoidosis patients represent up to 2% of lung transplant recipients worldwide; median survival is around 5 years. Sarcoidosis is the most common disease to recur in transplanted lung, with reported recurrence rates of 35–60%, but it appears to have a good prognosis, often being asymptomatic and self-limiting.

Conclusions

Having made a diagnosis of sarcoidosis, it is important to remember that around two-thirds of patients achieve spontaneous remission. Many patients will not, therefore, need treatment. Although it is difficult to predict which patients will develop long-term sequelae, those with acute onset of symptoms and stage 0 or I disease generally have the best prognosis. Those with multi-system involvement require joint management with the relevant specialists.

Treatment is not indicated for asymptomatic stage 0 or I pulmonary disease, or for patients with asymptomatic stage II or III disease with mildly impaired, stable lung function. Oral corticosteroids may be indicated for patients with progressive stage II, III, or IV disease. Absolute indications for systemic corticosteroid treatment include hypercalcaemia, neurological, cardiac, or ocular involvement.

Serum ACE levels are more useful for follow-up—especially when monitoring response to treatment—than they are in diagnosis. There is still limited evidence to guide clinicians on the optimum timing for starting treatment and for how to long to treat. Patients with repeated relapses may need long-term steroids with or without additional immunosuppression. Inhaled steroids may be of value for treating intractable cough.

References

1. Rybicki BA, Iannuzzi MC, Frederick MM, Thompson BW, Rossman MD, Bresnitz EA, et al. Familial aggregation of sarcoidosis: a case-control etiologic study of sarcoidosis (ACCESS). Am J Respir Crit Care Med. 2001;164(11):2085–91.
2. Scadding JG. Prognosis of intrathoracic sarcoidosis in England. Br Med J. 1961;2:1165–72.
3. Birnie DH, Sauer WH, Bogun F, Cooper JM, Culver DA, Duvernoy CS, et al. HRS expert consensus statement on the diagnosis and management of arrhythmias associated with cardiac sarcoidosis. Heart Rhythm. 2014;11(7):1305–23.
4. Lower EE, Harman S, Baughman RP. A randomized, double-blind placebo controlled trial of dexmethylphenidate hydrochloride (d-MPH) for sarcoidosis associated fatigue. Chest. 2008;133:1189–95.
5. Lower EE, Malhotra A, Surdulescu V, Baughman RP. Armodafinil for sarcoidosis-associated fatigue: a double-blind, placebo-controlled, crossover trial. J Pain Symptom Manag. 2013;45(2):159–69.
6. Wells AU, Hirani N. Interstitial lung disease guideline: the British Thoracic Society in collaboration with the Thoracic Society of Australia and New Zealand, and the Irish Thoracic Society. Thorax. 2008;63(Suppl V):v1–58.
7. Gibson GJ, Prescott RJ, Muers MF, Middleton WG, Mitchell DN, Connolly CK, et al. British Thoracic Society Sarcoidosis study: effects of long-term corticosteroid treatment. Thorax. 1996;51(3):238–47.
8. Cremers JP, Drent M, Bast A, Shigemitsu H, Baughman RP, Valeyre D, et al. Multinational evidence-based World Association of Sarcoidosis and Other Granulomatous Disorders recommendations for the use of methotrexate in sarcoidosis: integrating systematic literature research and expert opinion of sarcoidologists worldwide. Curr Opin Pulm Med. 2013;19:545–61.
9. Müller-Quernheim J, Kienast K, Held M, Pfeifer S, Costabel U. Treatment of chronic sarcoidosis with an azathioprine/prednisolone regimen. Eur Respir J. 1999;14:1117.
10. British Tuberculosis Association. Chloroquine in the treatment of sarcoidosis. A report from the Research

Committee of the British Tuberculosis Association. Tubercle. 1967;48(4):257–72.

11. Baltzan M, Mehta S, Kirkham TH, Cosio MG. Randomized trial of prolonged chloroquine therapy in advanced pulmonary sarcoidosis. Am J Respir Crit Care Med. 1999;160:192–7.

12. Doty JD, Mazur JE, Judson MA. Treatment of sarcoidosis with infliximab. Chest. 2005;127:1064–71.

13. Baughman RP, Drent M, Kavuru M, Judson MA, Costabel U, du Bois RM, et al. Infliximab therapy in patients with chronic sarcoidosis and pulmonary involvement. Am J Respir Crit Care Med. 2006;174:795–802.

14. Grossman JM, Gordon R, Ranganath VK, Deal C, Caplan L, Chen W, et al. American College of Rheumatology 2010 recommendations for the prevention and treatment of glucocorticoid-induced osteoporosis. Arthritis Care Res (Hoboken). 2010;62(11):1515–26.

15. Bone and Tooth Society, National Osteoporosis Society, Royal College of Physicians. Glucocorticoid-induced osteoporosis: guidelines for prevention and treatment. London: RCP; 2002.

16. National Institute for Health and Care Excellence. Osteoporosis: assessing the risk of fragility fracture. NICE clinical guideline 146. 2012. Available at: www.nice.org.uk.

17. Statement on sarcoidosis. Joint statement of the American Thoracic Society (ATS), the European Respiratory Society (ERS) and the World Association of Sarcoidosis and Other Granulomatous Disorders (WASOG) adopted by the ATS Board of Directors and by the ERS Executive Committee, February 1999. Am J Respir Crit Care Med. 1999;160(2):736–55.

Vasculitis and Rare Lung Diseases

17

Pasupathy Sivasothy and Muhunthan Thillai

Introduction

The European Respiratory Society's White Book defines a rare disease as a disorder affecting less than 1 in 2000 of the population [1]. The terms "rare lung disease" and "orphan lung disease" are frequently used interchangeably, but they are not identical. Orphan lung diseases are those that tend not to receive attention in the research community and for which there may be no specific treatment. Patients may experience delay in diagnosis or in accessing expertise in managing their condition, and may feel abandoned in the world of healthcare. Not all rare lung diseases will be orphan lung diseases and not all orphan lung diseases with be rare lung diseases (e.g. parasitic infections). This chapter will concentrate on the rare lung diseases listed in Table 17.1.

Pulmonary Vasculitis

The vasculitides are a heterogeneous group of multisystem diseases that are characterised by a triad of inflammation, damage to the vessel wall,

Table 17.1 The principal rare lung diseases

Pulmonary vasculitis
Granulomatosis with polyangiitis (Wegener's)
Microscopic polyangiitis
Eosinophilic granulomatosis with polyangiitis (Churg–Strauss)
Behçet's disease
Takayasu's arteritis
Autoimmune diseases
Anti-basement membrane syndrome
Pulmonary alveolar proteinosis
IgG4 related lung disease
Disorders of genetic origin
Lymphangioleiomyomatosis associated with tuberous sclerosis
Multiple cystic lung disease in Birt–Hogg–Dubé syndrome
Other rare diseases
Thoracic endometriosis
Langerhan's cell histiocytosis
Idiopathic pulmonary haemosiderosis

Adapted from Gibson GJ, Loddenkemper R, Lundbäck B, Sibille Y, editors. Rare and orphan lung disease. In: European Lung White Book. Sheffield, UK: European Respiratory Society; 2013

and impaired blood flow with ensuing local tissue injury. The clinical presentation of these vasculitides is defined by the site, type, and size of the vessel and pathological pattern of vessel injury, as shown in Table 17.2.

In light of recent advances in the understanding of the aetiology and pathogenesis of these disorders, their nomenclature was modified at the International Chapel Hill Consensus

P. Sivasothy (✉)
Department of Medicine, Cambridge University Hospitals Foundation Trust, Cambridge, UK
e-mail: pasupathy.sivasothy@addenbrookes.nhs.uk

M. Thillai
Cambridge Interstitial Lung Disease Unit, Papworth Hospital, Cambridgeshire, UK

© Springer International Publishing AG, part of Springer Nature 2018
S. Hart, M. Greenstone (eds.), *Foundations of Respiratory Medicine*,
https://doi.org/10.1007/978-3-319-94127-1_17

Table 17.2 The features of the main pulmonary vasculitides

Vessel size	International Chapel Hill consensus conference definitions 2012
Small vessel	
Granulomatosis with polyangiitis (Wegener's) (GPA)	*Necrotizing granulomatous inflammation* usually involving the upper and lower respiratory tract, and necrotizing vasculitis affecting predominantly small to medium vessels
Eosinophilic granulomatosis with polyangiitis (Churg-Strauss) (EGPA)	*Eosinophil-rich and necrotizing granulomatous* inflammation often involving the respiratory tract, associated with asthma and eosinophilia. ANCA is more frequent when glomerulonephritis is present
Microscopic polyangiitis (MPA)	*Necrotizing vasculitis*, with few or no immune deposits, predominantly affecting small vessels. Necrotizing arteritis involving small and medium arteries may be present. Necrotizing glomerulonephritis is very common. Pulmonary capillaritis often occurs. *Granulomatous inflammation is absent*
Anti–glomerular basement membrane (anti-GBM) disease	*Vasculitis affecting glomerular capillaries, pulmonary capillaries,* or both, with deposition of anti-GBM autoantibodies. Lung involvement causes pulmonary haemorrhage, and renal involvement causes glomerulonephritis with necrosis and crescents
Large vessels	
Takayasu arteritis (TAK)	Arteritis, often granulomatous, predominantly affecting the aorta and/or its major branches. It can affect the *pulmonary arteries* causing pulmonary hypertension. Onset usually in patients younger than 40 years
Variable vessel	
Behcet's disease (BD)	Vasculitis occurring in patients with Behcet's disease that can affect arteries or veins. Behcet's disease is characterized by recurrent oral and/or genital aphthous ulcers accompanied by cutaneous, ocular, articular, gastrointestinal, and/or central nervous system inflammatory lesions. Small vessel vasculitis, thromboangiitis, *thrombosis,* arteritis, and *arterial aneurysms* may occur

Adapted from Jennette JC, Falk RJ, Bacon PA, Basu N, Cid MC, Ferrario F, et al. 2012 Revised International Chapel Hill Consensus Conference Nomenclature of Vasculitides. Arthritis Rheum. 2013;65(1):1–11

Conference 2012 [2]. Histological descriptive terms were used to replace eponyms. The principle pulmonary vasculitides are associated with anti-neutrophilic cytoplasmic antibody (ANCA) and called the ANCA-associated vasculitides (AAV). These consist primarily of granulomatosis with polyangiitis (GPA, previously known as Wegener's granulomatosis), eosinophilic granulomatosis with polyangiitis (EGPA, Churg-Strauss Syndrome) and microscopic polyangiitis (MPA).

are utilised, the latter giving rise to the higher value. The annual incidence of vasculitis is estimated at 11–20 per million. Although the incidence of AAV is similar across Europe, there is an increased incidence of GPA and EGPA in northern Europe and increased incidence of MPA in southern Europe. There is a seasonal and cyclical incidence of GPA, with it being more common in the winter and seeming to have a peak incidence every 3–4 years.

Epidemiology

The prevalence of vasculitis is estimated to be between 90 and 278 per million, depending on whether clinic- or population-based surveys

Aetiology

The precise aetiology of the ANCA-associated vasculitides is unknown. Infections (commonly *S. aureus, E. coli* and *Klebsiella*) have been implicated in GPA. Chronic carriers of *S. aureus* who express toxic shock toxin 1 have an increased frequency of relapses. Molecular mimicry between bacterial antigens and ANCA (*E. coli, S. aureus*), toll-like receptor activation (*S. aureus*) and idiotype-anti idiotype mechanism with bacterial antigens (*S. aureus* and *Klebsiella*) have been shown to be associated with ANCA-associated vasculitis.

A genome-wide association study found anti-proteinase 3 ANCA (PR3 ANCA) was associated with HLA-DP and the genes encoding α_1-antitrypsin (SERPINA1) and proteinase 3 (PRTN3). This supported the clinical observation that patients with ZZ α_1-antitrypsin deficiency have a 100-fold increased risk of developing GPA. Anti-myeloperoxidase ANCA (MPO ANCA) is associated with HLA-DQ.

Occupational exposure to silica, quartz, organic solvents, arable crops, and livestock farming has been associated with AAV. In addition, drugs which have been linked with the development of AAV include propylthiouracil, hydralazine, carbimazole, D-pencillamine, phenytoin, allopurinol, and sulphonamides.

Pathogenesis

The pathogenesis of MPA is now well understood. In murine *in vivo* studies MPO ANCA has been shown to be pathogenic. When MPO-deficient mice were immunized against MPO and their splenocytes or IgG were transferred to normal recipient mice, the recipients went on to develop pulmonary capillaritis and glomerulonephritis, which was histologically identical to MPA.

Further evidence to support the pathogenicity of MPO ANCA in the development of MPA comes from the clinical observation that a pregnant woman with active MPO-ANCA positive MPA gave birth to a child with pulmonary haemorrhage and glomerulonephritis. The neonate's blood contained IgG MPO ANCA, and it was presumed that passive placental transfer of maternal IgG MPO ANCA caused the disease.

Clinical Approach to Patients with Suspected AAV

The presentation of vasculitis can be variable, making early diagnosis and treatment a challenge. There are no accepted specific diagnostic criteria for vasculitis, but there are classification criteria aimed at differentiating them from each other, as seen in Table 17.2. There is frequently a history of prodromal symptoms of fevers, malaise, night sweats, flitting arthritis, weight loss, headache, and polymyalgia in the preceding 6 months. The main pulmonary vasculitides are reviewed below, and recommended investigations are listed in Table 17.3.

Table 17.3 Investigations for vasculitis

Investigation for vasculitis[a]	
All patients	
Blood tests	FBC, U&E, CRP
Urine dipstick and microscopy	
CXR	
Selected tests depending on presentation	
Blood tests	ANCA
	Blood culture
	Hepatitis B and C
	HIV
	Anti-GBM
	Rheumatoid factor, ANA, anti-phospholipid antibody
	Cryoglobulin and complement
Radiology	HRCT thorax
Pulmonary physiology	Spirometry with flow volume loop
Bronchoscopy	To exclude infection and confirm alveolar haemorrhage; rarely mucosal biopsy and transbronchial biopsies are useful
Biopsy of relevant tissue	Kidney, lung, or nasal
Neurological	Nerve conduction test
Cardiology	Echocardiogram

[a]Full blood count (FBC) looking for neutrophilia, eosinophilia, or a drop in haemoglobin, together with urea and electrolytes (U&E) looking for renal damage, should be routinely undertaken. Vasculitis is found with infections, and blood cultures to exclude bacteraemia (especially due to sub-acute endocarditis) should be considered. Mixed cryoglobulinaemia is invariably found with hepatitis C. Auto-antibody screen to exclude other connective tissue diseases should be carried out if indicated

Table 17.4 The main imitators of vasculitis

Infections	
Acute	Mycotic aneurysms associated with septicaemia, sub-acute endocarditis
Chronic	TB, HIV, syphilis, hepatitis
Malignancy	Haematological—lymphoma, myeloma, leukaemia
	Atrial myxoma
Hypercoaguable states	Anti-phospholipid syndrome
	Thrombotic thrombocytopenic purpura
Hereditary	Ehler-Danlos
	Marfan's
Other	Cocaine abuse
	Cholesterol emboli

It is important to exclude infection and other mimics of vasculitis because treatment of vasculitis entails the use of immunosuppressive drugs, and the consequences of not recognising infection may be devastating. The main mimics of vasculitis are listed in Table 17.4.

Granulomatosis with Polyangiitis (Wegener's)

Granulomatosis with polyangiitis (GPA) is classically characterised by the triad of upper respiratory tract, lower respiratory tract, and renal involvement. However, up to 25% of patients will have a limited form of GPA, with only upper and lower respiratory tract involvement. Tissue damage is characterised by necrotizing granulomatous inflammation affecting predominantly small to medium vessels.

It is a disease which predominantly occurs in the third to the fifth decade of life. It is rare in children. A second peak of incidence is found with increasing age. GPA has a prevalence of 24–145 per million, with an annual incidence of 8.4 per million population.

Clinical Features: Upper Airways

GPA invariably involves the upper airways. Ear, nose, and throat symptoms are the most common symptoms at initial presentation, and are present in over 90% of patients during their disease history. Rhinosinusitis associated with epistaxis and nasal crusting is present in 70% of patients at initial presentation. Hearing loss will develop in 15–25% of patients, due to inflammation of either the middle ear or Eustachian tube. Nasal disease can progress to nasal septal perforation, and saddle nose deformity due to vascular necrosis of cartilage. Nasal crustation can cause impaired nasal breathing and chronic cough.

Clinical Features: Lower Airways

Granulomatous involvement of the trachea and bronchi can lead to stenosis in 10–30% of patients. This is more common in female patients. Subglottic narrowing is the most common site of involvement, and is invariably associated with active nasopharyngeal disease. Symptoms arising from airway narrowing are variable and may include exertional dyspnoea, "wheeze," change in voice, haemoptysis, and persistent cough. At the time of bronchoscopy only 26% of airway narrowing is due to acute inflammation, with fibrous mature scarring as the predominant cause of the narrowing.

Lung parenchymal involvement may present with cough, haemoptysis, or recurrent infective symptoms, or may be silent. Radiographic abnormalities are noted in more than 70% of patients at some point during their disease. These range from single to multiple lung nodules found in 20–50% of patients. Cavitation of lung nodules will occur in two-thirds of cases. Pulmonary infiltrates, consolidation, intrathoracic lymphadenopathy, atelectasis, pleural thickening, and pleural effusions have all been described (Fig. 17.1a–d).

Extrapulmonary Features

Renal presentation of disease can be insidious. Microscopic haematuria is frequently overlooked, and a dipstick examination of the urine for

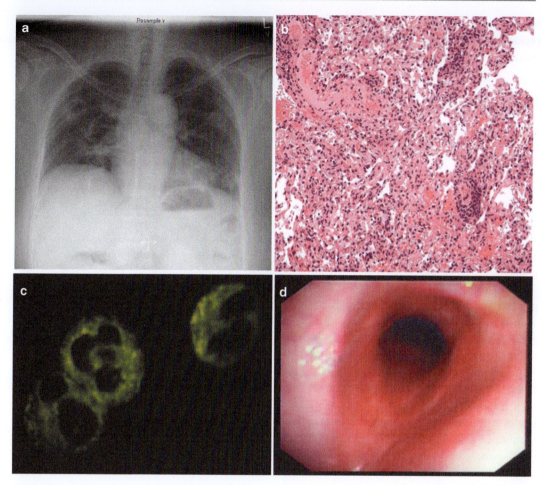

Fig. 17.1 (**a–d**) Granulomatosis with polyangiitis. (**a**) A chest radiograph in a patient with multiple lung nodules with both cavitatory and solid appearance. (**b**) CT guided biopsy undertaken due to concern of metastatic carcinoma shows small and medium vessel vasculitis with necrosis with the giant cells. (**c**) Immunofluoresence shows C-ANCA staining pattern with cytoplasmic staining. (**d**) Subglottic stenosis is shown with involvement of the vocal cords inferiorly

blood and protein should always be undertaken. Involvement of the eye may present with visual disturbance, pain, grittiness, and dryness in up to 30% of patients. Granulomatous inflammation of the orbits can cause proptosis in up to 15% of patients. Conjunctivitis, episcleritis, and scleritis may also occur.

Palpable purpura, skin ulcers, and haemorrhagic lesions have all been described as dermatological presentations. Neurological, cardiac, and gastroenterological presentations with mononeuritis multiplex, heart failure or arrhythmias, and gastrointestinal bleeding, respectively may occur in GPA, but are less common than in EGPA.

Microscopic Polyangiitis (MPA)

MPA is characterised by a necrotizing vasculitis, with few or no immune deposits, predominantly affecting small vessels. Necrotizing glomerulonephritis is very common. Pulmonary capillaritis frequently occurs. Although some of its features overlap with GPA, it is distinguished by the absence of granulomatous inflammation and lack of upper respiratory tract involvement. In its most severe manifestation it is a cause of pulmonary-renal syndrome.

It is more common in men and is typically but not invariably associated with ANCA positivity. It has a peak incidence in the sixth decade. It has a prevalence of six to seven per million, and an annual incidence of one per million in Northern Europe.

Clinical Features

There is typically a prodromal illness with fever, weight loss, arthralgia, myalgia, and fatigue that precedes the diagnosis. Pulmonary involvement includes diffuse alveolar hemorrhage, pleurisy, and pleural effusions. Presenting symptoms are dyspnea, cough, or hemoptysis, and can occur in up to 30% of patients. Recurrent and chronic sub-clinical alveolar haemorrhage has been associated with pulmonary fibrosis, and carries a poor prognosis.

Renal involvement is present in over 90% of patients. Crescentic glomerulonephritis and focal segmental glomerulonephritis with fibrinoid necrosis are typically seen. Microscopic haematuria with proteinuria is commonly found.

Gastro-intestinal involvement has been reported in 30–40% of patients. It can present with abdominal pain, diarrhoea, ischaemia, or bowel perforation. Neurological (mononeuritis multiplex, cerebral vasculitis); dermatological (leukocytoclastic vasculitis); musculoskeletal (arthritis); ophthalmic (retinal vasculitis); and cardiological (myocarditis and pericarditis) involvement have all been described.

Eosinophilic Granulomatosis with Polyangiitis (Churg-Strauss Syndrome)

Eosinophilic granulomatosis with polyangiitis (EGPA) is characterised by eosinophil-rich and necrotizing granulomatous inflammation, often involving the respiratory tract, associated with asthma. It has a prevalence of 10–13 per million in Northern Europe. In asthma sufferers it has a significantly higher prevalence of 67 per million (1 in 15,000). There is no sex predominance for EGPA, and it can present between the ages of 15 and 75, with a median age of presentation of 50.

The diagnosis of EGPA poses a challenge due to overlap with hypereosinophilic syndromes.

The European Respiratory Society has proposed the following for the diagnosis of EGPA:

- Asthma (with or without pulmonary opacities)
- Blood eosinophilia $>1.5 \times 10^9$ or >10% of circulating leucocytes or proven tissue eosinophilia with blood eosinophilia of $>0.75 \times 10^9$
- Vasculitis (or surrogates)
  - Necrotising vasculitis (biopsy proven of any organ)
  - Alveolar Haemorrhage (defined as bloody bronchoalveolar lavage with compatible radiology)
  - Mononeuritis multiplex
  - Necrotising glomerulonephritis
  - Palpable purpura
  - Haematuria associated with casts or haematuria and 2+ proteinuria
  - Myocardial infarction with proven coronary arteritis
  - ANCA-associated with at least one of the following
    Myocarditis or pericarditis
    Abdominal pain associated with diarrhoea
    Peripheral neuropathy

It has been noted that a subgroup of patients exists with hypereosinophilic asthma who have systemic manifestations (pericardial effusion, skin rash, neuropathy) without evidence of vasculitis and who are ANCA negative. Longitudinally over time these patients may go on to develop a vasculitis. The term "hypereosinophilic asthma with systemic manifestation" has been coined to describe them.

Clinical Features

Three phases in the development of EGPA have been suggested. A *prodromal phase* in which asthma (including cough-variant asthma) has been present for several years. This phase is often associated with rhinosinusitis and nasal polyposis. This is followed by an *eosinophilic phase* in which there is a peripheral eosinophilia with tissue infiltration which can be initially labelled simple pulmonary eosinophilia, eosinophilic gastroenteritis, or chronic eosinophilic pneumonia. Finally, after several years, there is a *vasculitis phase* with organ involvement including (a) the nervous system, most commonly with mononeuritis multiplex; (b) the cardiac system with myocarditis, pericarditis, and coronary arteritis; (c) gastroenterological system with ischaemia and bleeding; and (d) dermatologically with subcutaneous nodules, palpable purpura, and haemorrhagic lesions.

It has been suggested that there are two types of EGPA: (1) ANCA-associated EGPA with mononeuritis multiplex, pulmonary haemorrhage, cutaneous vasculitis, and rarely renal disease; and (2) ANCA-negative EGPA with nasal polyposis, pulmonary infiltrates, cardiac disease, and eosinopilic gastroenteritis. The latter is associated with a poorer prognosis. There is, however, considerable overlap between the two.

There is a reported association of leukotriene antagonists with Churg Strauss Syndrome. Studies now suggest this is related to corticosteroid withdrawal after initiating therapy, rather than direct drug toxicity.

ANCA Patterns with AAV

ANCA testing is frequently undertaken in two steps. An initial immunofluoresence test is undertaken looking for either a cytoplasmic (C-ANCA) or peri-nuclear staining pattern (P-ANCA). Then, if positive, an enzyme-linked immunosorbent assay (ELISA) is undertaken. The primary antigen in C-ANCA is the serine protease 3, PR3-ANCA, and in P-ANCA is myeloperoxidase, MPO-ANCA. In addition, other C-ANCA and P-ANCA antigens, including antibodies to bacterial permeability inhibitor (BPI) associated with cystic fibrosis and h-LAMP-2 (associated with necrotising glomerulonephritis), have been described.

Patients with GPA have a positive ANCA in up to 96% of cases, with 88% being PR3 ANCA positive. In contrast, patients with MPA have a positive ANCA in up to 98% of cases, with 79% being MPO-ANCA positive. In the case of EGPA, up to 64% of patients will be ANCA positive, with MPO-ANCA accounting for the majority of cases.

ANCA-positive ELISA results can be found incidentally, but may herald the development of vasculitis. A period of observation is recommended in patients with positive results without evidence of vasculitis.

Medical Management and Treatment of AAV

Until the advent of cyclophosphamide and corticosteroid therapy, vasculitis carried a poor prognosis, with 90% 2-year mortality in the 1960s. In the subsequent years a series of pivotal clinical studies altered the management and prognosis of vasculitis. These studies and the staging criteria of the disease proposed by the European vasculitis study group (EUVAS) have helped develop guidelines on the management of vasculitis. The staging criteria are:

- *Limited disease.* Disease confined to the upper airways that is usually applied to GPA.
- *Early generalised disease.* This signifies disease without threatened end organ function. Nodular and cavitatory lung disease fall into this category.
- *Active generalised disease.* This denotes disease with threatened end organ function. This is usually applied to threatened renal damage.
- *Severe disease.* This signifies impending end organ failure and dysfunction. Examples include diffuse alveolar haemorrhage and severe renal failure
- *Refractory disease.* Disease that has failed to enter remission despite appropriate therapy.

The European League Against Rheumatism (EULAR) in 2009 and the British Rheumatology Society (BSR) in 2013 published guidelines on the management of small- to medium-vessel vasculitis and large-vessel vasculitis [3–5]. Their recommendations for the management of small- to medium-vessel vasculitis have been modified in Table 17.5. The key recommendations are:

Table 17.5 Treatment of AAV based on site and severity of disease

Clinical class	Localised	Early systemic	Generalised systemic	Severe	Refractory
Constitutional symptoms	−	+	+	+	+
Renal function	Creatinine <120 µmol/L	Creatinine <120 µmol/L	Creatinine <500 µmol/L	Creatinine >500 µmol/L	Any
Threatened organ function	−	−	−	+	+
Induction	Single agent (CS, AZA, MXT)	CYC + CS or MTX + CS	CYC + CS or CS+ RTX	CYC+ CS+ PE	CYC + CS + PE ± RTX
Recommended dosage	CS (1 mg/kg/day) tapered down to 0.25 mg/kg/day by 12 weeks AZA 1–2 mg/kg/day MTX 20–25 mg/week Oral CYC 1.5–2 mg/kg/day PE seven exchanges within first 2 weeks RTX 2× 1 g infusion 2–4 weeks apart with six monthly repeat				
Maintenance	Once remission is achieved with CYC or RTX transition to maintenance with AZA 1–2 mg/kg or MTX 20–25 mg/week should be considered The duration of maintenance therapy should be 12–24 months				

CS Corticosteroid, AZA Azathioprine, MTX methotrexate, CYC Cyclophosphamide, PE Plasma exchange, RTX Rituximab

- That patients with primary small- and medium-vessel vasculitis should be managed in collaboration with, or at, centres of expertise.
- ANCA testing (including indirect immunofluorescence and ELISA) should only be performed in the appropriate clinical context.
- A positive biopsy is strongly supportive of vasculitis, and it is recommended that the procedure is used to assist diagnosis and further evaluation for patients suspected of having vasculitis. These include CT-guided lung biopsy or open lung biopsy if the diagnosis cannot be made from tissue elsewhere.
- The use of a structured clinical assessment, urine analysis, and other basic laboratory tests at each clinical visit for patients with vasculitis is recommended.
- Patients with ANCA-associated vasculitis should be categorised according to different levels of severity to assist treatment decisions.
- It is recommended that a combination of cyclophosphamide (intravenous or oral) and glucocorticoids or rituximab and corticosteroids (if cyclophosphamide is contraindicated) is used for remission induction in generalised primary small- and medium-vessel vasculitis.
- It is recommended that a combination of methotrexate and glucocorticoid (as a less toxic alternative to cyclophosphamide) is used for the induction of remission in non-organ threatening or non-life threatening ANCA-associated vasculitis.
- Assessment for *Staphylococcus aureus* nasal carriage should be carried out and if detected, eradication therapy with nasal mupirocin should be carried out.

Predictors of Relapse in Treatment of AAV

Studies have shown that the risk factors for relapse in AAV include (a) a diagnosis of GPA; (b) ENT disease; (c) PR3 ANCA; (d) persistent ANCA despite treatment; (e) an increase in ANCA titres; (f) immunosuppression reduction (i.e. azathioprine, methotrexate or mycophenolate withdrawal); (g) lower total cyclophosphamide exposure; and (h) corticosteroid withdrawal.

Detection and Protection Against Adverse Effects of Treatment

Mesna Treatment for Oral Cyclophosphamide

Epidemiological studies have shown the cumulative dose of cyclophosphamide (>30 g) is associated with uroepithelial carcinoma. Mesna protects by scavenging the urotoxic acrolein metabolite of cyclophosphamide. Patients who are smokers can develop uroepithelial toxicity at a lower cumulative dose than non-smokers, and should therefore be screened for non-vasculitis-related haematuria.

Pneumocystis jirovecii Prophylaxis Treatment

Early studies have shown the risk of *Pneumocystis jirovecii* pneumonia can be as high as 20%. This is more frequently observed when high-dose corticosteroids therapy is used. It is recommended that trimethoprim/sulphamethoxazole be used either as 960 mg alternate days or 480 mg od. At this low dose it appears safe to use in conjunction with methotrexate, but it is advised to omit prophylaxis on the day that methotrexate is taken because of concerns about myelotoxicity.

Immunoglobulin Level Monitoring for Patients on Rituximab

Rituximab therapy leads to B lymphocyte depletion and secondary hypogammaglobulinaemia. Immunoglobulin levels and lymphocyte subclasses should be checked prior to each therapy with rituximab. If recurrent infections and hypogammaglobulinaemia occur, immunoglobulin replacement therapy should be considered.

Prognosis of AAV

The prognosis of AAV prior to corticosteroids and cyclophosphamide was a 1-year mortality of 80% and 2-year mortality of 90%. These figures have now reversed, with over 90% of patients now achieving remission. A study following up 535 patients with newly diagnosed GPA or MPA entered into EUVAS clinic trials found an increased mortality ratio of 2.6 compared to the general population. Survival at 1 year, 3 years, and 5 years was 88%, 85%, and 78% respectively. Predictors of poor survival at presentation were advanced renal failure, increasing age, a high Birmingham vasculitis assessment score (BVAS), high white blood cell (WBC) count, and a low haemoglobin.

In a separate study, the French Vasculitis Study Group reviewed the data of 1108 patients in their database. They reported a 5-year survival of 72.5% (MPA), 86.1% (EGPA), and 86.9% (GPA). They described a five factor score where each of the following scored 1 point (1) age > 65 years; (2) cardiac symptoms; (3) gastrointestinal involvement; (4) renal insufficiency with a stabilized creatinine >150 μmol/L; and (5) the absence of ENT symptoms, which are protective in GPA and EGPA. Scores of 0, 1, and ≥2 were associated with 5-year survival of 91%, 79%, and 60% respectively.

Other Pulmonary Vasculitides

Behçet's Disease

Behçet's disease is a rare multisystem disease characterised by vasculitis affecting variable sized arteries and veins [6]. It is associated with the clinical triad of recurrent oral ulceration, recurrent genital ulceration, and uveitis. It is seen more commonly in men of Mediterranean and Middle Eastern origin. The highest prevalence is in Turkey, where there is a prevalence of 100 per million population. There is an association with HLA-B51 (in 50–70% of patients) and GIMAP (GTPase immune-associated proteins) family of proteins, indicating genetic factors in its aetiology. The mechanism of the pathogenesis of the disease remains unclear.

Clinical Features

Diagnosis is made when oral ulceration together with two of the following four criteria are present: (1) cutaneous lesions; (2) genital ulceration; (3) ocular lesions (retinitis or uveitis); and (4) pathergy (an exaggerated erythematous papular response to a small needlestick).

Pulmonary manifestations frequently found include pulmonary artery aneurysms, pulmonary artery thrombosis, pulmonary infarction, consolidation, mosaic perfusion, pleural effusions, and pleural nodules. There is a rarer pulmonary variant of Behçet's disease called Hughes Stovin syndrome, which is characterised by multiple pulmonary aneurysms· peripheral venous thrombosis, recurrent fever, haemoptysis, and cough, without oral and genital ulceration.

Radiological Investigations

The most common finding on chest radiographic and CT findings are lung masses attributed to a pulmonary artery aneurysm (Fig. 17.2). After the aorta, the pulmonary artery is the second most common site of large vessel arterial involvement. In Behçet's disease, pulmonary artery aneurysms are more common than thromboembolic disease. Pulmonary artery aneurysms can regress after medical treatment with steroid and/or immunosuppressive agents.

Treatment

There are no randomised large population-based clinical trials to provide evidence for pulmonary disease treatment recommendations in this rare disease. The presence of pulmonary artery aneurysms requires a combination of cyclophosphamide and corticosteroids. The aneurysms frequently regress with the use of steroids. There are case reports where aneurysms associated with recurrent bleeding have been managed with embolization.

Takayasu's Arteritis

Takayasu's arteritis is a rare, often granulomatous, large-vessel vasculitis, predominantly

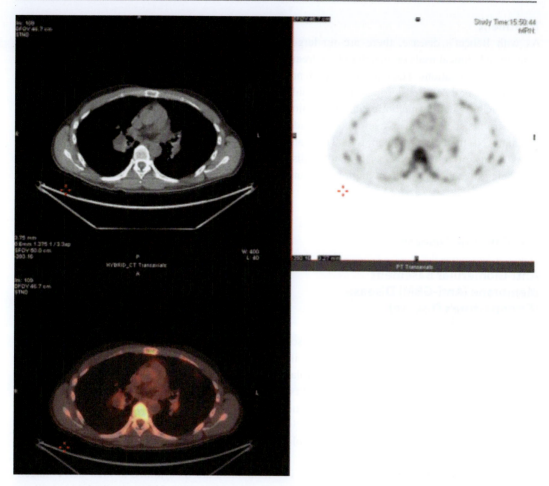

Fig. 17.2 A CT-PET showing large vessel saccular aneurysm of the right pulmonary artery with uptake of FDG, typically seen in Behcet's disease. These aneurysms will regress with therapy. Although tissue confirmation is rarely feasible in life, post-mortem samples show both vasculitis and thrombosis in the wall and lumen of the vessels

affecting the aorta and/or its major branches. It can sometimes affect the pulmonary arteries, causing pulmonary hypertension. Onset usually occurs in patients younger than 40 years. It is more common in females.

Clinical Features

Non-specific constitutional symptoms, such as fever, weight loss, arthralgias, myalgias, and malaise, together with exertional dyspnea (75% of patients), haemoptysis (42% of patients), palpitations and chest pain (49% of patients), can occur. Physical examination is usually unhelpful, but absent or diminished pulses and discrepancy in blood pressures have been noted in 49% of patients.

Radiological Investigations

Histological diagnosis of pulmonary artery Takayasu's disease is unusual, and a clinico-radiological diagnosis is usually made. The radiological features seen on CT, magnetic resonance imaging, and pulmonary angiography include irregularity, narrowing, and occlusion of the pulmonary arteries. CT-PET and dual-energy CT can show increased uptake in the walls of the pulmonary arteries, reflecting active granulomatous inflammation.

Treatment

As with Behçet's disease, there are no large, randomised clinical trials on which to base treatment recommendations. The majority of patients respond to oral corticosteroids and steroid-sparing agents such as methotrexate or azathioprine. In resistant disease cyclophosphamide and anti-TNF therapy have been used. There are case reports of refractory vessel stenosis disease being treated with balloon angioplasty and stenting.

Autoimmune Diseases

Anti-Glomerular Basement Membrane (Anti-GBM) Disease (Goodpasture's Disease)

This rare disease is characterized by the association of pulmonary haemorrhage, extracapillary glomerulonephritis, and anti-glomerular basement membrane antibodies [7]. It was first described in 1919 by Ernest Goodpasture, who reported pulmonary haemorrhage and rapidly progressive glomerulonephritis in an 18-year-old patient with 'flu.

The annual incidence in Northern Europe is estimated at 1 per million. The age of onset is associated with two peaks, the first one in the third decade of life, and a further smaller peak in the sixth to seventh decade of life. There is a seasonal incidence of anti-GBM, with it being more common in the spring and early summer. Mechanical damage to the kidney by lithotripsy and ureteric obstruction has been associated with development of anti-GBM disease.

Alveolar haemorrhage occurs predominantly in younger men. In the older peak, isolated renal disease is more common with no sex predominance. Alveolar haemorrhage is invariably associated with cigarette smoking or exposure to inhaled hydrocarbons. Pulmonary haemorrhage in the absence of renal disease is rare. An overlap syndrome between ANCA vasculitis and anti-GBM disease has been described. Up to 32% of patients who test positive for anti-GBM antibodies will also test positive for ANCA.

MPO-ANCA is the most frequently associated is this scenario.

Pathogenesis

Evidence for the role of anti-GBM antibodies in the development of Goodpasture's disease came from the classical adoptive transfer experiments. Antibodies from humans with Goodpasture's disease were transferred to monkeys, which developed glomerulonephritis and alveolar haemorrhage with antibodies binding to the glomerular basement membrane. Additional evidence came from patients undergoing renal transplantation for Goodpasture's disease. Those who still had circulating antibodies present at the time of transplantation went on to develop disease in the donor kidney. Furthermore, antibody removal by plasmapheresis is associated with recovery from alveolar haemorrhage and renal failure.

The basement membrane is an extracellular structure composed primarily of collagen, laminin, and proteogylcans. Type IV collagen forms a matrix on which other components integrate. Type IV collagen comprises three sub units: $\alpha3$, $\alpha4$, and $\alpha5$, assembled into a monomer. These monomers are then joined at their non-collagen C terminal domain (NC1) via disulphide bridges to form hexamers. Studies have shown anti-GBM antibodies are directed against Type IV collagen, and specifically the NC1 domain of $\alpha3$ chain [8].

In addition to evidence for antibody-mediated disease, there is evidence showing auto-reactive T cells play a part in the development of disease. Anti-GBM disease has a positive association with the human leukocyte antigen HLA-DR15 haplotype, particularly the DRB1*1501 allele, and negative associations with HLA-DR1 and DR7, which are viewed as protective.

Anti-GBM antibodies are frequently found in the general population in low titres. The difference between healthy normal individuals and those with anti-GBM disease is that the antibodies are restricted to IgG2 and IgG4 in healthy individuals, compared to IgG1 and IgG3 in patients with anti-GBM disease. It is thought that the ability of different subclasses to bind to

Fc receptors is implicated in the pathogenesis of disease with IgG1 and IgG3.

Clinical Features

Patients frequently have a prodromal constitutional systemic illness similar to that seen in vasculitis, with symptoms of fever, sweats, loss of appetite, and arthralgia. They may suffer dyspnoea in the absence of alveolar haemorrhage due to anaemia.

Pulmonary haemorrhage presenting with haemoptysis has historically been the predominant symptom associated with disease. This is now changing with the reduction of smoking, especially among young men. It usually heralds renal involvement in the ensuing months. Infections are frequently associated with the onset of anti-GBM disease as in the original description with influenza.

Renal disease can occur in isolation (more commonly in the older peak incidence) or in conjunction with pulmonary haemorrhage. It is usually rapid in evolution. Initially microscopic haematuria with casts is present and it can progress rarely in severe disease to macroscopic haematuria. Patients may present with oliguria or anuria with volume overload and symptoms of uraemia.

Investigations

Radiology

The chest radiograph is abnormal in up to 80% of patients. It classically shows central diffuse infiltrative shadowing with peripheral sparing. In addition, ill-defined nodules and consolidative changes have been reported. CT findings mirror that of the chest radiograph, with perihilar ground glass changes with peripheral sparing (Fig. 17.3a–d).

Pulmonary Function Testing

An increase in K_{CO} (corrected gas transfer coefficient) is described as the most sensitive and specific test for alveolar haemorrhage. The

mechanism for this is that the free haemoglobin in the alveoli is able to bind inspired carbon monoxide and increase K_{CO} values.

Serology and Tissue Biopsy

The presence of circulating anti-GBM antibodies and tissue biopsy evidence of anti-GBM antibodies fixed to glomerular or alveolar basement membrane is used to make a diagnosis.

Differential Diagnosis for Pulmonary Renal Syndrome

The main causes of pulmonary renal syndromes are the vasculitides, especially MPA. There is overlap between MPA and anti-GBM disease. In this setting, antibodies to both ANCA (mainly MPO) and anti-GBM are found simultaneously. Patients tend to have lower levels of anti-GBM antibodies and are managed as MPA vasculitis. Other causes of pulmonary renal syndrome are listed in Table 17.6.

Treatment of Anti-GBM Disease

Unlike the pulmonary vasculitides, there are no large randomised trials upon which to base treatment decisions. The treatment of choice is corticosteroids (1 mg/kg/day), cyclophosphamide (2 mg/kg/day), and plasmapheresis (daily 4 L plasma exchange with 5% albumin for 14 days or until anti-GBM antibodies are undetectable). Smoking cessation in smokers is encouraged.

Prognosis

In contrast to pulmonary vasculitides, relapse is rare in anti-GBM disease. When relapse does occur, it may be related to the development of overlap disease with AAV. Predictors for mortality are high anti-GBM antibody titres and the presence of ANCA. Predictors of kidney survival are the serum creatinine on presentation, the need for dialysis, and the percentage of crescents seen on renal biopsy.

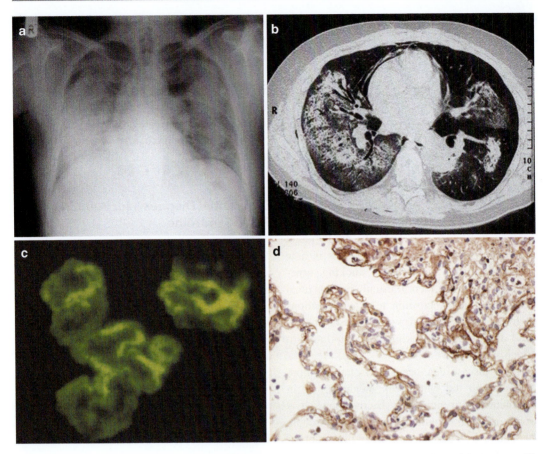

Fig. 17.3 (a–c) A case of diffuse alveolar haemorrhage due to Anti-glomerular basement membrane (GBM) disease with overlap with microscopic polyangiitis. (a) Shows a typical chest radiograph with peripheral sparing of the lung fields. (b) A CT confirms with perihilar ground glass changes with peripheral sparing. (c) Immunofluoresence shows P-ANCA staining pattern with peri-nuclear staining. ELISA showed this was due to antibodies to myeloperoxidase (MPO). (d) Lung biopsy shows alveolar basement membrane staining brown showing the presence of anti-GBM antibodies

Table 17.6 The differential diagnosis of pulmonary renal syndrome

Pulmonary vasculitides	Microscopic polyangiitis[a]
	Granulomatosis with polyangiitis[a]
	Eosinophilic granulomatosis with polyangiitis[a]
	Behcets disease[a]
	Henoch Schonlein[a]
Secondary vasculitis	Systemic lupus erythematosus[a]
	Anti-glomerular basement membrane disease[a]
	Polymyositis[a]
	Rheumatoid arthritis[a]
	Drug induced vasculitis
	Post infective (pneumonia with glomerulonephritis)
Other causes	Paraquat poisoning
	Renal thrombosis with pulmonary emboli
	Pulmonary oedema with renal failure

[a]Associated with a rapidly progressive glomerulonephritis

Pulmonary Alveolar Proteinosis

Pulmonary alveolar proteinosis (PAP) is a rare lung disease, with an annual incidence of 0.2 cases per million. It is characterised by the accumulation of lipoproteinaceous material within the alveoli due to impaired surfactant clearance by macrophages [9].

There are three main types of PAP: (1) Primary autoimmune PAP; (2) secondary PAP related to various conditions including haematological malignancy, infection, and inhalation of hydrocarbons or mineral dusts; and (3) inherited genetic. The following section will concentrate on autoimmune PAP.

Pathogenesis

The serendipitous finding that knockout mice deficient in granulocyte monocyte colony stimulating factor (GMSCF) developed a disease process histologically similar to PAP has been the basis of understanding the mechanism of disease in PAP.

Type II pneumocytes secrete surfactant proteins (A, B, C, and D) and lipids into the alveoli. Surfactant reduces alveolar surface tension and prevents alveolar collapse at the end of expiration. Alveolar macrophages play a pivotal role in the clearance of surfactant proteins and lipids. GMCSF controls the migration, differentiation, and function of alveolar macrophages. In primary auto-immune PAP there are high concentrations of neutralising anti-GMCSF IgG antibodies. These antibodies bind GMCSF, preventing macrophage clearance of surfactant, and reduce their anti-infection abilities. Anti-GMCSF antibodies have been shown to be pathogenic in adoptive transfer experiments.

Clinical Presentation

The presentation of PAP is non-specific, with dyspnoea and cough being the most common symptoms. The presence of chest pain, fever, and sweats may indicate concomitant infection. Clinical examination may reveal cyanosis, clubbing, and crepitations on auscultation.

Investigations

Radiology

The characteristic chest radiograph in PAP shows diffuse symmetrical pulmonary infiltrates with sparing of the costophrenic angles and apices. Less frequently, diffuse opacities are found ranging from ground glass to reticular nodular shadowing to consolidation with air bronchograms.

The CT appearances in PAP are characteristic, showing a "crazy paving" geographical appearance. This is defined as a smooth septal line thickening superimposed on underlying ground glass changes. The extent of ground glass changes correlates with severity, as judged by pulmonary function tests and hypoxaemia (Fig. 17.4).

Although characteristic of PAP, "crazy paving" is found in a variety of other conditions including infection, malignancy, and inhalational lung injury.

Pulmonary Function Tests

Pulmonary function testing typically shows a restrictive defect with reduced diffusing capacity. There is usually desaturation on a 6-min walk, and depending on severity, resting hypoxaemia on room air.

Laboratory and Invasive Investigations

Lactate dehydrogenase is frequently elevated between two to three times the upper limit of

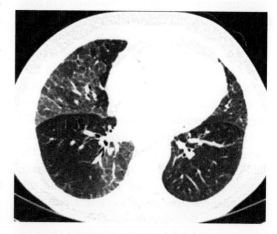

Fig. 17.4 Diffuse basal interstitial change with areas termed "crazy paving" in the right lung seen in a case of pulmonary alveolar proteinosis (PAP)

normal. It has been suggested that it may be a useful to monitor disease control in PAP. Anti-GMCSF antibodies are found in autoimmune PAP. In addition, anti-GMCSF antibodies have been described in acute myeloid leukaemia and healthy normal individuals. A threshold of >19 ug/ml has been found to have a good predictive value for autoimmune PAP.

The returns from bronchoalveolar lavage (BAL) in autoimmune PAP have a macroscopically milky appearance. Cytological analysis reveals periodic acid Schiff (PAS) staining material, predominantly lymphocytic, with foamy macrophages and hyaline material. The BAL should be sent for microbiological cultures, since up to 5% of patients will also have an opportunistic infection. In the majority of cases, a combination of radiology and BAL is all that is needed to make a diagnosis. Rarely, lung biopsy in the form of transbronchial or thoracoscopic lung biopsy may be needed.

Treatment

The clinical course of autoimmune PAP is not easily predicted. In case series, up to 28% of patients have spontaneously improved.

Lung Lavage

As with other rare lung diseases, there are no large, randomised control trials on which to base treatment recommendations. Whole (or less frequently, segmental) lung lavage is undertaken in most patients except those who improve spontaneously. This is generally undertaken in an ICU or theatre setting. The patient is intubated with a double lumen endotracheal tube and paralysed. Single-lung ventilation is undertaken with a FiO_2 of 1.0. The non-ventilated lung is lavaged with warm saline (37 °C) in 0.5–1.0 L aliquots. The fluid is then removed by suctioning. Sequential aliquots are instilled and removed until the return changes from milky to clear. Up to 40 L of saline may be required. Not all the lavage will be removed, and the patient will need to be ventilated for 2–3 h post-procedure for respiratory

support as it is cleared. During the procedure, manual chest percussion has been used to increase the return. Although it has been reported that both lungs have been lavaged sequentially at the same sitting, our practice is to perform this on the contralateral lung 24–48 h later. There is an improvement of symptoms, pulmonary function tests, and hypoxaemia with whole-lung lavage. In over half of patients, it may be need repeating on more than one occasion.

GMCSF Therapy

Although whole-lung lavage is considered the standard of care, it is not easily available, and alternative treatments have been trialled. These include subcutaneous and inhaled GMCSF therapy. Small uncontrolled or retrospective studies have shown improvements on par with whole-lung lavage, but clinical improvement is achieved over a longer time period. A recent meta-analysis of GMCSF therapy studies showed it was only effective in 59% of patients, and so its role is unclear. One approach is to consider supplementary drug treatment following whole-lung lavage.

Rituximab and Plasmapheresis

Refractory PAP not responsive to whole-lung lavage and GMCSF have been treated on compassionate grounds with plasmapheresis and rituximab, on the basis both of these therapies would reduce circulating anti-GMCSF levels and improve disease in a similar manner to anti-GBM disease. There are small open-label studies with rituximab, which showed improvements in the primary outcome oxygenation and secondary outcomes pulmonary function and radiology. At present, rituximab and plasmapheresis cannot be recommended outside clinical trials or for refractory disease on compassionate grounds.

IgG4-Related Disease

IgG4-related sclerosing disease (IgG4-RD) is a relatively newly described condition [10]. It was initially reported in association with autoimmune pancreatitis in the 1990s. Over the subsequent years it has been associated with biliary duct, salivary gland, renal tract, and aortic, as well as pulmonary disease. Multiorgan involvement is common with IgG4-related disease.

IgG4-RD is more common in men than women (2.8:1). It typically develops in the seventh decade of life, but has been described in patients between the ages of 15 and 75.

Pathological Findings

The diagnosis of IgG4-RD is primarily a histopathological one. It relies on the presence of elevated IgG4 positive plasma cells in tissue together with characteristic pathological features found on biopsy. These are: (a) dense lymphoplasmacytic infiltrate; (b) fibrosis, arranged at least focally in a storiform pattern (whorled matted or spoke-like appearance); and (c) obliterative phlebitis.

Other features associated with IgG4-RD include phlebitis without obliteration of the lumen, and increased tissue eosinophils. The presence of granulomas and excess neutrophils are inconsistent with a diagnosis of IgG4-RD.

A raised serum IgG4 level of >140 mg.dl^{-1} is found in 70–90% of patients with IgG4-RD and 5% of the normal population, and cannot alone be used to make the diagnosis of IgG4-RD. Normal serum IgG4 levels can also be found in a minority of patients with biopsy-proven IgG4-RD.

Pathogenesis of IgG4-Related Disease

The mechanism of IgG4-RD is unclear. Evidence from studies in autoimmune pancreatitis has suggested various mechanisms. Associations with HLA DRB1*0405 and HLA DQB1*0401 indicate genetic susceptibility factors. Th2 cells and cytokines including T cytokines and transforming growth factor-β are thought to play important roles in IgG4-positive plasma cell tissue infiltration and the development of fibrosis.

Molecular mimicry has been postulated as possible mechanism. Stimulation of toll-like receptors have been shown to induce the production of IgG4, giving rise to the theory various bacteria could give rise to increased IgG4 production by stimulating the innate immune system.

Clinical Presentation of Pulmonary IgG4-RD

The symptoms of pulmonary IgG4-RD are nonspecific. They range from cough, haemoptysis, exertional dyspnoea, and chest pain through to being asymptomatic. Pulmonary disease may be an incidental finding whilst investigating disease elsewhere in up to half of patients. Constitutional symptoms (fever, sweats, and weight loss) are unusual.

Investigations

Radiology

The features found on CT include mediastinal lymphadenopathy (found >40% of all patients with Ig4-RD); solid nodular lesions occasionally with spiculations, giving concern initially of underlying malignancy; pleural thickening and nodularity (found in ~25% of patients with pulmonary disease); alveolar interstitial disease ± honeycombing; bronchiectasis; pleural effusions (rare); airway stenosis (rare); and fibrosing mediastinitis (case reports only).

Pulmonary Function Tests

Pulmonary function tests reflect the broad clinic-radiological features of disease presentation, with both restrictive and obstructive pictures found.

Laboratory and Invasive Investigations

The serum Ig4 level is raised in the majority of patients with IgG4-RD, but it is not specific or sensitive enough to make a diagnosis of disease on its own.

Bronchoalveolar lavage has been undertaken with transbronchial lung biopsy to diagnose disease. The BAL has been shown to have a raised IgG4 levels in comparison to patients with sarcoidosis. As this correlates with raised serum levels, IgG4 measurements in lavage fluid do not help in confirming the diagnosis.

Tissue diagnosis from surgical lung biopsy, CT-guided lung or pleural biopsy, or transbronchial biopsy are key to making a diagnosis of IgG4-RD.

Differential Diagnosis

The differential diagnoses of IgG4-RD include sarcoidosis (mediastinal lymphadenopathy is common in both), malignancy (solid nodules with spiculation are found in IgG4-RD), Castleman's disease (mediastinal lymphadenopathy and masses seen with both), lymphomatoid granulomatosis and idiopathic interstitial pneumonia (similar radiological lung parenchymal disease pattern).

Treatment of IgG4-RD

In the absence of randomised clinical trial to guide the management of IgG4-RD (due to disease rarity), corticosteroid therapy in the form of prednisolone 0.5–1 mg/kg/day has emerged as the mainstay for treatment from case series involving organ threatening disease, which in the lung usually means symptomatic parenchymal or pleural disease. No specific treatment is required in non-organ threatening disease, such as lymphadenopathy alone.

The majority of patients respond well to corticosteroid therapy, but relapses are not uncommon. In this scenario there are reports of successful use of azathioprine, methotrexate, and mycophenolate in combination with corticosteroids. In refractory disease, rituximab has been used on the basis that reduction of IgG4 levels will induce remission. This has not invariably been the case. The response to treatment has been shown to be less successful in those with well-developed fibrosis.

Idiopathic Pulmonary Haemosiderosis

Pulmonary haemosiderosis is a consequence of repeated alveolar haemorrhage. Idiopathic pulmonary haemosiderosis (IPH) has to be differentiated from other causes of recurrent alveolar haemorrhage resulting in haemosiderosis. The diagnosis of IPH is made by exclusion of secondary causes, which include the imitators of vasculitis (Table 17.4) and causes of pulmonary-renal syndrome (Table 17.6). It is characterised by (a) diffuse haemorrhage within alveolar spaces; (b) haemosiderin-laden macrophages best seen with Perl's reaction with Prussian Blue stain; (c) interstitial thickening with hyperplasia of type II pneumocytes and fibrosis; and (d) the absence of capillaritis, vasculitis, granulomas, or other vascular malformations.

IPH is a rare disease, with an annual incidence of 0.2–1.0 per million [11]. Up to 20% of cases present in adult life, but the majority are children under the age of 10. In adults most cases present in the late teens to third decade of life. There is an equal sex incidence in children, and slight male preponderance in adults.

Pathogenesis

Alveolar haemorrhage is associated with dyspnoea, haemoptysis, and radiological pulmonary infiltrates. Following haemorrhage, alveolar macrophages clear the erythrocytes from the alveoli. In the process they convert haemoglobin's iron into haemosiderin within 72 h. The haemosiderin-laden macrophages stay within the lung for 4–8 weeks.

The mechanism of alveolar damage leading to IPH is unknown, and has to be differentiated from immune-mediated damage by auto-antibodies to the basement membrane in anti-GBM disease and blood vessels in ANCA-associated vasculitis, together with immune complex-mediated damage, e.g. SLE, cryoglobulinaemia, and Henoch-Schonlein purpura.

There are reports of IPH occurring in families, suggesting either a genetic or environmental cause. There is a single study linking IPH associated with coeliac disease to HLA B8*. There are associations of IPH with cow's milk allergy (Heiner's Syndrome) and coeliac disease. In these conditions, circulating immune complexes with alveolar deposition of IgA and IgG has been seen in some patients. Treatment with either milk- or gluten-free diets have resulted in improvement or remission of disease in these cases.

The role of fungal infections related to the fungus *Stachybotrys atra* and other moulds, including aspergillus and alternaria, has been postulated. It was suggested that the fungal toxin trichotecen, which inhibited angiogenesis, impaired the development of alveolar membranes in the children, causing haemorrhage. This link has been questioned in other studies.

Clinical Presentation of IPH

A triad of haemoptysis, anaemia, and pulmonary infiltrates with no other cause is described in IPH. The disease presentations can be variable, ranging from chronic development to fulminant acute disease. Symptoms include cough, haemoptysis, dyspnoea, and fatigue. Haemoptysis may be absent in children, and is invariably present in adults. Clinical examination in the acute setting may find tachypnea, pallor, tachycardia, wheeze, fever, and crackles. In chronic disease, clubbing with fibrotic crackles may develop.

Investigations

Radiology
There are no specific radiological features of IPH. Chest radiographs may show bilateral pulmonary infiltrates, which recedes and leaves reticular changes. The CT scan mirrors these changes, with diffuse infiltrative changes predominantly in the lower lobes that clear leaving a reticular-nodular pattern. Chromium isotope[51]

or technetium Tc^{99} pertechnetate-labeled red cell nuclear medicine scans have been undertaken to show alveolar haemorrhage. Normal lungs do not take up red cells, but when active alveolar haemorrhage is present in IPH there is leakage and retention within the alveoli.

Pulmonary Functions Tests
In acute IPH, a raised diffusing capacity for carbon monoxide and airflow obstruction have been described. In chronic IPH, a restrictive picture with a low or normal diffusing capacity for carbon monoxide can develop.

Laboratory and Invasive Investigations
Microcytic hypochromic anaemia may be found on the full blood count. Eosinophilia and neutrophilia may be present. The ferritin level may be normal or elevated due to alveolar release from clearance of erythrocytes, and does not reflect tissue iron stores.

It is important to exclude the presence of secondary causes of pulmonary haemosiderosis. ANCA, anti-GBM antibodies, rheumatoid factor, anti-phospholipid antibody, anti-nuclear antibody, and cryoglobulins should be screened. In light of the association of IPH with coeliac disease and milk allergy, anti-gliadin antibodies together with serum precipitins to casein and lactalbumin should be performed.

Bronchoscopy and lavage is important to confirm the presence of haemosiderin-laden macrophages and exclude infection. Tissue, ideally from surgical lung biopsy, is needed for diagnosis. It allows for the exclusion of vasculitis and capillaritis as the cause of pulmonary haemosiderosis.

Treatment and Prognosis

Corticosteroids have been shown in case series to be effective. A survey of prescribing in acute and chronic IPH showed a variation of practice across the world. The mainstay in all centres was corticosteroid therapy with hydroxychloroquine, azathioprine, and cyclophosphamide used (in descending order of use) as steroid-sparing agents. In two reported cases of lung transplantation, the disease recurred in the allograft.

The reported survival from a predominantly children-based cases series is 2–4 years from diagnosis. The prognosis in IPH for adults appears better than for children. This is thought to be related to their slower and milder disease presentation.

Cystic Lung Diseases

Cystic lung diseases have a characteristic radiological appearance on CT [12] and unlike the presence of cysts in the liver or kidneys, those in the lungs are always reflective of an underlying pathology. There are a number of causes of this phenomenon, and the main ones are listed in Table 17.7. Cysts can be differentiated from bullae or cavities, as true cysts are thin walled (less than 2–3 mm thick) and have areas of low attenuation (Fig. 17.5a–c). Bullae do not have thin walls, whereas cavities are thick-walled, gas-filled spaces which develop in areas of the lung which have consolidation, masses, or nodules. The more common appearances of cysts in the lungs include centrilobular emphysema, chronic

Table 17.7 The main causes of cystic lung disease as seen on CT scan

Centrilobular emphysema
Chronic hypersensitivity pneumonitis
Atypical infection causing pneumatocoeles
Langerhans cell histiocytosis (LCH)
Lymphoid interstitial pneumonia (LIP)
Lymphangioleiomyomatosis (LAM)
Birt Hogg Dubé syndrome
Desquamative interstitial pneumonia

Cystic appearances can be seen in centrilobular emphysema, chronic hypersensitivity pneumonitis and infection but the remainder are rarer causes of 'true cysts' in the lung. Adapted from Beddy P, Babar J, Devaraj A. A practical approach to cystic lung disease on HRCT. Insights imaging. 2011 Feb;2(1):1–7

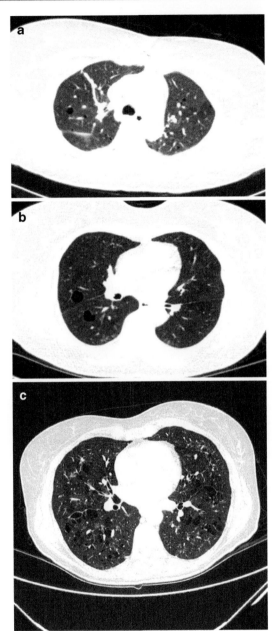

Fig. 17.5 (a–c) (a) Scattered thin-walled cysts (up to 11 mm) in both lungs with persistent diffuse ground glass change in a case of cystic lung disease due to Birt Hogg Dubé syndrome. (b) Thin-walled cysts in the right lung with background ground glass and areas of extreme apical sparing due to LIP. (c) Scattered spiculated nodules and cysts in a patient with PLCH. There is some co-existing emphysema

hypersensitivity pneumonitis, and infections leading to pneumatocoeles. The following section covers the most important, rarer causes of "true" cystic lung disease.

Langerhans Cell Histiocytosis (LCH)

Pathogenesis

Langerhans cell histiocytosis (LCH) is a rare multisystem disorder due to the abnormal proliferation of a type of myeloid dendritic cell called a Langerhans cell [13]. The disorder is of unknown aetiology. Although a few historical studies have supported the theory of a viral aetiology, the consensus now is that the disease is a chronic inflammatory reactive condition, or even a neoplastic process. The disease can affect a number of organs including primarily the bones (causing lytic bone lesions), lymph nodes, the skin, the central nervous system, GI system, and the lungs. The multifocal form of the condition primarily affects children, with a peak incidence of 1 in 200,000 in children between 5 and 10 years old. The pulmonary form of disease occurs in approximately 10% of all cases, and this most often occurs in adults. The condition affecting the lungs has previously had a number of terms, including eosinophilic lung granulomas and histiocytosis X.

Clinical Presentation of Pulmonary LCH

Although the vast majority of cases of pulmonary LCH are associated with cigarette smoking, there is no strong evidence as to a direct cause. The condition affects both sexes equally, and most often presents between the ages of 20 and 40. Patients may present with non-specific respiratory symptoms (including cough, shortness of breath, pleuritic chest pain, haemoptysis, fever), with a spontaneous pneumothorax, with features of pulmonary hypertension in advanced disease or as an incidental finding on a CT scan.

Investigations

Chest radiographs may be non-specific, and hence the hallmark radiological test is the CT scan. The early stage of disease reveals nodules only. These progress to the classical findings of thin-walled cysts and nodules, which are found mainly in the middle and upper lobes. There may also be associated interstitial thickening. The cysts themselves have a characteristic appearance of unequal sizes and shapes. This appearance with middle and upper lobe predominance may help differentiate them from other cystic conditions. If classical, these changes seen on CT in a young smoker may be enough to make the diagnosis. If a tissue diagnosis is warranted, bronchoscopy with transbronchial lung biopsies can be performed, but this has a high false-negative rate. Surgical lung biopsy is the definitive choice and reveals a proliferation of CD1a-positive Langerhans cells.

Treatment

The mainstay of treatment is conservative, with smoking cessation crucial to improving prognosis. Supportive treatments including oxygen therapy, pulmonary rehabilitation, and treatment of pulmonary hypertension may be needed. A number of small studies have reviewed novel treatments, but none are in routine use. Glucocorticoids may help in selected cases (e.g. those with significant interstitial or nodular change), but there is no real evidence to support their widespread use in all patients. Lung transplantation may be an option in more severe cases.

Lymphangioleiomyomatosis

Pathogenesis

Pulmonary lymphangioleiomyomatosis (LAM) is a rare lung disorder of unknown cause [14]. The resulting cystic changes can be very destructive to normal lung tissue. Cyst formation is often found in conjunction with smooth muscle proliferation, and is associated with a number of extra-pulmonary features including renal angiomyolipomas, meningiomas, and cystic changes within lymph nodes.

Clinical Presentation of Pulmonary LAM

LAM predominantly affects women of childbearing age. They are more likely to be non-smokers and premenopausal. Up to 30% of patients have associated tuberous sclerosis with the findings of intellectual disability, seizures, and multiple benign soft tissue tumours. Patients predominantly present with shortness of breath, but can also present with a range of respiratory symptoms including pleuritic chest pain, cough, haemoptysis, chylothorax, and spontaneous pneumothorax.

Investigations

Chest radiographs may be normal in early disease and progress to reveal reticular nodular opacities in more advanced cases. CT scans generally reveal a large number of thin-walled cysts in both lungs which are often uniformly shaped and affect all lung fields (unlike LCH), but tend to spare the extreme apices. Bronchoscopy with transbronchial biopsy may be diagnostic in over 50% of cases, but when they are not, patients will need a surgical biopsy for a definitive diagnosis. This shows a characteristic cell morphology and protein staining.

Treatment

Treatment tends to be supportive, with supplemental oxygen, treatment of infections, management of pulmonary hypertension, and pulmonary rehabilitation. Targeted treatments have been used in a small number of patients, and the mainstay of this is the mTOR inhibitor sirolimus, which has been shown to improve a number of respiratory indicators (including 6-min walk testing, diffusion capacity, quality of life scores) but is generally reserved for patients with progressive disease due to the side effects of the drug. Lung transplantation for advanced disease may be an option.

Lymphoid Interstitial Pneumonia

Lymphoid interstitial pneumonia (LIP) is a rare benign interstitial lung disease which results from a lymphocytic infiltrate into the alveolar spaces and the lung interstitium [15]. The aetiology is unknown, but it is associated with collagen vascular disorders such as Sjogren's syndrome and other autoimmune diseases (including rheumatoid arthritis and SLE). It is also seen in patients who are HIV-positive. The condition can affect a specific part of the lung only, or become diffuse throughout both lungs. It is most often seen in middle-aged and older women, who present predominantly with shortness of breath. Respiratory examination often reveals crackles in the chest. CT scans reveal cystic changes, ground glass changes, and pulmonary nodules, but these features are not specific, and hence most patients will need a surgical lung biopsy which shows characteristic extensive lymphyocytic infiltration into the alveolar spaces. Treatment is both supportive and targeted towards treating the underlying condition (e.g. immunosuppression in patients with rheumatoid). Patients who are asymptomatic may need monitoring only. There is a small risk of patients with LIP progressing to lymphoma, and this may warrant long-term radiological follow-up.

Birt Hogg Dubé Syndrome

Birt Hogg Dubé syndrome is a rare cystic lung condition with an autosomal dominant inheritance [16]. It is due to a mutation in the gene encoding folliculin. Patients predominantly present with skin fibrofolliculomas, and the cystic changes in the lungs may be an incidental finding. When they do present with lung disease, a spontaneous pneumothorax may be the first finding, but some patients do present with non-specific symptoms including shortness of breath and cough. CT of the chest reveals thin-walled cystic lesions, and the condition is associated with renal tumours, which warrants ultrasound or CT scans of the abdomen every 2–3 years. A definitive diagnosis can be made through genetic testing for mutations in the folliculin gene, and current testing can detect up to 90% of mutations. There is no specific treatment for the lung, and management tends to be supportive only.

References

1. Rare and orphan lung disease. In: Gibson GJ, Loddenkemper R, Lundbäck B, Sibille Y, editors. European lung white book. Sheffield, UK: European Respiratory Society; 2013.
2. Jennette JC, Falk RJ, Bacon PA, Basu N, Cid MC, Ferrario F, et al. 2012 revised international Chapel Hill consensus conference nomenclature of vasculitides. Arthritis Rheum. 2013;65(1):1–11.
3. Ntatsaki E, Carruthers D, Chakravarty K, D'Cruz D, Harper L, Jayne D, et al. BSR and BHPR guideline for the management of adults with ANCA-associated vasculitis. Rheumatology (Oxford). 2014;53(12):2306–9.
4. Mukhtyar C, Guillevin L, Cid MC, Dasgupta B, de Groot K, Gross W, et al. EULAR recommendations for the management of primary small and medium vessel vasculitis. Ann Rheum Dis. 2009;68(3):310–7.
5. Mukhtyar C, Guillevin L, Cid MC, Dasgupta B, de Groot K, Gross W, et al. EULAR recommendations for the management of large vessel vasculitis. Ann Rheum Dis. 2009;68(3):318–23.
6. Chae EJ, Do KH, Seo JH, Park SH, Kang JW, Jang YM, et al. Radiologic and clinical findings of Behçet disease: comprehensive review of multisystemic involvement. Radiographics. 2008;28(5):e31.
7. Kluth DC, Rees AJ. Anti-glomerular basement membrane disease. J Am Assoc Nephrol. 1999;10:2446–53.
8. Pedchenko V, Bondar O, Fogo AB, Vanacore R, Voziyan P, Kitching AR, et al. Molecular architecture of the Goodpasture autoantigen in anti-GBM nephritis. N Engl J Med. 2010;363(4):343–54.
9. Borie R, Danel C, Debray MP, Taille C, Dombret MC, Aubier M, et al. Pulmonary alveolar proteinosis. Eur Respir Rev. 2011;20(120):98–107.
10. Stone JH, Zen Y, Deshpande V. IgG4-related disease. N Engl J Med. 2012;366:539–51.
11. Ioachimescu OC, Sieber S, Kotch A. Idiopathic pulmonary haemosiderosis revisited. Eur Respir J. 2004;24:162–70.
12. Beddy P, Babar J, Devaraj A. A practical approach to cystic lung disease on HRCT. Insights Imaging. 2011;2(1):1–7.
13. Zinn DJ, Chakraborty R, Allen CE. Langerhans cell histiocytosis: emerging insights and clinical implications. Oncology (Williston Park). 2016;30(2):122–32. 139.
14. Harari S, Torre O, Cassandro R, Moss J. The changing face of a rare disease: lymphangioleiomyomatosis. Eur Respir J. 2015;46(5):1471–85.
15. Kokosi MA, Nicholson AG, Hansell DM, Wells AU. Rare idiopathic interstitial pneumonias: LIP and PPFE and rare histologic patterns of interstitial pneumonias: AFOP and BPIP. Respirology. 2016;21(4):600–14.
16. Menko FH, van Steensel MA, Giraud S, Friis-Hansen L, Richard S, Ungari S, et al. Birt-Hogg-Dubé syndrome: diagnosis and management. Lancet Oncol. 2009;10(12):1199–206.

Pulmonary Embolism

Dejene Shiferaw and Shoaib Faruqi

Introduction

Deep venous thrombosis (DVT) and pulmonary embolism (PE) are manifestations of the same pathological process of venous thromboembolism (VTE). DVT describes the formation of thrombus in a deep vein, usually in one of the legs. In PE, a common and potentially fatal condition, the pulmonary arteries become obstructed by emboli that usually dislodge from a DVT. Concurrent DVT can be detected by venography in 70% of patients presenting with PE [1]. Compression venous ultrasonography (CUS), which has largely replaced venography, reveals DVT in one-third to one-half of patients with PE [1, 2]. PE is less likely when a thrombus is confined to calf veins, while up to 50% of patients with proximal DVT will go on to develop PE. Lack of an identifiable associated DVT in patients with PE is well recognised, and possible explanations include *de novo* thrombosis in the pulmonary arteries or right heart, complete dislodgement of thrombi from peripheral veins, or false-negative CUS.

Patients with PE can present with a wide range of presenting symptoms. PE is often classified depending on risk factors, haemodynamic status of the patient, and time of onset of symptoms. PE associated with a transient risk factor (e.g. lower limb surgery) is termed "provoked," and without an associated risk factor, "unprovoked." Haemodynamically unstable or "high risk" (massive) PE is associated with sustained hypotension. Patients with haemodynamically stable PE range from those with small asymptomatic PE (low-risk PE) to those with right ventricular strain and/or evidence of myocardial necrosis, referred to as sub-massive PE/intermediate-risk PE. Depending on anatomical location, PE can also be described as saddle, lobar, segmental, or sub-segmental (Figs. 18.1, 18.2, 18.3, 18.4 and 18.5).

Epidemiology

Though VTE is one of the most common cardiovascular diseases, it is almost impossible to determine the exact overall incidence, as it is often asymptomatic, misdiagnosed, or unrecognized at death. Population studies approximate the annual incidence of VTE to be 100–200 cases per 100,000. The overall incidence of VTE is higher in males compared with females (56 vs. 48 per 100,000 respectively). The incidence of VTE increases with age, particularly in women,

D. Shiferaw · S. Faruqi (✉)
Department of Respiratory Medicine, Hull and East Yorkshire Hospitals NHS Trust, Castle Hill Hospital, Cottingham, UK
e-mail: Shoaib.Faruqi@hey.nhs.uk

© Springer International Publishing AG, part of Springer Nature 2018
S. Hart, M. Greenstone (eds.), *Foundations of Respiratory Medicine*,
https://doi.org/10.1007/978-3-319-94127-1_18

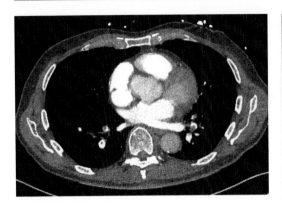

Fig. 18.1 CT pulmonary angiogram (CTPA) demonstrating bilateral segmental and sub-segmental pulmonary emboli

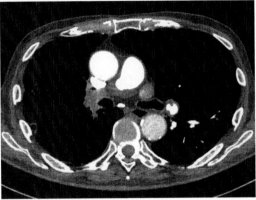

Fig. 18.4 CTPA showing complete occlusion of the right main pulmonary artery and a filling defect on the left. See V/Q scan images from the same patient (Fig. 18.8)

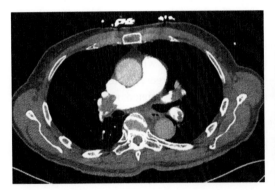

Fig. 18.2 CTPA showing large-volume bilateral pulmonary emboli

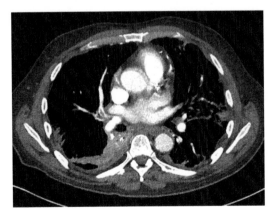

Fig. 18.3 CTPA demonstrating pulmonary embolism within the right middle lobe pulmonary artery and its segmental branches. There is evidence of consolidation within the posterior right lung

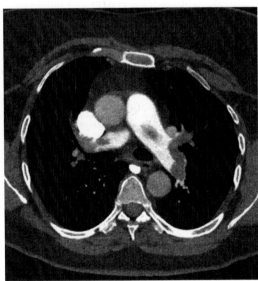

Fig. 18.5 CTPA demonstrating a "saddle" embolus; embolus in the main pulmonary artery extending into both the left and right pulmonary arteries

with incidence of >500 per 100,000 in those over age 75.

Untreated, the risk of death from PE is high. Studies published before 1960 reported mortality rates of 23–87%. The International Cooperative Pulmonary Embolism Registry (ICOPER) showed that the 90-day mortality rate for patients with acute PE and systolic blood pressure <90 mmHg (massive PE) at presentation (108 patients) was 52.4%, versus 14.7% in the remainder of the cohort [3]. The Germany-based Management Strategy and Prognosis of Pulmonary Embolism Registry (MAPPET) of 1001 patients with acute PE showed that in-hospital mortality was 8.1% for hemodynamically stable patients versus 25% for those presenting with cardiogenic shock, and 65% for those requiring cardiopulmonary resuscitation [4].

Several prognostication models have been developed to predict patient outcomes, based both solely on clinical parameters as well as inclusive of investigations. The PE Severity Index (PESI) and its simplified version (sPESI) are the best validated models [5, 6]. In a recent meta-analysis, the overall 30-day mortality rate was 2.3% (1.7–2.9%) in the low-risk group and 11.4% (9.9–13.1%) in the high-risk group for PESI (9 studies); and 1.5% (0.9–2.5%) in the low-risk group and 10.7% (8.8–12.9%) in the high-risk group for sPESI (11 studies). Both the PESI/sPESI and other models identify hypotension as the most important predictor of adverse prognosis. As well as identifying high-risk patients, these scores can reliably identify patients at a low risk of dying from PE who can potentially be managed as an outpatient [7].

Pathogenesis and Pathophysiology

The pathogenesis of VTE is similar to that underlying the generation of a thrombus. Virchow's triad identifies the three primary factors predisposing to thrombus formation: venous stasis, endothelial injury, and a hypercoagulable state. A predisposing factor can be identified in up to 80% of patients with VTE. Identification of risk factors for VTE aids in making a clinical diagnosis of VTE as well as guiding decisions about duration of anticoagulation and the need for thromboprophylaxis. Risk factors include increasing age, prolonged immobility, malignancy, major surgery, multiple trauma, previous VTE, and heart failure. The predictive value of these risk factors is not equal, and the European Society of Cardiology (ESC) guidelines classify them into strong, moderate, and weak risk factors (Table 18.1) [8]. PE usually arises from thrombus originating in the deep veins of the lower limbs; however, they may rarely originate

Table 18.1 Predisposing factors for VTE (adapted from ESC PE guidelines)

Strong risk factors (Odds ratio >10)	Moderate risk factors (Odds ratio 2–9)	Weak risk factors (Odds ratio <2)
• Lower limb fracture • Hospitalization for heart failure or atrial fibrillation/flutter (within 3 months) • Hip or knee replacement • Major trauma • Previous VTE • Spinal cord injury	• Arthroscopic knee surgery • Auto-immune disease • Central venous lines • Oral contraceptive therapy/hormone replacement therapy • Acute severe infections • Inflammatory bowel disease • Cancer (high risk in metastatic disease) • Stroke • Post-partum period • Superficial vein thrombosis • Thrombophilia	• Bed rest >3 days • Diabetes mellitus • Hypertension • Immobility due to sitting (e.g. prolonged car or air travel) • Increasing age • Laparascopic surgery • Obesity • Pregnancy • Varicose veins

Adapted from Konstantinides SV, Torbicki A, Agnelli G, et al. 2014 ESC Guidelines on the diagnosis and management of acute pulmonary embolism: the Task Force for the Diagnosis and Management of Acute Pulmonary Embolism of the European Society of Cardiology (ESC). Endorsed by the European Respiratory Society (ERS). Eur Heart J. 2014 Nov 14;35(43):3033–69, 3069a–3069k

from the pelvic, renal, or upper extremity veins, or the right heart. Most PEs are multiple and involve the lower lobes more frequently than the upper lobes.

The haemodynamic effect of PE depends on the extent to which it obstructs the pulmonary circulation, the duration over which that obstruction develops, and the underlying cardiopulmonary reserve of the patient. Due to the large reserve capacity of the pulmonary circulation, pulmonary artery pressure increases significantly only if more than 30–50% of the its total cross-sectional area is occluded by thromboemboli. The main haemodynamic effect of PE is a reduction in the cross-sectional area of the pulmonary vascular bed through direct physical obstruction, hypoxemia, and release of pulmonary artery vasoconstrictors. This leads to an increase in pulmonary vascular resistance and right ventricular afterload. Right ventricular dilation and myocyte stretch affects myocardial contractility via the Frank-Starling mechanism, while neurohumoral activation leads to inotropic and chronotropic stimulation. These compensatory mechanisms improve blood flow through the pulmonary circulation and temporarily stabilize systemic blood pressure, but are limited, as the thin-walled RV is unable to generate a mean pulmonary artery pressure above 40 mmHg acutely. Smaller thrombi typically travel more distally and occlude smaller vessels in the lung periphery. These induce an inflammatory response adjacent to the parietal pleura and often give rise to pleuritic chest pain.

Clinical Presentation

There are no clinical signs or symptoms specific for PE. The most common presenting symptom is dyspnoea (see below), followed by pleuritic chest pain and cough. Tachypnoea is the commonest physical sign (see "PE Physical Signs" on next page), evident in more than half of the patients with PE [9]. However, many patients, including those with large PE, have mild and non-specific symptoms or are asymptomatic. Hence,

maintenance of high level of clinical suspicion of PE based on the presence of risk factors is crucial in making a diagnosis.

> **PE Symptoms in Patients Presenting with Confirmed PE**
> Patients presenting with suspected PE, but in whom PE was subsequently excluded, have a similar spectrum of symptoms and signs, indicating that making a clinical diagnosis of PE is unreliable: [9]
>
> - Dyspnoea at rest or on exertion (73%)
> - Pleuritic chest pain (44%)
> - Cough (37%)
> - Orthopnea (28%)
> - Calf or thigh pain and/or swelling (44%)
> - Wheezing (21%)
> - Haemoptysis (13%)

> **PE Physical Signs** [9]
> - Tachypnoea(54%)
> - Calf or thigh swelling, erythema, oedema, tenderness, palpable cords (47%)
> - Tachycardia (24%)
> - Crackles (rales) (18%)
> - Decreased breath sounds (17%)
> - Lound P2 (15%)
> - Raised JVP (14%)
> - Fever, mimicking pneumonia (3%)
> - Circulatory collapse (8%)

Patients with massive PE may have features of right heart failure, manifesting as elevated jugular venous pressure (JVP), S3 gallop, a parasternal heave, cyanosis and shock. A transition from tachycardia to bradycardia, or development of a right bundle branch block pattern suggests right heart strain and impending shock. In a patient presenting with hypotension and elevated JVP, PE should be excluded unless there is an alternative explannation.

Diagnostic Approach

Making a diagnosis of PE is often a challenge, as the symptoms and signs are not specific. Consideration of the likelihood of the diagnosis and excluding other differentials is partly achieved by history taking, physical examination, and a chest X-ray. If PE remains a possibility, the two-level Wells score is recommended to determine the likelihood of PE (Table 18.2) [10]. Patients with suspected PE and "unlikely" two-level Wells PE score should be offered plasma D-dimer testing (Fig. 18.6). Those with positive D-dimer will need further investigation. Patients with suspected PE and "likely" two-level PE Wells score should not be offered D-dimer testing, but diagnostic imaging should be done immediately (Fig. 18.6).

Table 18.2 Two-level PE Wells Score

Clinical feature	Points
Clinical signs and symptoms of DVT (minimum of leg swelling and pain with the palpation of deep veins)	3
An alternative diagnosis is less likely than PE	3
Heart rate > 100 beats per minute	1.5
Immobilisation for more than 3 days or surgery in the previous 4 weeks	1.5
Previous DVT/PE	1.5
Haemoptysis	1
Malignancy (on treatment, treated in the last 6 months, or palliative)	1
Clinical probability simplified score	
PE likely	More than 4
PE unlikely	4 or less

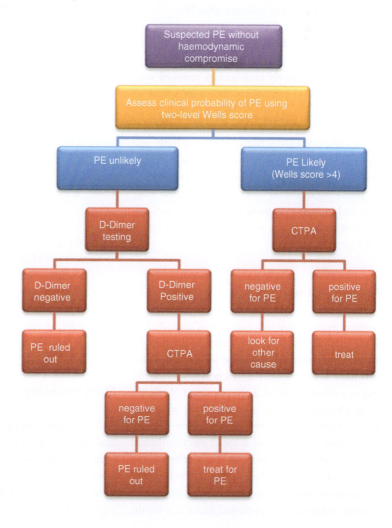

Fig. 18.6 Diagnostic algorithm for suspected PE in a haemodynamically stable patient

Treatment should not be delayed while waiting for investigations.

Investigations

Arterial Blood Gas (ABG)

ABG analysis, either alone or in combination with other clinical variables, is of limited diagnostic utility in suspected PE.

While the commonest abnormality is hypoxia and hypocapnia (due to hyperventilation), a normal ABG will not rule out PE. Significant pulmonary arterial obstruction is likely to cause severe hypoxia and increase the Alveolar-arterial (A-a) gradient. However, it is not uncommon to find a normal A-a gradient in patients with PE.

The presence and extent of hypoxaemia in patients with PE is highly variable and correlates poorly with the embolic load. When an artery is occluded, this is partly matched by reduced ventilation (due to the bronchoconstrictor effect of low alveolar CO_2). This reduction in airflow to unperfused lung reduces wasted ventilation. Blood is diverted away from embolised lung, and there is a wider distribution of Va/Q ratios and a shift to a higher Va/Q, reflecting the increase in the physiological dead space, while the low Va/Q units and reduction in mixed venous PO_2 secondary to reduced cardiac output contribute to arterial hypoxaemia.

Plasma D-Dimer

D-dimer is a degradation product of cross-linked fibrin, and plasma levels are elevated in all acute thrombotic disorders. D-dimer should be tested only after assessing the pre-test probability of PE, and in patients with unlikely two-level Wells PE score. D-dimer may be measured by a variety of assay types including quantitative, semi-quantitative, and qualitative rapid enzyme-linked immune sorbent assay (ELISAs); quantitative and semi-quantitative latex; and whole blood assays. Quantitative and semi-quantitative rapid ELISA D-dimer assays are the preferred method, with the

highest sensitivity (>95%) and negative likelihood ratio. British Thoracic Society (BTS) guidelines recommend each hospital to provide information on sensitivity and specificity of its D-dimer test. A D-dimer level of <500 ng/ml using rapid ELISA assays (quantitative or semi-quantitative rapid ELISA) is generally regarded as normal.

In a patient with unlikely pre-test probability, a negative D-dimer test reliably excludes PE. Meta-analysis has shown that 3-month thromboembolic risk was <1% in patients left untreated with a negative test [11]. In patients with likely pre-test probability of PE, a negative D-dimer is not enough to exclude PE. In patients with high clinical suspicion of PE and a normal D-dimer, the prevalence of PE could be as high as 19–28%. As these patients have a high probability of VTE, they should undergo diagnostic imaging and do not need D-dimer testing.

D-dimer has low specificity and limited diagnostic value in the elderly, pregnancy, and patients with cancer, renal dysfunction, and acute illnesses. Despite low specificity, the sensitivity remains high in these groups of patients. Age-adjusted D-dimer levels (cut-off = age × 10 ng/ml for patients older than 50 years) have been shown to increase specificity while maintaining sensitivity above 97%. Age-adjusted cut-off values may allow a reduction of unnecessary diagnostic imaging in elderly patients, although this strategy is not yet validated or incorporated into routine medical practice.

Sensitivity of D-dimer is also not high enough for safe exclusion of PE in patients presenting after 2 weeks of symptom onset, and those on oral or parenteral anticoagulation treatment. In these patients, diagnostic imaging is required to reliably exclude or confirm acute PE.

Electrocardiography (ECG)

ECG is often abnormal in patients with PE, but findings are neither sensitive nor specific for the diagnosis. The most common ECG abnormalities seen in patients with PE are sinus tachycardia and non-specific ST-T changes. The classical signs of right heart strain are usually seen in patients with

PE associated with significant haemodynamic compromise. These include tall-tented P wave in lead II (P pulmonale), rightward axis deviation, and right bundle branch block. The classic S1Q3T3 pattern is also a sign of acute cor pulmonale and reflects right heart strain. However, it is rarely seen, and is of little clinical value in the absence of clinical suspicion of PE.

ECG abnormalities often resolve rapidly within a few days, but minor changes such as T-inversion in V1-3 may persist for months. The importance of an ECG lies in excluding other potential differentials such as acute myocardial infarction and pericarditis.

Chest X-Ray (CXR)

The main advantage of CXR in the work-up of patients suspected of PE is to rule out other causes of dyspnoea and hypoxia like pneumothorax, pneumonia, left ventricular failure, large pleural effusion, and lobar collapse. However, PE might coexist with these conditions and it is important to reconsider PE if patients are not responding to treatment.

Plain radiograph abnormalities occasionally seen in PE include: enlarged pulmonary artery (Fleischner sign), peripheral wedge of airspace opacity which implies lung infarction (Hampton hump), regional oligaemia (Westermark's sign), pleural effusion, and 'knuckle' sign (abrupt tapering or cut-off of a pulmonary artery secondary to embolus). A normal CXR in a patient with severe acute dyspnoea and hypoxemia, in the absence of bronchospasm or cardiac shunting, is strongly suspicious for PE.

Echocardiography (Echo)

Routine use of echo is not recommended in the regular diagnostic work-up of a haemodynamically stable patient with suspected PE. Echo findings of haemodynamically significant PE include right ventricular (RV) dilatation, RV hypokinesia/dysfunction, and pulmonary hypertension. However, these findings are neither sensitive nor specific, and hence a negative study cannot exclude PE.

If the patient is too unstable for CTPA, echo can be used to make a presumptive diagnosis of PE. A normal echo in a haemodynamically unstable patient virtually excludes PE as a cause, and an alternative diagnosis should be sought.

Diagnostic Imaging

Computed Tomography Pulmonary Angiography (CTPA)

Since the advent of multidetector CT (MDCT) angiography, CTPA is the first-choice diagnostic imaging modality in patients with suspected PE. The PIOPED II study demonstrated 83% sensitivity and 96% specificity with CTPA in detecting acute PE. It also showed that the predictive value of MDCTA varied substantially when the pre-test probability was taken in to account. A negative CTPA had a high negative predictive value (NPV) for PE in patients with a low (96%) or intermediate (89%) clinical probability of PE. NPV of PE in patients with negative CTPA and high clinical probability was lower, at 60%. Therefore, a negative CTPA should be interpreted with caution if the clinical suspicion remains high. Interpretation of filling defects in keeping with sub-segmental PE may vary, and a compression ultrasound of the lower limb may be considered in this situation to guide therapy. Conversely, the positive predictive value (PPV) of CTPA was high in patients with intermediate (92%) or high (96%) clinical pre-test probability.

In adequately risk-stratified populations, the diagnostic yield of CTPA is around one-fifth, and this drops as low as one-tenth if risk stratification is not properly done. CTPA may provide an alternative diagnosis such as pneumonia and, less welcomed, pulmonary nodules. Despite the diagnostic utility, CTPA request should be made after appropriate risk stratification [12].

CTPA findings of right ventricular dysfunction include: bowing of the interventricular septum, contrast medium reflux into inferior vena cava, and increased right ventricle to left ventricle diameter ratio on axial sections (Fig. 18.7).

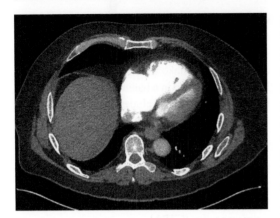

Fig. 18.7 CTPA in a patient with acute PE, showing evidence of right heart dilation

Ventilation Perfusion (V/Q) Scan

V/Q scan is a safe and established diagnostic test for PE, which is associated with few allergic reactions. Due to high false-positive rate, it is best applied in patients with a normal chest X-ray and no significant symptomatic concurrent cardiorespiratory disease. The high incidence of non-diagnostic/intermediate probability test results means PE is diagnosed or excluded only in a minority of patients. In recent years V/Q scan has largely been replaced by CTPA.

The PIOPED study confirmed the effectiveness of high probability and normal perfusion scans to confirm and exclude PE, respectively. A normal perfusion scan has a NPV close to 100% and effectively excludes PE. Also, a high probability scan has a PPV >90% and confirms PE in patients with moderate or high probability of PE (Fig. 18.8).

Unfortunately, a large proportion of patients (up to 46% in some studies) with suspected PE do not fall in to either high or normal study category and require further imaging. The use of single-photon emission tomography (SPECT) may increase the diagnostic yield of V/Q scans.

V/Q scan may be useful in pregnant patients, those with severe allergy to IV contrast media, and those with renal failure. V/Q scan has the additional benefit of low radiation and may be considered the first-line test for young female patients, as the radiation dose to breast tissue is significantly lower than that of CTPA. Standardized reporting criteria must be used, and non-diagnostic result should always be followed by further imaging.

Lower Limb Ultrasonography

Usually PE originates from DVT in the lower limbs. Compression venous ultrasonography (CUS) of the lower limbs, an inexpensive and non-invasive test, has largely replaced venography in diagnosing VTE. CUS has sensitivity of >90% and specificity of around 95% for DVT in symptomatic patients. CUS demonstrates DVT in 30–50% of patients with PE, so as more than half of patients with confirmed PE could have a negative CUS, it should not be used as the only imaging modality to exclude PE. CUS of the lower limbs can be used as an initial test in those with clinical signs of DVT, as an initial test in all patients to reduce the need for lung imaging—e.g. pregnant women—and after non-diagnostic isotope scanning. Identification of DVT is sufficient to warrant anticoagulation treatment without further imaging.

Pulmonary Angiography

Contrast-enhanced pulmonary angiography is no longer regarded as the "gold standard" for diagnosing PE, as the less-invasive CTPA offers similar diagnostic accuracy with fewer complications. Pulmonary angiography is invasive, expensive, and carries significant risks—especially in patients with haemodynamic compromise or respiratory failure. In a study of 1111 patients, the procedure-related mortality was 0.5%, major non-fatal complications occurred in 1%, and minor complications in 5% [13].

Magnetic Resonance Pulmonary Angiography

Although technically appealing due to absence of radiation, currently MRA has little or no role in diagnosing PE. This is due to a combination of low sensitivity, high proportion of inconclusive results, and low availability in most centers.

Thrombophilia Screening

Large cohort studies have shown that testing for heritable thrombophilia does not predict the likelihood of recurrence in unselected patients with symptomatic venous thrombosis. Hence, routine testing for heritable thrombophilia in unselected patients presenting with a first episode of VTE is not recommended. Testing for heritable

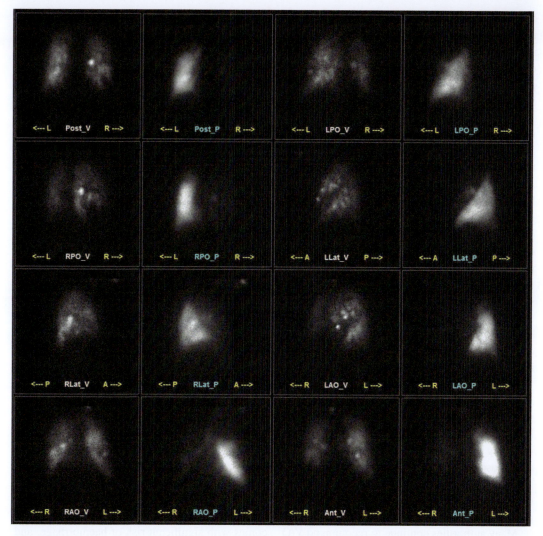

Fig. 18.8 Ventilation Perfusion (V/Q) Scan showing absent perfusion in the right lung and left upper lobe due to pulmonary embolism (this is in keeping with a complete occlusion of the right main pulmonary artery, as seen on CTPA from the same patient in Fig. 18.4)

thrombophilia in selected patients, such as those with a strong family history of unprovoked recurrent thrombosis, may influence the decision regarding duration of anticoagulation. However, there is no validated recommendation as to how such patients should be selected.

VTE in Pregnancy

Pregnancy-associated VTE remains one of the main direct causes of maternal mortality in the developed world. The risk of VTE is four to fivefold higher in pregnant women than in non-pregnant women of the same age, although the absolute risk remains low, at around 1 in 1000 pregnancies. VTE can occur at any stage of pregnancy, but the highest risk is during the post-partum period, with a 20-fold increased risk of VTE.

The diagnostic work-up of pregnant women suspected of acute VTE differs from that established for the non-pregnant population.

The role of D-dimer testing in the investigation of acute VTE in pregnancy remains controversial. Plasma D-dimer levels rise progressively during pregnancy, and are elevated in most healthy pregnant women towards late third trimester and early post-partum period, thus reducing further the specificity of a positive test. The other limiting factor is the absence of a validated pre-test probability score in pregnancy to use alongside D-dimer testing.

The clinical use of a negative D-dimer in pregnant women is also not straightforward. Current guidelines from the Royal College of Obstetricians and Gynaecologists (RCOG) and American Thoracic Society recommend that D-dimer should not be used to exclude PE in pregnancy [14]. In contrast, the European Society of Cardiology recommends testing D-dimer levels, stating that a normal level can exclude PE in pregnancy just as for other patients.

Current RCOG guidelines suggest compression duplex ultrasound scan only for women suspected of PE with symptoms and signs of DVT. Those without signs and symptoms of DVT do not require ultrasound Doppler routinely, instead a V/Q scan or CTPA should be performed.

The choice of technique for definitive diagnosis (V/Q vs. CTPA) will depend on local availability and individual hospital protocol. CTPA has potential advantages over V/Q scan, including being readily available, delivering a low radiation dose to the foetus, and the fact that it can identify other pathology. This benefit is offset by the increased radiation dose to breast tissue compared to V/Q scanning.

Many authorities continue to recommend V/Q scanning as the first-line investigation in pregnancy because of its high negative predictive value and its substantially lower radiation dose to the pregnant breast tissue. However, if the initial CXR is abnormal, CTPA is the preferred initial test.

Management

Initial Assessment and Supportive Measures

Acute right ventricular failure secondary to pulmonary emboli leads to under-filling of the left ventricle and resultant systemic hypotension, and is the commonest cause of death in massive pulmonary embolism. Fluid resuscitation needs to be based on the patient's volaemic status, as aggressive fluid therapy may be detrimental for RV function (beyond a certain point, further stretch of the RV would lead to a fall in cardiac output as per the Frank-Starling principle). Pending definitive treatment, such as thrombolysis, ionotropic support may be necessary if the patient has refractory hypotension despite adequate fluid resuscitation. Though hypoxaemic respiratory failure is quite frequent in PE, this is usually correctable with oxygen, which should be provided.

Thrombolytic Treatment

The first randomised trial evaluating urokinase compared to heparin was published over 40 years ago [15]. Significant acceleration in the resolution rate of pulmonary thromboemboli at 24 h, as shown by pulmonary arteriograms, lung scans, and right-sided pressure measurements, was demonstrated. No significant differences in recurrence rate of pulmonary embolism or in 2-week mortality were observed.

Since this study, several others have substantiated this finding of faster clot dissolution and haemodynamic improvement compared with standard anticoagulation. However, thrombolysis comes with significant risk of haemorrhage, and benefits have to be balanced against risks. In a recent meta-analysis of studies on systemic thrombolysis in acute PE, a major haemorrhage rate of 9.7% and intracranial or fatal haemorrhage rate of 1.7% were reported [16].

Thrombolysis for High-Risk PE

Patients with systolic blood pressure (SBP) <90 mmHg or a drop in SBP $\geq$ 40 mmHg for greater than 15 min are at high risk of 30-day mortality [8]. This drop in blood pressure should not be accounted for by other factors such as hypovolaemia, sepsis or cardiac arrhythmia.

The case fatality rate in "High-Risk PE" exceeds the rate of intracranial, fatal, or major haemorrhage. The only study which randomised patients with PE in cardiogenic shock ("High-Risk PE") to thrombolysis (streptokinase with heparin) or standard anti-coagulation (heparin) was terminated early: all four thrombolysed patients survived, whereas the control group all died [17].

Analysis of large databases of acute PE patients both from the United States and from Europe suggest that in haemodynamically unstable patients, thrombolytic therapy is associated with a lower risk of death than no thrombolytic therapy, whereas the converse was reported in normotensive patients. The in-hospital all-cause case fatality rate in unstable patients with thrombolytic therapy was 15% versus 47% without thrombolytic therapy. Only 30% of unstable patients with acute PE received thrombolysis, suggesting that even in this high-risk group there was under-use of thrombolysis.

Thrombolysis for Intermediate Risk/Sub-Massive PE

Several studies have evaluated the prognostic value of associated DVT, rise in blood cardiac injury markers, and features of right ventricular dysfunction on CT scan and echocardiography, which in general confer worse prognostic outcomes. The use of a composite score, including these parameters, helps predict 30-day mortality. Based on the clinical predictive scores (PESI or sPESI), presence of RV dysfunction, and elevation of cardiac biomarkers, ESC guidelines further divide those patients with confirmed PE but not in cardiogenic shock into intermediate and low risk. The tests used to assess RV dysfunction are at the physician's discretion. However, some degree of assessment of RV dysfunction can be assessed by RV dilatation seen on CTPA. Serum cardiac biomarkers (e.g. troponins) are elevated in around half of all patients with PE, which puts them in the intermediate-risk category. This is despite the fact that the vast majority of patients assessed via the PESI/s-PESI will fall into a low-risk group.

As patients with intermediate risk/submassive PE have a poorer prognosis, the question is whether thrombolysis would be useful in this group. Despite trials showing more rapid haemodynamic improvement and clot resolution, there is no clear mortality benefit. The Pulmonary Embolism Thrombolysis (PEITHO) trial [18] was designed to investigate the efficacy and safety of thrombolytic therapy with a weight-based dose of intravenous tenecteplase, in addition to standard anti-coagulation. One thousand and six patients with intermediate-risk PE (RV dysfunction, confirmed by echocardiography or CT angiography, and myocardial injury confirmed by a positive troponin) were enrolled. Although there was clear and early benefit on haemodynamic decompensation in the thrombolysis group, all-cause 7-day and 30-day mortality rates were low and not significantly different between the treatment groups (1.2% vs. 1.8% and 2.4 vs. 3.2% for tenecteplase and placebo respectively). Major bleeding and haemorrhagic stroke were substantially more frequent in the tenecteplase group (11.5% and 2.4%, 2%, and 0.2% respectively). The risk of major bleeding was higher in those over the age of 75. Thus, the haemodynamic benefits of thrombolysis came at a cost of significantly increased major (particularly intracranial) haemorrhage.

The trial gives us the mortality rates for intermediate-risk PE, which are low. It also tells us the risks of major bleeding with thrombolysis, which are similar to those reported in meta-analyses and are not insignificant. The trial data suggest that it is safe to treat intermediate-risk patients with standard anticoagulation and to closely monitor for later deterioration, and subsequently intervene with thrombolysis if "high risk" criteria are met.

Percutaneous directed low-dose thrombolysis has been shown to be effective approach in DVT. It is an interesting hypothesis that peripherally administered low-dose thrombolysis would be equally effective from the haemodynamic perspective, whilst at the same time minimising the risk of bleeding, in the context of acute PE. Trial data suggest that "low dose" alteplase is equally efficacious as standard dose, and perhaps has lower bleeding risks, not dissimilar to anticoagulation alone. Low-dose systemic thrombolysis merits further evaluation in larger trials with clinically meaningful end-points.

Table 18.3 Contraindications for systemic thrombolytic therapy

Absolute contraindications	Relative contraindications
History of haemorrhagic stroke or stroke of unknown origin at any time	Transient ischaemic attack in preceding 6 months
Ischaemic stroke in preceding 6 months	Oral anticoagulant therapy
Known active bleeding	Pregnancy or within 1 week post partum
Gastrointestinal bleeding within the last month	Non-compressible punctures
Recent major trauma/surgery/head injury (within preceding 3 weeks)	Traumatic resuscitation
Central nervous system damage or neoplasms	Advanced liver disease
	Active peptic ulcer
	Infective endocarditis

Agents Used for Systemic Thrombolysis

The pharmacological agents used in thrombolysis and the recommended regimes, as well as important absolute and relative contraindications (Table 18.3) for thrombolytic therapy are listed below.

Streptokinase 250,000 U as a loading dose over 30 min, followed by 100,000 U/h over 12–24 h. Accelerated regime: 1.5 million Units over 2 h.

Urokinase 4400 U/kg as a loading dose given over a period of 10 min at a rate of 90 mL/h, followed by continuous infusion of 4400 U/kg/h at a rate of 15 mL/h for 12 h. Accelerated regime: 3 million Units over 2 h.

Recombinant Tissue Plasminogen Activator (tPA) 100 mg as a continuous infusion over 2 h. A 15-mg bolus can be administered first, followed by 85 mg administered over 2 h. Heparin drip must be discontinued during the infusion. Low dose: 0.6 mg/kg up to a maximum dose 50 mg.

Catheter-Based Therapies

Catheter-directed therapies (CDTs) involve inserting a catheter percutaneously into the pulmonary arterial circulation and providing "directed therapy." These therapies include "low-dose" fibrinolytic instillation, clot fragmentation, and clot aspiration. Though several techniques and devices have been described, the lack of prospective randomised controlled data to support efficacy precludes recommendation in guidelines. The common techniques used are ultrasound-assisted thrombolysis (USAT) and catheter-directed thrombolysis (CDT). Ultrasound-assisted thrombolysis requires a specific catheter with a cable

that transmits high-frequency ultrasound signals. These ultrasound signals are supposed to loosen fibrin strands, and thereby increase thrombus penetration by the thrombolytic agent, theoretically increasing efficacy of thrombolysis. However, ultrasound on its own has not been used in any of these trials, and is not likely to be effective. A recent registry-based study reported the outcomes of 101 patients prospectively receiving CDT. Clinical success, as defined by improvement in haemodynamic and pulmonary vascular parameters as well as survival to hospital discharge, was met in 24 of 28 with massive PE, and 71 of 73 with sub-massive PE. However, despite the "maximal" care offered, there was still significant mortality reported, and there was no comparator arm. Importantly, no significant haemorrhagic complications were reported, and USAT was not noted to be superior to standard catheter-directed administration of low-dose fibrinolytic. This approach to therapy, especially in those at high risk of haemorrhagic complications, merits further evaluation.

Surgery

Emergency surgical embolectomy for massive pulmonary embolism is rarely performed, particularly with the advent of readily available thrombolysis. The indications are not firmly established, but may be considered with massive PE, where thrombolysis is contraindicated or unsuccessful and where death is likely. Mortality is high, particularly when performed on patients who are peri-cardiorespiratory arrest. Elective pulmonary thromboendarterectomy for chronic thromboembolic pulmonary hypertension is a highly effective operation in appropriately selected cases, and is discussed in more detail in Chap. 19.

Anticoagulation

Early anticoagulation is indicated in patients with suspected or confirmed PE to prevent early death and recurrence of VTE. Anticoagulation should be given for a minimum of 3 months, but some patients with high risk of recurrence and low risk of bleeding may benefit from indefinite anticoagulation. Therapy should be initiated as soon as possible to achieve therapeutic anticoagulation. This is usually achieved by administering parenteral unfractionated heparin (UFH), low-molecular weight heparin (LMWH), or Fondaparinux. Parenteral treatment should overlap initiation of oral Vitamin K antagonists (VKA) and precede by 5–10 days the direct oral anticoagulants (DOACs) Dabigatran and Edoxaban. Apixaban and Rivaroxaban can be started directly without the need for preceding parenteral treatment, or 1–2 days thereafter.

Parenteral Anticoagulation

LMWH or Fondaparinux are preferred over unfractionated heparin for initial anticoagulation of VTE, as they are associated with lower risks of bleeding, heparin-induced thrombocytopenia (HIT), and osteopenia, whilst being equally efficacious. LMWH has greater bioavailability than unfractionated heparin and can be administered by subcutaneous injections at a fixed dosage. Intravenous unfractionated heparin may be chosen for high-risk patients who might need thrombolysis or embolectomy, in haemodynamically stable patients with renal failure, and those with a high risk of bleeding. The rationale behind this is that in the event of a bleed, the UFH infusion could be discontinued and, if need be, reversed. However, often LMWH is given at initial presentation and is probably equally safe in haemodynamically compromised patients.

LMWHs have a longer duration of action and do not require regular laboratory monitoring and dose adjustment, unlike unfractionated heparin. Although laboratory monitoring is not usually required, the anti–factor Xa level should be checked in patients with renal insufficiency, morbid obesity, and pregnancy because the pharmacokinetic properties, efficacy, and safety of LMWHs are not well established in these situations. For pregnant women, LMWH is continued until the end of pregnancy, as warfarin is teratogenic and contraindicated during pregnancy. For patients with an active malignancy, most guidelines recommend LMWH over VKA. A Cochrane systematic review of ten randomized controlled trials concludes that LMWH is significantly more effective than VKA in decreasing recurrence of a VTE, but not mortality [19]. It may also be difficult to maintain good INR control while patients are on chemotherapy.

Heparin-induced thrombocytopenia (HIT) is a potentially serious immunological complication of unfractionated heparin or less commonly, LMWH. A low platelet count ($<150 \times 10^9$/L or 30% drop from baseline) develops 5–14 days after heparin is started and may occur in isolation or with new venous and arterial thromboses. HIT is caused by IgG antibodies against complexes of platelet factor 4 and heparin. These complexes bind to platelet and monocyte receptors, releasing pro-coagulants and generating thrombin. New venous thrombosis, often in the leg, may occur in about 30% of cases and may be complicated by venous gangrene. Heparin must be stopped and direct thrombin inhibitors (argatroban, danaparoid) substituted until the platelet count recovers and warfarin started.

Oral Anticoagulation

Vitamin K antagonists such as warfarin have been the standard treatment up until the development of new direct-acting oral anticoagulants.

Vitamin K Antagonists
The anticoagulant effect of VKAs such as warfarin is mediated by inhibition of the enzyme epoxide reductase in the liver. This enzyme normally reduces vitamin K to its active form, which is necessary for the synthesis of Vitamin K-dependent clotting factors II, VII, IX, and X, as well as endogenous anticoagulant proteins C and S. Protein C has a short half-life (8 h) and is depleted before the other vitamin K-dependent clotting factors, leading to an initial pro-coagulant

effect. This effect is ameliorated by concurrent parenteral treatment with UFH, LMWH, or Fondaparinux, and parenteral anticoagulation should be continued for at least 5 days and until the international normalized ratio (INR) is more than two for two consecutive days.

Direct Oral Anticoagulants (DOACs)

Dabigatran, a direct thrombin inhibitor, and Factor Xa direct inhibitors (Apixaban, Rivaroxaban and Edoxaban) are effective in preventing recurrence of VTE. Phase III clinical trials have demonstrated non-inferiority, both in terms of efficacy and safety, compared to the standard treatment. The rivaroxaban and apixaban studies excluded patients treated with heparin for more than 48 h, whereas initial treatment consisted of open-label parenteral anticoagulation in the other two (median of 9 and 7 days in the dabigatran and edoxaban trials, respectively). Based on the rapid onset of the DOACs, concurrent parenteral therapy is not needed. Thus these therapies introduce the option of managing patients without parenteral anticoagulation, and indeed as outpatient-based therapy for those with low-risk PE.

DOACs are associated with significantly less bleeding episodes (major, fatal, intracranial, clinically relevant non-major, and total) as compared to warfarin. Another major advantage is that they do not require therapeutic monitoring. Equal efficacy and a relative dearth of drug interactions provide a compelling argument in favour of the DOACs. The lack of an agent for rapid reversal of anticoagulation was a potential drawback of all the DOACs until recently. Idarucizumab, a monoclonal antibody that binds dabigatran has been shown to be effective, and has been approved for use. Andexanet alfa, a recombinant modified human factor Xa decoy protein, has been shown to substantially reduce anti-factor Xa activity in patients with acute major bleeding associated with factor Xa inhibitors, with effective haemostasis occurring in 79%.

The Role of Inferior Vena Cava (IVC) Filter in Addition to Anticoagulation

Retrievable IVC filter insertion in acute PE should be considered if anticoagulation is contraindicated, or temporary cessation of anticoagulation within 1 month is envisaged. A randomized controlled trial of IVC filter insertion involving 400 patients with proximal deep vein thrombosis, with or without pulmonary embolism, showed that placement of a permanent IVC filter in addition to anticoagulation significantly reduced the risk of recurrent PE compared with anticoagulation alone. However, this benefit was counterbalanced by increased risk of recurrent DVT, and a lack of impact on all-cause mortality [20]. Another trial found that placement of an IVC filter for 3 months did not reduce PE recurrence or mortality in anticoagulated patients with PE and DVT who had additional risk factors for recurrent VTE. The latest American College of Chest Physicians (ACCP) guidelines recommend against IVC filter insertion in patients with PE receiving anticoagulation, although they recognize that there is uncertainty regarding the risk and benefits in patients with hypotension.

Outpatient Management of PE

The PESI and sPESI scores (Table 18.4) are the most extensively validated prognostic scores to predict outcome in PE. These have been shown to accurately identify "low risk" PE. In an open-label, randomized non-inferiority trial, acute PE patients with PESI risk classes I or II were safely and effectively managed as outpatients, as compared to standard in-patient care. Similar results of outpatient-based treatment have been demonstrated using other scoring criteria. A meta-analysis on this subject concluded that independent of the risk stratification methods used, the rate of adverse events associated with outpatient PE treatment is low, and low-risk patients with acute PE can safely be treated as outpatients if home circumstances are adequate [21].

Duration of Anticoagulation

The aim of anticoagulant treatment in patients with PE is to prevent recurrence of VTE. However, the optimal duration of oral anticoagulant treatment after a first episode of pulmonary embolism

Table 18.4 Pulmonary Embolism Severity Index (PESI) and simplified PESI (sPESI) indices

PESI		s-PESI	
Variable	Points	Variable	Points
Age	1 per year	Age > 80 years	1
Male sex	10		
History of cancer	30	History of cancer	1
History of heart failure	10	History of heart failure or chronic lung disease	1
History of chronic lung disease	10		
Pulse rate > 110 beats min^{-1}	20	Pulse rate > 110 beats min^{-1}	1
Systolic blood pressure < 100 mmHg	30	Systolic blood pressure < 100 mmHg	1
Respiratory rate ≥ 30 breaths min^{-1}	20		
Body temperature < 36 °C	20		
Altered mental status (disorientation, confusion or somnolence)	60		
Arterial oxygen saturation < 90%	20	Arterial oxygen saturation < 90%	1
Risk classification		*Risk classification*	
Class I (<65 points): Very low risk		0 points: Low risk	
Class II (66–85 points): Low risk		≥1 point: High risk	
Class III (86–105 points): Intermediate risk			
Class IV (106–125 points): High risk			
Class V (>125 points): Very high risk			

Collectively, patients in PESI classes I and II are classified as low-risk. A sPESI score of 0 indicates low risk. Online risk calculators are available

remains uncertain. VKAs, LMWH, and DOACs are highly effective in preventing recurrent VTE during treatment, but they do not attenuate the risk of subsequent recurrence after discontinuation of treatment, irrespective of duration. Clinical trials have shown that the risk of recurrence after 6 or 12 months of anticoagulation is similar to that of after 3 months of anticoagulation once treatment is stopped. Patients with unprovoked PE should be anticoagulated for at least 3 months. After this period, indefinite anticoagulation should be considered for patients with a first unprovoked proximal VTE and a low risk of bleeding.

Indefinite treatment reduces the risk for recurrent VTE by about 90%, but it carries a 1% or higher annual risk of major bleeding. Hence the risk-to-benefit ratio of long-term anticoagulation should be evaluated regularly if prolonged treatment is considered. The morbidities associated with VTE, such as chronic venous insufficiency and chronic thrombo-embolic pulmonary arterial hypertension, and mortality associated with PE need to be balanced against the risk of major and fatal haemorrhage. Clearly, if there is a transient risk factor for VTE, then anticoagulation longer than 3 months should not be necessary, a view endorsed by all current guidelines. On the other hand, in those with an ongoing risk factor, such as an active malignancy, indefinite anticoagulation would be reasonable.

Following the first episode of acute unprovoked VTE, the risk of recurrence is up to 10% in the first year after withdrawal of anticoagulant treatment. Although not rigorously studied prospectively, the risk of long-term recurrence over 5–10 years is estimated in the range of 30–50% in this group. There are several well recognized risk factors for recurrence, the most important being a previous episode of VTE. A negative D-dimer test 1 month after withdrawal of VKA seems to be a protective factor for recurrence of VTE (RR 0.4). Indeed, serial testing of D-dimer might be useful, as well, to predict recurrence. Risk factors for bleeding include older age (particularly >75 years), previous gastrointestinal bleeding, previous stroke (either haemorrhagic or ischaemic), chronic renal or hepatic disease, concomitant antiplatelet therapy, presence of other serious acute or chronic illness, poor anticoagulation control, and sub-optimal monitoring of anticoagulant therapy. Utilizing clinical parameters, algorithms such as the Vienna prediction model and the DASH model have been proposed to estimate the risk of recurrence of VTE. The decision about indefinite anticoagulation should be based on the individual risks of VTE recurrence and bleeding, with their associated morbidity and mortality.

References

1. Hull RD, Hirsh J, Carter CJ, Jay RM, Dodd PE, Ockelford PA, et al. Pulmonary angiography, ventilation lung scanning, and venography for clinically suspected pulmonary embolism with abnormal perfusion lung scan. Ann Intern Med. 1983;98(6): 891–9.
2. Kearon C, Ginsberg JS, Hirsh J. The role of venous ultrasonography in the diagnosis of suspected deep venous thrombosis and pulmonary embolism. Ann Intern Med. 1998;129(12):1044–9.
3. Goldhaber SZ, Visani L, De Rosa M. Acute pulmonary embolism: clinical outcomes in the International Cooperative Pulmonary Embolism Registry (ICOPER). Lancet. 1999;353:1386–9.
4. Kasper W, Konstantinides S, Geibel A, Olschewski M, Heinrich F, Grosser KD, et al. Management strategies and determinants of outcome in acute major pulmonary embolism: results of a multicenter registry. J Am Coll Cardiol. 1997;30:1165–71.
5. Aujesky D, Obrosky DS, Stone RA, Auble TE, Perrier A, Cornuz J, et al. Derivation and validation of a prognostic model for pulmonary embolism. Am J Respir Crit Care Med. 2005;172(8):1041–6.
6. Jimenez D, Aujesky D, Moores L, Gómez V, Lobo JL, Uresandi F, et al. Simplification of the pulmonary embolism severity index for prognostication in patients with acute symptomatic pulmonary embolism. Arch Intern Med. 2010;170(15):1383–9.
7. Aujesky D, Roy PM, Verschuren F, Righini M, Osterwalder J, Egloff M, et al. Outpatient versus inpatient treatment for patients with acute pulmonary embolism: an international, open-label, randomised, non-inferiority trial. Lancet. 2011;378(9785):41–8.
8. Konstantinides SV, Torbicki A, Agnelli G, Danchin N, Fitzmaurice D, Galiè N, et al. 2014 ESC guidelines on the diagnosis and management of acute pulmonary embolism. Eur Heart J. 2014;35(43):3033–69. 3069a–3069k.
9. Stein PD, Beemath A, Matta F, Weg JG, Yusen RD, Hales CA, et al. Clinical characteristics of patients with acute pulmonary embolism: data from PIOPED II. Am J Med. 2007;120(10):871–9.
10. Wells PS, Anderson DR, Rodger M, Stiell I, Dreyer JF, Barnes D, et al. Excluding pulmonary embolism at the bedside without diagnostic imaging: management of patients with suspected pulmonary embolism presenting to the emergency department by using a simple clinical model and d-dimer. Ann Intern Med. 2001;135(2):98–107.
11. Carrier M, Righini M, Djurabi RK, Huisman MV, Perrier A, Wells PS, et al. VIDAS D-dimer in combination with clinical pre-test probability to rule out pulmonary embolism. A systematic review of management outcome studies. Thromb Haemost. 2009;101(5):886–92.
12. Faruqi S, Kishore N, Bodington R, Meghjee S, Thirumaran M. The diagnostic yield of CTPA: pulmonary embolism, alternative diagnoses and incidental findings. Acute Med. 2016;15(3):130–3.
13. Stein PD, Athanasoulis C, Alavi A, Greenspan RH, Hales CA, Saltzman HA, et al. Complications and validity of pulmonary angiography in acute pulmonary embolism. Circulation. 1992;85(2): 462–8.
14. Thromboembolic disease in pregnancy and the puerperium: acute management (green-top guideline No. 37b). London: Royal College of Obstetricians and Gynaecologists; 2015. Available at: https://www.rcog.org.uk/globalassets/documents/guidelines/gtg-37b.pdf.
15. [No authors listed]. The urokinase pulmonary embolism trial: a national cooperative study. Circulation. 1973;47(2 Suppl):II1–108.
16. Marti C, John G, Konstantinides S, Combescure C, Sanchez O, Lankeit M, et al. Systemic thrombolytic therapy for acute pulmonary embolism: a systematic review and meta-analysis. Eur Heart J. 2015;36(10):605–14.
17. Jerjes-Sanchez C, Ramírez-Rivera A, de Lourdes García M, Arriaga-Nava R, Valencia S, Rosado-Buzzo A, et al. Streptokinase and heparin versus heparin alone in massive pulmonary embolism: a randomized controlled trial. J Thromb Thrombolysis. 1995;2(3):227–9.
18. Meyer G, Vicaut E, Danays T, Agnelli G, Becattini C, Beyer-Westendorf J, et al. Fibrinolysis for patients with intermediate-risk pulmonary embolism. N Engl J Med. 2014;370(15):1402–11.
19. Akl EA, Kahale L, Barba M, Neumann I, Labedi N, Terrenato I, et al. Anticoagulation for the long-term treatment of venous thromboembolism in patients with cancer. Cochrane Database Syst Rev. 2014;7:CD006650.
20. Decousus H, Leizorovicz A, Parent F, Page Y, Tardy B, Girard P, et al. A clinical trial of vena caval filters in the prevention of pulmonary embolism in patients with proximal deep-vein thrombosis. Prévention du Risque d'Embolie Pulmonaire par Interruption Cave Study Group. N Engl J Med. 1998;338:409–15.
21. Piran S, Le Gal G, Wells PS, Gandara E, Righini M, Rodger MA, et al. Outpatient treatment of symptomatic pulmonary embolism: a systematic review and meta-analysis. Thromb Res. 2013;132(5): 515–9.

Pulmonary Hypertension

Peter M. Hickey, Robin Condliffe, Allan Lawrie, and David G. Kiely

Clinical Features

Introduction

Pulmonary hypertension is a heterogeneous group of conditions, defined at cardiac catheterisation by a mean pulmonary arterial pressure (mPAP) of ≥ 25 mmHg. Identifying the form of pulmonary hypertension is key, as it defines prognosis and treatment. It was subclassified initially by the World Health Organisation in 1973, but significantly changed with advancement in understanding and recognition of similar histological characteristics in patients with different associated medical conditions [1]. The current accepted classification was updated during the fifth World Symposium in Nice, France in 2013 (Table 19.1) [2]. Pulmonary hypertension is currently classified into five groups (Table 19.1). It ranges from rare conditions—such as pulmonary arterial hypertension (PAH) in Group 1, to chronic thromboembolic pulmonary hypertension (CTEPH) in Group 4, for which there are specific treatments—to more commonly seen mild elevations in pulmonary artery pressure in the setting of cardiac (Group 2) and respiratory disease (Group 3), where treatment is currently aimed at treating the underlying cardiac and respiratory disease (Fig. 19.1) [3].

Where pulmonary artery pressure elevation is severe, discriminating between different forms of pulmonary hypertension can be challenging. Systematic evaluation and awareness of risk factors for different forms of pulmonary hypertension is helpful in informing diagnostic strategies. Advances in diagnostic imaging have improved the classification of patients, although increasingly, patients are being seen who may not have a classic phenotype.

Over the last two decades there has been a rapid advancement in our knowledge, understanding, and management of patients with pulmonary hypertension. For those with PAH over 40, randomised controlled trials have been conducted and multiple new therapies have been licensed (Fig. 19.2). For patients with CTEPH the

P. M. Hickey (✉)
Pulmonary Vascular Research Group,
Department of Infection, Immunity and Cardiovascular Disease (IICD), University of Sheffield,
Sheffield, South Yorkshire, UK
e-mail: peterhickey@nhs.net

R. Condliffe
Pulmonary Vascular Disease Unit, Royal Hallamshire Hospital, Sheffield Teaching Hospitals NHS Trust,
Sheffield, South Yorkshire, UK

A. Lawrie
Pulmonary Vascular Research Group, Department of Infection, Immunity and Cardiovascular Disease,
University of Sheffield, Sheffield, South Yorkshire, UK

D. G. Kiely
Pulmonary Vascular Disease Unit, Royal Hallamshire Hospital, Sheffield Teaching Hospitals NHS Trust,
Sheffield, South Yorkshire, UK

© Springer International Publishing AG, part of Springer Nature 2018
S. Hart, M. Greenstone (eds.), *Foundations of Respiratory Medicine*,
https://doi.org/10.1007/978-3-319-94127-1_19

Table 19.1 Classification of pulmonary hypertension

Classification
1. Pulmonary arterial hypertension
1.1. Idiopathic
1.2. Heritable
1.2.1. BMPR-2 mutation
1.2.2. Other mutation
1.3. Drugs and toxin induced
1.4. Associated with
1.4.1. Connective tissue disease
1.4.2. Human immunodeficiency virus (HIV) infection
1.4.3. Portal hypertension
1.4.4. Congenital heart disease
1.4.5. Schistosomiasis
1′. Pulmonary veno-occlusive disease and/or pulmonary capillary haemangiomatosis
1′.1. Idiopathic
1′.2. Heritable
1′.2.1. E1F2AK4 mutation
1′.2.2. Other mutations
1′.3. Drugs, toxins and radiation induced
1′.4. Associated with
1′.4.1. Connective tissue disease
1′.4.2. HIV infection
1″. Persistent pulmonary hypertension of the newborn
2. Pulmonary hypertension due to left heart disease
2.1. Left ventricular systolic dysfunction
2.2. Left ventricular diastolic dysfunction
2.3. Valvular disease
2.4. Congenital/acquired left heart inflow/outflow tract obstruction and congenital cardiomyopathies
2.5. Congenital/acquired pulmonary veins stenosis
3. Pulmonary hypertension due to lung disease and/or hypoxia
3.1. Chronic obstructive pulmonary disease
3.2. Interstitial lung disease
3.3. Other pulmonary diseases with mixed obstructive and restrictive pattern
3.4. Sleep-disordered breathing
3.5. Alveolar hypoventilation disorders
3.6. Chronic exposure to high altitudes
3.7. Developmental lung diseases
4. Chronic thromboembolic pulmonary hypertension and other pulmonary artery obstructions
4.1. Chronic thromboembolic pulmonary hypertension
4.2. Other pulmonary artery obstructions
4.2.1. Angiosarcoma
4.2.2. Other intravascular tumours
4.2.3. Arteritis
4.2.4. Congenital pulmonary arteries stenosis
4.2.5. Parasites (hydatidosis)
5. Pulmonary hypertension with unclear and/or multifactorial mechanisms
5.1. Haematological disorders: Chronic haemolytic anaemia, myeloproliferative disorders, splenectomy
5.2. Systemic disorders: Sarcoidosis, pulmonary histiocytosis, lymphangioleiomyomatosis
5.3. Metabolic disorders: Glycogen storage disease, Gaucher disease, thyroid disorders
5.4. Others: Pulmonary tumoural thrombotic microangiopathy, fibrosing mediastinitis, chronic renal failure (with or without dialysis), segmental pulmonary hypertension

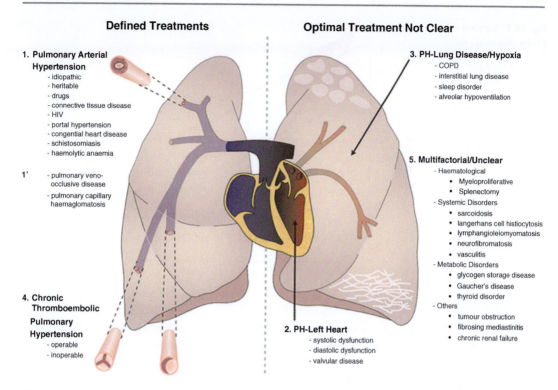

Fig. 19.1 PH classification and treatment grouping [3]. Reproduced from Kiely DG, Elliot CA, Sabroe I, Condliffe R. Pulmonary hypertension: diagnosis and management. BMJ. 2013 Apr 16;346:f2028. With permission from BMJ Publishing Group Ltd

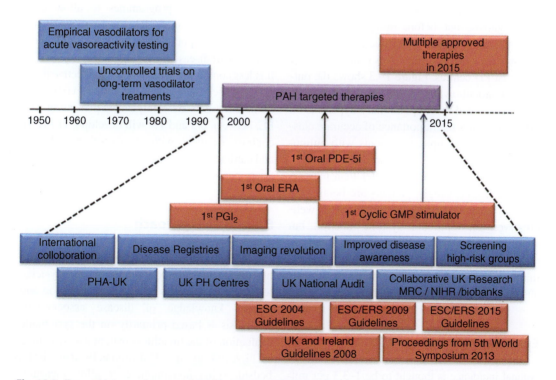

Fig. 19.2 Recent history and progress in pulmonary hypertension

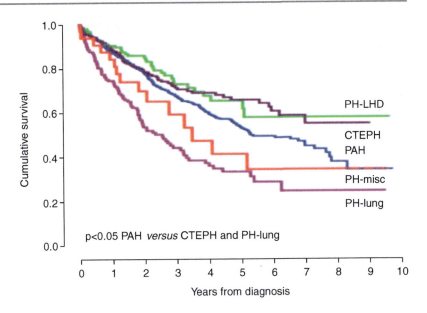

Fig. 19.3 Survival in PH by subgroup [4]. Reproduced with permission of the European Respiratory Society ©: European Respiratory Journal. Oct 2012, 40 (4) 874–880; doi: https://doi.org/10.1183/09031936.00137511

development of surgical techniques such as pulmonary endarterectomy offers a potential cure, and more recently, balloon pulmonary angioplasty has resulted in significant improvements in patient outcomes. Despite a significant improvement in life expectancy, pulmonary hypertension remains a life-limiting condition for many patients.

Echocardiography most commonly suggests the diagnosis, but before initiating treatment, patients require systematic evaluation. In the UK and in many other countries, this is undertaken at specialist PH centres. Figure 19.3 shows the outcome of patients evaluated at a specialist PH centre for suspected severe pulmonary hypertension [4]. It illustrates the importance of accurate classification. For example, in patients with pulmonary hypertension with left heart disease (LHD), the outcome is significantly better than patients with PAH. Increasingly, patients are being seen with severe pulmonary hypertension with well-preserved left ventricular systolic function, but significant diastolic dysfunction. It is important that these patients are carefully assessed and not misdiagnosed as having PAH, where prognosis and treatments are significantly different.

Epidemiology

Annual incidence is thought to be 1–3.3 per million of population for idiopathic pulmonary hypertension (iPAH), previously known as primary pulmonary hypertension, and 1.75–3.7 per million for CTEPH [3]. Overall, PAH has been quoted as having a prevalence of 15–52 per million population [3, 5]. iPAH is therefore a rare condition, but awareness of conditions associated with PAH is important, as they allow for the introduction of specific screening programmes to allow early diagnosis. For example, PAH is seen in systemic sclerosis (9%), portal hypertension (2–6%), congenital heart disease (5–10%) and HIV (0.5%) [3]. It is less commonly seen in other connective tissue diseases such as SLE (1%) and mixed connective tissue disease (2–5%). In patients presenting with PE, between 0.5 and 7% will develop CTEPH. In contrast, in patients with severe respiratory disease and cardiac disease, mild elevations in pulmonary artery pressure are common.

Diagnostic Approach

Diagnosis of pulmonary hypertension requires a high index of suspicion, requiring the physician to have an awareness of this rare condition and also a knowledge of disease associations. Diagnosis is based primarily on the systematic evaluation of the breathless patient and screening of high-risk groups. Unfortunately, there is no bedside sphygmomanometer to allow measurement of pulmonary hypertension. Given the non-specific nature of symptoms, it may masquerade as multiple other conditions, most of which are more common, such as asthma. PAH most commonly presents with progressive exertional breathlessness, but as it progresses, patients can present with symptoms of right heart dysfunction such as pre-syncope, syncope, oedema, and ascites. It is important to recognise that particularly in a young patient, ankle oedema is a very late feature of pulmonary hypertension. Patients are also prone to tachyarrhythmias, with right atrial enlargement pre-disposing to atrial flutter as the most common arrhythmia. Haemoptysis is also seen in congenital heart disease (CHD) and pulmonary embolic disease (usually from bronchial arteries) and other very rare forms of pulmonary hypertension, such as pulmonary capillary haemangiomatosis [3]. Breathlessness in patients with a high prevalence of PAH, such as connective tissue disease, should result in prompt investigation for pulmonary hypertension.

History

A detailed history is key in identifying risk factors for various forms of pulmonary hypertension. PH associated with left heart disease (PH-LHD) is often accompanied by a history of multiple cardiovascular risk factors, such as atrial fibrillation, diabetes, and hypertension. Pulmonary hypertension associated with respiratory disease is often accompanied by a history of chronic lung disease, or features consistent with a diagnosis of obstructive sleep apnoea or obesity hypoventilation syndrome. However, it is important not to attribute severe breathlessness to very mild abnormalities of lung function. In one-third of patients with CTEPH, there is no history of a previous thromboembolic event, so investigation of unexplained pulmonary hypertension should include an assessment for this.

PAH is associated with a history of progressive breathlessness. Patients have often had frequent consultations and multiple investigations in both primary and secondary care before the diagnosis is made. The average delay from initial presentation to diagnosis remains approximately 2 years. As the disease progresses, history may include

dizziness or syncope related to embarrassment of left heart filling, or features of right ventricular failure such as oedema and ascites. Patients may complain of chest pain due to myocardial hypoperfusion in the setting of right ventricular hypertrophy, or compression of the coronary artery by an enlarged pulmonary artery [3].

Physical Examination

Physical examination should look both for features of pulmonary hypertension and also for associated diseases. Features of pulmonary hypertension include a prominent pulmonary component of the second heart sound, raised JVP, systolic murmur of tricuspid regurgitation, oedema, and/or ascites. General examination may reveal kyphoscoliosis or other chest wall deformity, or marked obesity suggestive of an underlying obesity hypoventilation syndrome. Clubbing or cyanosis may be present, and suggest the presence of underlying congenital heart disease. Clubbing may also be a feature of lung or liver disease. Respiratory examination may reveal the crackles of interstitial lung disease, or bronchiectasis, or wheeze from obstructive lung diseases. Features of connective tissue diseases should be carefully looked for including sclerodactyly, telangiectasia, or other skin changes [6]. It is not unusual for patients to present with pulmonary hypertension and undiagnosed connective tissue disease, or for PAH to predate the development of a connective tissue disease.

Investigations

A diagnostic approach to investigating patients with suspected pulmonary hypertension is shown in Fig. 19.4 [3]. Investigations will depend on the history and the most likely cause for symptoms, in addition to the speciality reviewing the patient (e.g. cardiology or respiratory). For unexplained breathlessness, lung function and CXR will usually be performed in respiratory clinic, and BNP, ECG, and echocardiography in cardiology clinics. These investigations may identify an alternative cause of breathlessness or chest pain, or suggest pulmonary hypertension. If breathless-

Fig. 19.4 Diagnostic approach to suspected pulmonary hypertension [3]. Reproduced from Kiely DG, Elliot CA, Sabroe I, Condliffe R. Pulmonary hypertension: diagnosis and management. BMJ. 2013 Apr 16;346:f2028. With permission from BMJ Publishing Group Ltd

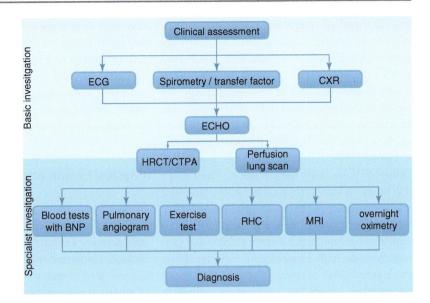

ness remains unexplained and the patient has not had an echocardiogram, then this should be considered. Depending on availability, some physicians perform cardiopulmonary exercise testing for unexplained breathlessness. Characteristic abnormalities in pulmonary hypertension include reduced peak oxygen consumption (peak VO$_2$), low oxygen pulse (VO$_2$/HR; a surrogate measurement for stroke volume), low end-tidal pCO$_2$, high ventilatory equivalents for carbon dioxide (VE/VCO$_2$), and prolonged desaturation. If severe pulmonary hypertension is suggested by these investigations, the patient should be referred for specialist assessment and, depending on the clinical presentation, CTPA and lung perfusion scanning can be considered. Subsequent assessment, including cardiac catheterisation and further imaging and testing for conditions such as hypoventilation (where indicated) would then be required to confirm the presence of pulmonary hypertension and identify the cause and severity of the disease (Table 19.2).

Chest X-ray and ECG are abnormal in up to 90% of patients with iPAH. Abnormalities to look for include cardiomegaly, right atrial or ventricular hypertrophy and enlarged central pulmonary arteries [9]. ECG findings include right axis deviation, right ventricular hypertrophy, right ventricular strain, and prominence of P-waves (Fig. 19.5) [6].

Spirometry and gas transfer may reveal evidence of underlying lung disease. In PAH the TLco is usually reduced (usually 60–80% predicted), although it can be normal. Patients with iPAH with more severe disease have lower TLco. A TLco <50% should alert the physician to the presence of an underlying connective tissue disease (TLco is lower in PAH-systemic sclerosis compared to iPAH, reflecting an additional abnormality to gas diffusion even in the absence of interstitial lung disease). In patients with PH, a normal or elevated TLco should raise the suspicion of a left to right shunt. The most common spirometric abnormality in iPAH is mild restriction.

Echocardiography is usually the first test to suggest the diagnosis of pulmonary hypertension. It gives information about cardiac structure and function, but also allows estimation of the systolic pulmonary artery pressure. It may give evidence as to the underlying cause of pulmonary hypertension if there is evidence of left heart disease, or congenital defects. Estimation of pulmonary artery pressure is based on the peak velocity of the tricuspid regurgitant (TR) jet, which is found in more than 90% of patients with significant PH. It is calculated using a modified Bernoulli equation (see below). Although this does correlate with invasive measures of PAP, measurements are operator dependent and may

Table 19.2 Investigations

Investigation	Characteristic findings	Notes
ECG	Right heart strain	Normal ECG does not exclude PH. Left axis deviation common in left heart disease
CXR	Cardiomegaly, enlarged pulmonary arteries	Look for features of underlying respiratory diseases
Spirometry	Reduced TLco. Usually 50–80% predicted in IPAH. If <50% predicted consider coexisting respiratory or connective tissue disease	Look for evidence of underlying respiratory diseases
Echocardiography	Right ventricular impairment. Congenital abnormalities. Estimation of sPAP. Paradoxical septal motion. If sPAP >60 mmHg and no paradoxical motion suggests elevated left sided pressures	Often initial screening investigation. Look for underlying left heart disease (valvular heart disease, large left atrium)
CTPA	Enlarged pulmonary artery. Dilated right ventricle. Posterior deviation of interventricular septum. Right ventricular hypertrophy. Features of CTEPH—Mural thrombus, stenosis, intraluminal webs. Pulmonary ground glass change common in PAH. CT may suggest cause of PAH eg oesophageal dilation in systemic sclerosis	Look for features of underlying cardiac or respiratory disease. Can also be used to assess disease severity in PAH. Pericardial and pleural effusions associated with more severe disease
Nuclear medicine: Q scan	Perfusion defects in CTEPH, may also be seen in respiratory disease	High sensitivity for CTEPH. Normal scan excludes CTEPH
Cardiac magnetic resonance (CMR) imaging	Detailed anatomical structure of cardiac chambers. Detailed metrics available to assess cardiac function. Can be used to assess disease severity and follow-up	Emerging modality, with evidence for use in diagnosis of PH, and subsequent disease monitoring. No single MR measure can confidently exclude PH although if MR normal if PH present, it is likely to be mild [7]
MR-angiography and 3D-MR perfusion maps	MRA can be used with CTPA and Q scanning to assess surgical accessibility of CTEPH. 3D MR perfusion maps can be used as a Q scan to exclude CTEPH	3D-MR perfusion scans helpful to rule out CTEPH [8]. Some patients may not tolerate CMR imaging (<5%). Has benefit of no radiation exposure
Right heart catheter	Allows measurement of pressure, cardiac output, estimate of left sided pressure and measurement of saturations of blood	Gold standard test to measure pressure but should not be used in isolation; results need to be carefully interpreted in conjunction with other tests. Falsely high PAWP may be due to over-wedging of balloon but also seen in CTEPH. Helpful for quantifying left to right shunts

CTEPH chronic thromboembolic pulmonary hypertension, *PAWP* pulmonary artery wedge pressue, *sPAP* systolic pulmonary artery pressure

be inaccurate in patients with severe TR [9]. Other features seen on echocardiography include measures of right ventricular function, and paradoxical septal motion suggestive of increased right ventricular pressure. It should be recognised that estimation of sPAP is more accurate in patients with cardiac disease compared to respiratory disease. In patients with COPD, echocardiography frequently overestimates sPAP and during exacerbations this can result in sPAP >30 mmHg higher than normal [10].

Modified Bernoulli Equation

$$sPAP = 4 \times \left[TR\, V_{max} \right]^2 + RAP$$

Blood testing should include screens for connective tissue diseases and HIV.

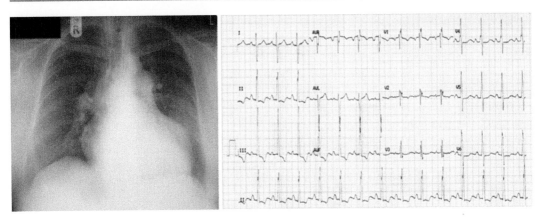

Fig. 19.5 CXR demonstrating enlarged right atrium, prominent pulmonary vessels, pruning of peripheral pulmonary vessels. ECG demonstrating right axis deviation, increased P-wave amplitude, inferior and anterior ST depression

Overnight oximetry ± transcutaneous CO_2 measurement is useful in selected cases to screen for sleep disordered breathing.

Isotope perfusion scanning has high sensitivity for CTEPH, and a normal scan excludes this disease. Furthermore, increased renal isotope uptake may suggest right to left shunting [11]. This investigation also has the advantage over CTPA that abnormalities seen in CTEPH can be more easily be appreciated by the non-specialist.

CTPA and *HRCT* provide detailed structural information. In PH, an assessment should be made of vessels, cardiac and mediastinal structures, and the lung parenchyma. CTPA may be the first investigation to suggest pulmonary hypertension, allowing evaluation of pulmonary artery size (should be smaller than corresponding aorta), right atrial and ventricular size, and septal deviation (Fig. 19.6). Assessment of vessels may demonstrate abnormal pulmonary venous drainage. Assessment of the lung parenchyma may identify interstitial lung disease or emphysema. Interestingly, ground glass change is frequently seen in PAH (over 30% of cases). Therefore, in patients who have CT scans performed for unexplained breathlessness, the presence of ground glass changes should raise the possibility of underlying PH, which may be supported by an enlarged pulmonary artery or (if contrast is given) a dilated right ventricle with displacement of the interventricular septum into the left ventricle. CTEPH is characterised by a mosaic perfusion pattern of the lung parenchyma, pulmonary arterial occlusions, stenoses and intraluminal webs, but can be easily missed by non-specialist radiologists.

Cardiac MR provides considerable structural and functional information. It is increasingly used as a diagnostic tool and, due to its superior ability to assess the right ventricle compared to echocardiography, it can be used for serial assessments. A number of features may suggest the presence of pulmonary hypertension, such as the presence of RV dilation and hypertrophy, reduced pulsatility of the pulmonary artery, and following an injection of gadolinium contrast late enhancement can be seen at the ventricular hinge points. Following an injection of gadolinium, perfusion maps can be obtained to look for defects, and an angiogram can be constructed, right to left shunts can be identified, and uptake into the myocardium can also be assessed.

Right heart catheterisation is used to confirm the diagnosis of PH by direct measurement of pulmonary arterial pressure. Further measurements are taken to assess for likely underlying cause, including cardiac output, and an estimate of left atrial pressure by pulmonary arterial wedge pressure (PAWP; sometimes also described as PCWP or PAOP). Measurements of

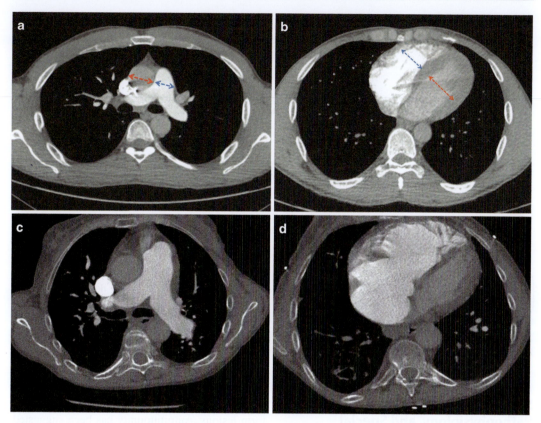

Fig. 19.6 CTPA imaging: (**a**) Normal pulmonary artery dimensions, (**b**) Normal RV + LV dimensions, (**c**) Dilated pulmonary trunk, (**d**) Dilated RA, RV with posterior displacement of interventricular septum [12]. Reproduced in part from Rajaram S, Swift AJ, Condliffe R, Johns C, Elliot CA, Hill C, et al. CT features of pulmonary arterial hypertension and its major subtypes: a systematic CT evaluation of 292 patients from the ASPIRE Registry. Thorax. 2015 Apr;70(4):382–7. With permission from BMJ Publishing Group Ltd

oxygen saturation allow for assessment of shunting, and the saturation of blood measured in the pulmonary artery can also be used to assess the severity of pulmonary hypertension. Vasoreactivity testing can also be carried out during right heart catheterisation, usually using inhaled nitric oxide. This can identify patients with iPAH likely to respond to high-dose calcium channel blockers. A positive test is defined as a reduction in PAP of at least 10 mmHg to less than 40 mmHg, without a fall in cardiac output [3]. A suggested approach to interpretation of data is given in Fig. 19.7. It should be noted that the PAWP can be an unreliable mea-surement. With the pulmonary artery catheter in position and the balloon up during measurement of PAWP, a blood sample can be taken. If a "true" wedge, this should be the same as the arterial saturation, given that the sample repre-sents blood taken from the pulmonary veins. It should also be noted that due to the non-cylin-drical nature of blood vessels in CTEPH, the PAWP may be difficult to measure and can be overestimated. The right heart catheter results therefore need to be carefully interpreted with the other investigations. In pulmonary hyperten-sion, like other conditions, one should never over-rely on a single investigation.

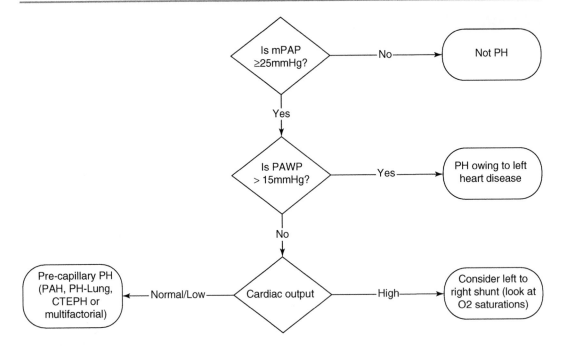

Fig. 19.7 Suggested approach for interpretation of RHC data

Subclassification of PH, Pathophysiology, and Special Circumstances

Group 1: PAH

PAH is a disease which affects small pulmonary arteries and pulmonary arterioles in the pre-capillary vascular bed. The disease involves thickening of vascular walls due to proliferation of smooth muscle cells. The vascular endothelium demonstrates abnormal proliferation, which with matrix proteins and fibroblastic proliferation forms plexiform lesions which obstruct the vascular lumen. Thrombosis *in situ* on the abnormal vascular endothelium can occur with or without the presence of abnormalities of clotting and platelet function (Fig. 19.8). The mechanism of these changes is as yet incompletely understood, but it is felt that a combination of auto-immune influence and upregulation of pro-inflammatory cytokines may be responsible. Thirty to fourty percent of patients with PAH have upregulation of pro-inflammatory cytokines such as IL-1 and IL-6, and inflammatory cells including lympho-

cytes and macrophages can be found in plexiform lesions. Autoimmunity has been suggested as potentially contributor, with the identification of reduced function of a subset of T-lymphocytes related to self-tolerance. A role for autoimmune-mediated chronic inflammation has been suggested as a potential contributor to the development of PAH [13].

Heritable PAH is associated with autosomal-dominant inheritance in almost all identified genetic mutations. Understanding the genetics is made more complicated by incomplete penetrance, with approximately 20% of individuals with a family history who carry the genetic mutation developing PAH, although the penetrance is higher in women. The best known group of mutations are those affecting the gene encoding bone morphogenetic protein receptor 2 (BMPR-2) a member of the TGF-β receptor superfamily. These mutations can be found in approximately 70% of cases of heritable PAH (HPAH), and in 10–40% of cases of iPAH. TGF-β pathways have been identified as important in the pulmonary vascular tree and control a range of cellular functions, including proliferation, migration,

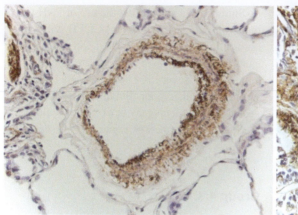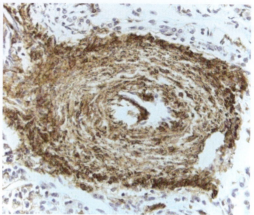

Fig. 19.8 Histological differences between pulmonary arteriole in normal (left) and pulmonary arterial hypertension (right). Staining for smooth muscle actin is indicated in brown [14]. Reprinted from Lawrie A, Waterman E, Southwood M, Evans D, Suntharalingam J, Francis S, et al. Evidence of a role for osteoprotegerin in the pathogenesis of pulmonary arterial hypertension. The American Journal of Pathology. 2008;172(1):256–64. With permission from Elsevier

differentiation, apoptosis, and control of extracellular matrix deposition [15]. In other cases known to have a heritable aetiology, mutations in activin receptor-like kinase type 1 (ALK1), endoglin, and further members of the TGF-β superfamily have been described [13]. ALK1 and endoglin mutations are known to cause hereditary haemorrhagic telangiectasia (HHT), and can rarely also lead to PAH [15].

Pulmonary hypertension is a relatively frequent complication of many connective tissue diseases, particularly systemic sclerosis, however it is also seen in lupus and mixed connective tissue disease. PH develops in approximately 10% of patients with systemic sclerosis. Histologically, PH develops in a similar manner to iPAH, with endothelial and smooth muscle proliferation, however fewer plexiform lesions are seen. PAH-CTD is associated with a poor prognosis, with 3-year survival of approximately 50%. Given the relatively high incidence of PH in systemic sclerosis particularly, screening of patients is recommended. European Respiratory Society guidelines recommend annual echocardiography in systemic sclerosis. Treatment is of the underlying connective tissue disease, but targeted pulmonary vascular treatment falls in line with that of iPAH [16]. In SLE, PH is seen in up to 1% of patients, and is usually PAH, although CTEPH can be seen. In mixed connective tissue disease, PAH appears more common (2–5%), whereas in rheumatoid arthritis, an isolated vasculopathy is only very rarely seen, and PH is usually only seen in the setting of significant interstitial lung disease or cardiac disease.

Group 2: PH-LHD

Left heart disease (LHD) is considered to be the most common cause of pulmonary hypertension, and is characterised by post-capillary disease (demonstrated by a raised PAWP) [17]. Given that there is usually no primary pre-capillary disease, pulmonary vascular resistance is often normal, with no abnormality in the gradient between PAP and PAWP (transpulmonary gradient). Elevated PAP in this situation is a result of increased left-sided filling pressures caused by left heart disease. Microvascular remodelling and type IV collagen deposition can be seen in relation to LHD, with consequent increase in PVR, and is thought to be related to increased stress on pulmonary capillary beds caused by chronic elevation of pulmonary venous pressure [17, 18]. Single cardiovascular risk factors are often seen in patients with PAH however, multiple cardiovascular risk factors often point towards PH-LHD [19].

Targeted pulmonary vasodilators are not recommended in PH-LHD. Treatment is of underlying left heart disease. In particular, treatment of valvular heart disease and optimisation of left ventricular systolic dysfunction may significantly improve pulmonary artery pressure elevation. Patients with heart failure with preserved ejection fraction or HFpEF will often have risk factors for LHD, and studies are currently ongoing of PAH therapies in selected patients with well preserved left ventricular systolic function. Echocardiography may demonstrate enlargement of the left atrium, often mild impairment of RV function, and despite high pulmonary artery pressures, usually an absence of paradoxical septal motion (reflecting the high left sided pressures).

Group 3: PH-Lung

PH can occur in any patient with any chronic lung disease. In patients with severe COPD, RV dysfunction is common, with 30% showing evidence of RV dilatation, and 19% affected by PH. In IPF awaiting lung transplantation, estimates suggest PH complicates between 31% and 85%, and in obesity hypoventilation estimates suggest PH in between 17% and 52% of cases. In patients with sleep-disordered breathing, it is unusual to see PH in the absence of restrictive lung function or elevated arterial pCO_2 [20]. PH can also be found in people living at high altitude (>3000 m), with chronic hypoxia leading to a disease process similar to iPAH.

The pathophysiology of PH in chronic lung disease is multifactorial. Hypoxia directly causes pulmonary vasoconstriction, and when chronic can lead to endothelial and smooth muscle proliferation and irreversible vascular remodelling driven by hypoxia-induced growth factors [20]. Chronic lung disease associated with parenchymal destruction or fibrosis can lead to increased vascular resistance through direct destruction of the capillary bed and inflammation-mediated vascular remodelling. In patients with emphysema, hyperinflation can compress the vascular bed and patients may also have widespread destruction of the capillary vascular bed.

Studies have shown that the use of PAH treatments in patients with severe COPD with either no or mild PH is not associated with any significant benefit, however studies are required in patients with severe PH seen in COPD and ILD where survival is poor. Small studies have suggested some patients may derive benefit, although there are some concerns regarding worsening of oxygenation.

Group 4: CTEPH

Chronic thromboembolic pulmonary hypertension is defined by RHC findings consistent with pre-capillary pulmonary hypertension, with evidence of organised flow limiting thrombus in pulmonary arteries after 3 months of therapeutic anticoagulation [21]. Two main pathogenic mechanisms are currently considered—the direct consequence of pulmonary thromboembolic events, and *in situ* thrombosis as a result of endothelial dysfunction, which would explain why a large proportion of patients with CTEPH have no history of acute PE. The incidence of CTEPH after acute PE is 0.5–7% [22]. CTEPH is the only form of pulmonary hypertension which can be considered to have a potentially curative treatment, which is surgical management with pulmonary endarterectomy. After investigation and diagnosis, an attempt should be made to classify patients into those with surgically accessible or inaccessible disease. As well as large vessel disease, patients with CTEPH are known to have a small vessel arteriopathy similar to that of iPAH, which correlates with progression of disease, and can be a limiting factor for operative outcomes. Patients who are not candidates for surgery may benefit from PH-specific targeted therapies [13]. A large international registry has recently published results on a large cohort of patients demonstrating that for patients with operable disease, surgery offers the best prospect of improved long-term outcomes [23]. Interestingly, those with surgical disease who do not undergo endarterectomy have survival significantly better than historically reported [4].

Special Circumstances

Pregnancy and PH

Pregnancy in any class of PH is associated with significant morbidity and mortality. Previous studies have suggested a mortality of up to 30%, although with targeted drug therapies and early delivery using regional techniques, recent reports have suggested improved outcomes, although the mortality remains very high. Patients are therefore counselled regarding the high risks and provided with contraceptive advice. For a small number of patients who present pregnant with PAH or wish to consider pregnancy despite the very high risk, management in a centre with experience of PH and pregnancy is advised.

In general, oestrogen contraceptives are avoided, and the use of a progesterone implant, intramuscular progesterone, intrauterine coil (should be inserted in a hospital environment due to the small risk of a vasovagal event) or oral progestogens can be used. Given the implications of contraceptive failure, a progesterone implant or coil are usually preferred, although this depends on the wishes of the woman. Emergency hormonal contraception is safe, but the dose may need to be increased in patients taking bosentan (an enzyme inducer).

PH and Anaesthesia

Pulmonary haemodynamics in pulmonary hypertension make anaesthesia a particularly hazardous time. It should be undertaken in a centre experienced at caring for patients with PH. All patients should be optimized in terms of targeted treatments to optimise pulmonary vascular resistance prior to consideration of anaesthesia. Anaesthetists need to carefully consider the effect and side effects of particular anaesthetic agents and the effects these will have on pulmonary haemodynamics. The goal is to maintain preload, systemic peripheral vascular resistance, and contractility to support RV output. Close monitoring is essential to prevent increases in pulmonary vascular resistance from hypoxia, hypercarbia, acidosis, agitation, pain, and hypothermia. Systemic blood pressure should be carefully maintained using agents such as vasopressin and phenylephrine to maintain RV

coronary perfusion pressures [24]. Increasingly, procedures are being performed using regional anaesthetic techniques.

Sepsis and PH

During stress events such as sepsis, systemic vascular resistance falls, prompting increased left ventricular output, but in PH this response is limited. Patients with PH therefore react very poorly to sepsis, and can rapidly develop septic shock and die unless sepsis is promptly recognised and managed aggressively. Early antibiotics and careful fluid management are crucial, and early assessment by critical care for inotropic support important in management. Titration of PH treatment may be necessary to optimize pulmonary vascular resistance.

Treatment

General Measures

PH patients should be encouraged to be active and exercise within their limits, and if available, should be encouraged to take part in supervised rehabilitation programmes. Pregnancy remains a high risk, and patients should be counselled and offered contraceptive advice. Influenza and pneumococcal vaccines are recommended.

Anticoagulation

Patients with CTEPH should be anticoagulated. In iPAH, data from retrospective studies and registries suggests that anticoagulation is associated with improved outcomes. More recently, a number of studies have suggested that their use in other forms of PAH such as systemic sclerosis may be associated with adverse outcome. The role of direct oral anticoagulants has yet to be established [25].

Oxygen

Supplementary oxygen has been shown to reduce vascular resistance in patients with PAH. Despite this, there is little supporting evidence for its routine use. The evidence for use of oxygen is extrapolated from data in COPD. The BTS Home Oxygen Guidelines (2015) suggest the use of long-term oxygen in patients with pulmonary hypertension when $PaO_2 < 8$ kPa [26].

Diuretics

Diuretics are routinely used in patients with pulmonary hypertension to treat decompensated right heart failure. There is no suggested standard regimen, but clinicians should titrate diuretics against a patient's weight and fluid balance. Regular monitoring is important to avoid dehydration and electrolyte imbalance.

Disease-Targeted Treatments

A number of randomized controlled trials have been performed in PAH and CTEPH. Historically, haemodynamics and 6MWT have formed the primary endpoints in studies lasting 12–16 weeks. More recently, composite endpoints including exercise capacity, haemodynamics, and time to clinical worsening have been used, with the duration of the studies significantly longer. Current treatments target three main pathways. More recently there has been a move towards early combination therapy with a phosphodiesterase inhibitor and endothelin receptor antagonist for patients in functional Class III (see Table 19.3 below) and there is increasing data that the use of triple therapy may be associated with improved outcomes. For patients in functional class IV, a parenteral prostanoid should be considered although this may not be appropriate for many patients.

Vasodilator Challenge and Calcium Channel Blockers

During right heart catheter, patients with iPAH should undergo vasoreactivity testing with a short-acting agent such as inhaled nitric oxide, although intravenous epoprostenol and adenosine have also been used. A positive response to vasodilator testing is defined as a fall in mean arterial pressure of 10 mmHg, to less than 40 mmHg,

Table 19.3 NYHA/WHO classification of functional status in pulmonary hypertension

1. No limitation of usual physical activity; ordinary physical activity does not cause increased dyspnoea, fatigue, chest pain, or near syncope
2. Mild limitation of physical activity: there is no discomfort at rest, but normal physical activity causes increased dyspnoea, fatigue, chest pain, or near syncope
3. Marked limitation of physical activity: there is no discomfort at rest, but less than ordinary activity causes increased dyspnoea, fatigue, chest pain, or near syncope
4. Unable to perform any physical activity and may have signs of right ventricular failure at rest: dyspnoea and/or fatigue may be present at rest and symptoms are increased by almost any physical activity

without a fall in cardiac output, and seen in only 10% of patients with iPAH. This group should be considered candidates for high-dose calcium channel blocker treatment. Approximately 50% will be long-term responders. Patients with PAH should not be treated empirically with calcium channel blockers in the absence of vasoreactivity testing, as patients may deteriorate rapidly.

Prostanoids

Prostacyclin is a naturally produced potent systemic and pulmonary vasodilator with antiproliferative and antiplatelet properties. It was the first PAH-specific drug to show convincing benefit on exercise capacity and survival, however it must be given by continuous infusion via a secure tunnel line [27]. Side effects common to many prostacyclin analogues include headaches, jaw ache, and flushing. Severe adverse effects such as rebound severe pulmonary vasoconstriction and acute right ventricular failure can occur with interruption of infusion. Other prostanoid analogues exist, such as iloprost (iv and nebulised) and treprostinil (oral, sc, iv, nebulised). Nebulised treatment requires multiple doses each day, and subcutaneous treatment is often limited by site pain.

Endothelin Receptor Antagonists

Naturally occurring endothelin is a potent vasoconstrictor, involved in both pulmonary vasoconstriction and stimulation of smooth muscle cell proliferation. Bosentan, a dual ET_A and ET_B endothelin receptor antagonist, was the first orally active treatment for PAH (excepting the small number of patients who benefit from high-dose calcium antagonists), and more recently ambrisentan and macitentan have been licensed for the treatment of PAH and work by antagonising the effect of endothelin. They have been shown to improve exercise capacity, functional class, and time to clinical worsening. Bosentan is an enzyme inducer and has a number of drug interactions, including with other PAH therapies. Liver function abnormalities are seen in approximately 10% of patients using this therapy at 1 year (although with monthly liver function monitoring, bosentan does not appear to be associated with significant irreversible liver damage) [13]. Newer agents such as ambrisentan and macitentan have a much lower frequency of liver function abnormalities and do not interact with other PAH therapies or oral contraceptives.

Phosphodiesterase-5 Inhibitors

Nitric oxide is a potent pulmonary vasodilator and inhibitor of cellular proliferation that is degraded by phosphodiesterase-5. Phosphodiesterase-5 inhibitors such as Sildenafil and Tadalafil have been shown to improve exercise capacity and functional class. They have interactions with nitrates, so the concomitant use is contraindicated [3].

Riociguat

Riociguat is a first-in-class soluble guanylate cyclase (sGC) stimulator, approved for the treatment of PAH or CTEPH which is either inoperable or persistent despite surgery. sGC is the receptor for endogenous nitric oxide (NO), and Riociguat both sensitizes the receptor to endogenous NO and stimulates it directly. Riociguat has been shown to improve exercise capacity and reduce pulmonary vascular resistance. Side effects include headache, GI upset, and dizziness, but it is generally well tolerated [28].

Selexipag

This is an orally active, selective IP receptor agonist targeting the prostanoid pathway, and has similar side effects to parenteral prostanoids. It has been shown to reduce the time to clinical worsening when used in addition to other PAH therapies. It offers the prospect of targeting 3 PAH pathways without the need for parenteral routes of administration.

Pulmonary Endarterectomy

Pulmonary endarterectomy is a procedure to remove chronic thromboembolic material from the pulmonary vasculature. It is the treatment of choice for surgically accessible CTEPH, resulting in significant improvements in functional class and survival. It should be remembered that although obstructing chronic thromboembolic material can be removed at PEA, outcome is also dependent on the presence of small vessel arteriopathy, and patients need to be carefully evaluated by experienced physicians. Peri-operative mortality is <5% in experienced centres [29].

Lung Transplantation

Lung transplantation is an important option for patients with PAH. It is indicated in patients with PAH or inoperable CTEPH when maximal medical treatment has failed. Both heart-lung block transplants and double-lung transplants can be performed. Most transplant recipients receive double-lung transplants. Survival was previously 52% at 5 years and 42% at 10 years, although recent reports suggest further improvements in outcome [30].

References

1. Hatano S, Strasser T. Primary pulmonary hypertension. In: Report on a WHO meeting, Geneva, 15–17 October 1973. Geneva: World Health Organization; 1975.
2. Simonneau G, Gatzoulis MA, Adatia I, Celermajer D, Denton C, Ghofrani A, et al. Updated clinical classification of pulmonary hypertension. J Am Coll Cardiol. 2013;62(25 Suppl):D34–41.
3. Kiely DG, Elliot CA, Sabroe I, Condliffe R. Pulmonary hypertension: diagnosis and management. BMJ. 2013;346:f2028.
4. Hurdman J, Condliffe R, Elliot CA, Davies C, Hill C, Wild JM, et al. ASPIRE registry: assessing the

Spectrum of pulmonary hypertension identified at a REferral Centre. Eur Respir J. 2012;39(4):945–55.

5. Ling Y, Johnson MK, Kiely DG, Condliffe R, Elliot CA, Gibbs JS, et al. Changing demographics, epidemiology, and survival of incident pulmonary arterial hypertension: results from the pulmonary hypertension registry of the United Kingdom and Ireland. Am J Respir Crit Care Med. 2012;186(8):790–6.

6. Edelman JD. Clinical presentation, differential diagnosis, and vasodilator testing of pulmonary hypertension. Semin Cardiothorac Vasc Anesth. 2007;11(2): 110–8.

7. Swift AJ, Rajaram S, Condliffe R, Capener D, Hurdman J, Elliot CA, et al. Diagnostic accuracy of cardiovascular magnetic resonance imaging of right ventricular morphology and function in the assessment of suspected pulmonary hypertension results from the ASPIRE registry. J Cardiovasc Magn Reson. 2012;14:40.

8. Rajaram S, Swift AJ, Telfer A, Hurdman J, Marshall H, Lorenz E, et al. 3D contrast-enhanced lung perfusion MRI is an effective screening tool for chronic thromboembolic pulmonary hypertension: results from the ASPIRE Registry. Thorax. 2013;68(7):677–8.

9. McCann C, Gopalan D, Sheares K, Screaton N. Imaging in pulmonary hypertension, part 1: clinical perspectives, classification, imaging techniques and imaging algorithm. Postgrad Med J. 2012;88(1039):271–9.

10. Arcasoy SM, Christie JD, Ferrari VA, Sutton MS, Zisman DA, Blumenthal NP, et al. Echocardiographic assessment of pulmonary hypertension in patients with advanced lung disease. Am J Respir Crit Care Med. 2003;167(5):735–40.

11. Worsley DF, Palevsky HI, Alavi A. Ventilation-perfusion lung scanning in the evaluation of pulmonary hypertension. J Nucl Med. 1994;35(5):793–6.

12. Rajaram S, Swift AJ, Condliffe R, Johns C, Elliot CA, Hill C, et al. CT features of pulmonary arterial hypertension and its major subtypes: a systematic CT evaluation of 292 patients from the ASPIRE registry. Thorax. 2015;70(4):382–7.

13. Montani D, Gunther S, Dorfmuller P, Perros F, Girerd B, Garcia G, et al. Pulmonary arterial hypertension. Orphanet J Rare Dis. 2013;8:97.

14. Lawrie A, Waterman E, Southwood M, Evans D, Suntharalingam J, Francis S, et al. Evidence of a role for osteoprotegerin in the pathogenesis of pulmonary arterial hypertension. Am J Pathol. 2008;172(1): 256–64.

15. Ma L, Chung WK. The genetic basis of pulmonary arterial hypertension. Hum Genet. 2014;133(5): 471–9.

16. Condliffe R, Howard LS. Connective tissue disease-associated pulmonary arterial hypertension. F1000Prime Rep. 2015;7:06.

17. Hussain N, Charalampopoulos A, Ramjug S, Condliffe R, Elliot CA, O'Toole L, et al. Pulmonary hypertension in patients with heart failure and preserved ejection fraction: differential diagnosis and management. Pulm Circ. 2016;6(1):3–14.

18. Guazzi M, Borlaug BA. Pulmonary hypertension due to left heart disease. Circulation. 2012;126(8):975–90.

19. Charalampopoulos A, Howard LS, Tzoulaki I, GinSing W, Grapsa J, Wilkins MR, et al. Response to pulmonary arterial hypertension drug therapies in patients with pulmonary arterial hypertension and cardiovascular risk factors. Pulm Circ. 2014;4(4):669–78.

20. Zangiabadi A, De Pasquale CG, Sajkov D. Pulmonary hypertension and right heart dysfunction in chronic lung disease. Biomed Res Int. 2014;2014:739674.

21. Lang IM, Madani M. Update on chronic thromboembolic pulmonary hypertension. Circulation. 2014;130(6):508–18.

22. Humbert M. Pulmonary arterial hypertension and chronic thromboembolic pulmonary hypertension: pathophysiology. Eur Respir Rev. 2010;19(115): 59–63.

23. Delcroix M, Lang I, Pepke-Zaba J, Jansa P, D'Armini AM, Snijder R, et al. Long-yerm outcome of patients with chronic thromboembolic pulmonary hypertension: results from an international prospective registry. Circulation. 2016;133(9):859–71.

24. Pritts CD, Pearl RG. Anesthesia for patients with pulmonary hypertension. Curr Opin Anaesthesiol. 2010;23(3):411–6.

25. Galie N, Humbert M, Vachiery JL, Gibbs S, Lang I, Torbicki A, et al. ESC/ERS Guidelines for the diagnosis and treatment of pulmonary hypertension. The Joint Task Force for the Diagnosis and Treatment of Pulmonary Hypertension of the European Society of Cardiology (ESC) and the European Respiratory Society (ERS). Endorsed by: Association for European Paediatric and Congenital Cardiology (AEPC), International Society for Heart and Lung Transplantation (ISHLT). Eur Respir J. 2015;46(4):903–75.

26. Hardinge M, Annandale J, Bourne S, Cooper B, Evans A, Freeman D, et al. British Thoracic Society guidelines for home oxygen use in adults. Thorax. 2015;70(Suppl 1):i1–43.

27. Barst RJ, Rubin LJ, Long WA, McGoon MD, Rich S, Badesch DB, Primary Pulmonary Hypertension Study Group, et al. A comparison of continuous intravenous epoprostenol (prostacyclin) with conventional therapy for primary pulmonary hypertension. N Engl J Med. 1996;334(5):296–301.

28. Garnock-Jones KP. Riociguat: a review of its use in patients with chronic thromboembolic pulmonary hypertension or pulmonary arterial hypertension. Drugs. 2014;74(17):2065–78.

29. Banks DA, Pretorius GV, Kerr KM, Manecke GR. Pulmonary endarterectomy: part I. Pathophysiology, clinical manifestations, and diagnostic evaluation of chronic thromboembolic pulmonary hypertension. Semin Cardiothorac Vasc Anesth. 2014;18(4): 319–30.

30. Fadel E, Mercier O, Mussot S, Leroy-Ladurie F, Cerrina J, Chapelier A, et al. Long-term outcome of double-lung and heart-lung transplantation for pulmonary hypertension: a comparative retrospective study of 219 patients. Eur J Cardiothorac Surg. 2010;38(3):277–84.

Transplantation

20

James L. Lordan

Introduction

Lung transplantation is an established therapeutic option for selected patients with end-stage respiratory disease failing to respond to conventional medical and surgical therapy. Lung transplantation is predominantly performed for survival benefit, but significant improvements in quality of life are achieved for the majority of lung transplant recipients [1].

The first human lung transplant was performed in 1963 by James Hardy, on a patient with severe emphysema and lung carcinoma, who died early of renal failure. Refinement of candidate selection, surgical technique, organ preservation, and immunosuppression led to the first successful heart-lung transplant in 1981 in a patient with idiopathic pulmonary arterial hypertension, followed by the first successful single-lung transplant (SLT) in 1983 in a patient with pulmonary fibrosis. Double-lung transplantation was performed in 1988 with a tracheal anastomosis, with later evolution to single sequential or bilateral lung transplantation (BLT), incorporating a mainstem bronchial anastomosis with reduced airway complications, which remains the lung transplant procedure of choice today.

J. L. Lordan
Cardiothoracic Block/Institute of Transplantation,
Freeman Hospital, Newcastle upon Tyne, UK
e-mail: Jim.Lordan@nuth.nhs.uk

Indications

The most common indications for lung transplantation reported in the ISHLT registry (January 1995 to June 2013) [2] are shown in Table 20.1. An understanding of the natural history of the individual conditions is essential to guide timing of listing for transplantation. The early referral and listing of patients for lung transplantation has been improved due to increased awareness of transplantation as an option of therapy, and the dissemination of respiratory disease-specific referral guidelines [3].

Selection of Lung Transplant Candidates: Referral and Listing Criteria

The selection of lung transplant recipients is an important factor affecting both early- and long-term survival post-transplantation and identifies patients most likely to benefit from transplantation [3]. The International Society of Heart and Lung Transplantation has published updated referral criteria in 2014 with specific disease-related recommendations to guide the timing of referral and listing for lung transplantation; to discuss the implementation of lung allocation scores by individual transplant centres; to identify intensive care strategies to bridge patients to transplantation with extra-corporeal membrane

Table 20.1 Indications for adult lung transplantation, single lung transplantation (SLT), bilateral lung transplantation (BLT), and total lung transplant procedures reported to the ISHLT registry from January 1995 to June 2014 [2]

Diagnosis	SLT (N = 16,226)	BLT (N = 29,457)	TOTAL (N = 45,683)
COPD/emphysema[a]	42.1%	26.7%	32.1%
Idiopathic pulmonary fibrosis	34.3%	18.5%	24.1%
Cystic fibrosis	1.4%	24.4%	16.2%
Alpha-1 AT def-emphysema[b]	4.9%	5.7%	5.4%
Idiopathic pulmonary arterial hypertension[c]	0.6%	4.2%	2.9%
Pulmonary fibrosis, other	4.7%	3.8%	4.1%
Bronchiectasis	0.4%	4.0%	2.7%
Sarcoidosis	1.9%	2.9%	2.5%
Re-transplantation: BOS	2.1%	1.5%	1.7%
Connective tissue disease	1.2%	1.6%	1.5%
Obliterative bronchiolitis (not retransplant)	0.7%	1.3%	1.1%
LAM	0.9%	1.1%	1.0%
Retransplant: Not-BOS	1.3%	0.8%	1.0%
Congenital heart disease[c]	0.6%	1.1%	0.9%
Cancer	0.0%	0.1%	0.1%
Other	3.1%	2.2%	2.6%

[a]Chronic Obstructive Pulmonary Disease (COPD)
[b]Alpha-1 Antitrypsin-deficiency assoc-COPD
[c]Pulmonary Hypertension, including idiopathic PAH and congenital heart disease [2]

oxygenation (ECMO) or Novalung technology in self-ventilating patients; and highlight expanded indications for lung transplantation.

In an era of expanding molecular medical and interventional therapeutic options, patients and clinicians may understandably see transplantation as a treatment of last resort, and be reluctant to engage with the process of lung transplantation. However, an early transplant referral will ensure a careful multi-disciplinary assessment, ensure comprehensive patient and carer education, facilitate overall adjustment to the prospect of lung transplantation, and essentially, improve or maintain physical conditioning and survival to a sufficient degree to benefit from transplantation.

General Considerations for Candidate Selection

The decision to list a candidate for transplantation identifies a candidate's reduced life expectancy from their underlying lung disease and a more favourable anticipated outcome with transplantation. The transplant candidate must be considered to be at a stage where this high-risk procedure is a necessity yet be strong enough physically and emotionally to survive the complex surgery and adhere to the demanding post-transplant immunosuppressive medical regimen. Specific criteria include: a candidate's high (>50%) risk of death within 2 years without transplantation, a high (>80%) likelihood of survival to 90 days post-transplantation, and an anticipated (>65%) prospect of survival to 5 years following successful transplantation.

Although age itself is not a contra-indication for transplantation, it is identified that older patients (age >65 years) have a poorer survival rate after lung transplantation, due to the more frequent presence of co-morbid diseases affecting early post-transplant recovery and longer term outcomes. Evaluation of a patient's biological age has facilitated listing for transplant in highly selected cases above this age cut-off.

Lung Transplant Assessment

The selection of suitable candidates is performed at the transplant centre, incorporating disease-specific factors, analysis of risk factors, and excluding any serious contraindications. Poor physical conditioning and severe organ dysfunction can be contraindications for transplantation in any age group. In selected cases, intensive physiotherapy and pulmonary rehabilitation can be implemented to improve the physical conditioning of patients with severe, advanced-stage chronic lung disease, sufficient to derive benefit from successful transplantation.

Contraindications

It is important to identify any specific co-morbid factors that adversely increase the risks of a poor outcome following transplantation. The presence of an absolute contraindication to transplantation, or the cumulative sum of relative co-morbid risk factors, may unfortunately preclude transplantation. This is important to ensure the optimum use of scarce donor organ resources and identify patients at highest likelihood of survival benefit from lung transplantation. A centre's resources, specific complex patient experience, transplant volume, and lung allocation criteria can impact on a centre's overall decision and timing to accept candidates with individual factors of increased risk, such as complex microbiological infections.

Absolute Contraindications

- Prior malignancy; a 5-year disease-free interval is recommended in the case of haematological malignancies, sarcoma, melanoma, or solid organ cancers (breast, bladder, bowel, or kidney). A 2-year interval may be appropriate in certain circumstances, for example, a non-melanoma skin malignancy with a low risk of recurrence.
- Irreversible organ dysfunction of brain, cardiac, renal, or liver. However, a dual organ transplantation can be considered in highly selected candidates (e.g. heart-lung or lung-liver transplantation).
- Coronary artery disease, in particular if not suitable for re-vascularisation, or other evidence of significant atherosclerosis-related end-organ disease or complications.

- Active or recurrent sepsis may preclude transplantation (e.g. uncontrolled urinary tract infections, renal calculi).
- Uncorrectable bleeding diathesis.
- Active or chronic infection. Inadequately controlled infection with highly virulent/resistant microbes (e.g. active *Mycobacterium tuberculosis* or *Burkholderia cenocepacia* infection).
- Chest wall deformity such as severe kyphoscoliosis; neuromuscular or diaphragm dysfunction.
- Body Mass Index >35 kg/m^2 (ideally BMI higher than 18 and less than 30)
- Poor adherence to a regimen of medical care.
- Ongoing psychiatric or psychological disease likely to impair post-transplant adherence to a regimen of care or affect long term outcome.
- Inadequate social support network.
- Physical frailty with poor rehabilitation potential.
- Active substance abuse or dependency (alcohol misuse, active cigarette smoking, nicotine, or illicit substances).

Relative Contraindications

- Age >65 with co-morbid factors.
- BMI 30–35 kg/m^2.
- Progressive cachexia (BMI <17 kg/m^2) unresponsive to nutritional supplementation, including percutaneous enteric gastrostomy or nasogastric feeding.
- Severe, symptomatic osteoporosis (particularly, if recent fractures).
- Previous thoracic surgery with pleuropulmonary adhesions or mediastinal shift.
- Mechanical ventilation.
- Highly virulent bacterial, fungal (mycetomas a concern, particularly if large, multiple, or close to pleural margin), or mycobacterial disease, in particular *M. Abscessus*.
- Extrapulmonary sepsis (e.g. uncontrolled urinary tract infections, renal calculi).
- Active hepatitis B or hepatitis C. Transplant may be considered in the absence of cirrhosis, portal hypertension, or absent virus replication (on blood virus PCR) on appropriate therapy in selected centres.

- Human immunodeficiency virus (HIV). Selected centres may consider transplantation if HIV disease controlled, HIV-RNA virus undetectable, and compliant with combination anti-retroviral therapy.
- *Mycobacterium abscessus*. There is a high risk of recurrence post-transplant with soft tissue pleuro-pulmonary or systemic infection. An ability to tolerate combination anti-mycobacterial treatment is important to confirm prior to lung transplantation, as prolonged/ongoing therapy is required post-transplant with associated morbidity.
- *Burkholderia* spp. or pan-resistant *Pseudomonas* colonisation, with absence of a bactericidal multiple-combination anti-microbial synergy testing regimen.
- *Burkholderia cenocepacia* (genomovar III) is considered an absolute contraindication in most centres due to risk of uncontrolled pulmonary, pleural, or systemic sepsis and poor post-transplant clinical outcomes.

Surgical Considerations

The development of pneumothorax is identified as a cause of acute serious clinical decline in advanced lung disease, supporting early intervention with intercostal drainage or pleurodesis if required for clinical stabilisation. Previous thoracic surgery is not uncommon in patients referred for lung transplantation. In the majority of cases, it does not preclude transplantation, but can be associated with increased risk of intra-operative bleeding, particularly if cardio-pulmonary bypass or ECMO is implemented with intra-operative anticoagulation, and potential sequelae including renal dysfunction, primary graft dysfunction, phrenic nerve damage, chylothorax, or requirement for re-exploration for bleeding. The presence of extensive pleuro-pulmonary or hilar adhesions with pleuro-pulmonary vascular collaterals may unduly increase the early surgical risks of transplantation due to bleeding or major early pleural sepsis, particularly in the setting of complex airway microbiology.

Disease Specific: Referral and Listing for Transplantation

Interstitial Lung Disease (ILD)

Both usual interstitial pneumonitis (UIP) and fibrotic non-specific interstitial pneumonitis (NSIP) are associated with a poor prognosis. Novel UIP/IPF treatment options, including pirfenidone and more recently nintedanib, have been reported to delay clinical progression, as measured by lung function, exacerbation reduction, exercise capacity, and possibly survival. Treatment is associated with significant medication-related adverse events, including gastro-intestinal upset, weight loss, liver function abnormalities, and photosensitivity. Disease progression is likely to occur, despite therapy, emphasising early consideration of lung transplantation. Single-lung transplant (SLT) has been performed for ILD over the decades, with acceptable long-term outcomes achieved. SLT remains an important opportunity to achieve transplantation for ILD patients, in the setting of limited donor organ availability and rapid clinical decline. The ISHLT has reported an increased use of bilateral lung transplantation (BLT) for patients with ILD, with early benefits in the setting of severe ILD-associated pulmonary hypertension. Bilateral lung transplantation offers some long-term benefits in the setting of lung allograft dysfunction, and is also the recommended procedure for COPD patients.

ILD: When to Refer for Lung Transplantation

- Diagnosis of usual interstitial pneumonitis (UIP) or fibrotic non-specific interstitial pneumonitis (NSIP)
- Inflammatory-related ILD with clinical progression despite a trial of anti-inflammatory therapy
- Dyspnoea and functional limitation
- Resting or exercise-related oxygen requirement
- Forced vital capacity (FVC) <80%, or diffusion capacity of the lung for carbon monoxide (DLCO) <40%

ILD: When to List for Lung Transplantation

- Decline in FVC ≥10% during 6 months of follow up
- Decline in DLCO ≥15% during 6 months of follow up
- Six minute walk test related O_2 desaturation <88%, an absolute distance <250 m, or a >50 m decline in walk distance over a 6 month follow up period.
- Pulmonary hypertension on echocardiogram or right heart catheterisation.
- Hospitalisation relating to clinical decline, pneumothorax, or acute exacerbation.

ILD-Specific Considerations

ILD can be associated with specific connective tissue diseases, with systemic manifestations. Specifically, scleroderma-related ILD or pulmonary arterial hypertension (PAH) can be complicated by systemic co-morbid factors adversely affecting listing for transplantation, including digital ulceration, myositis, renal crisis, or oesophageal dysmotility, with related potential for extra-oesophageal aspiration and pneumonia. Candidates are assessed for lung transplantation on an individual basis with respect to overall risks and predicted outcomes.

A combined upper zone emphysema and basal pulmonary fibrosis phenotype has been recently described with a rapid clinical decline and characterised by a markedly reduced DLCO, and deceptively well-preserved spirometry and static lung volumes, which might delay referral.

Cystic Fibrosis: Microbiological Issues Specific to Transplantation

In general, patients with cystic fibrosis are well prepared for transplantation referral, with established multi-disciplinary nutritional, diabetic, and microbiological input and adherence to a complex regime of care. The infectious disease issues related to potential lung candidates with CF are complex and challenging [4, 5]. Our knowledge and understanding of the effects of infections in the pre- and post-transplant periods is continually evolving. Advanced CF lung disease poses a specific challenge for transplantation, due to an associated complex microbiological profile, recurrent pulmonary sepsis, combination antibiotic requirements, and persistent colonisation of airways and sinuses by antimicrobial-resistant organisms. An increasing array of resistant bacterial, mycobacterial, and fungal species are being recognised as potential respiratory pathogens in CF, with a significant risk of early post-transplant deep surgical site infection. Excellence of surgical techniques, and peri-operative antibiotic prophylaxis to cover resistant isolates is optimised, including use of intra-operative taurolidine antiseptic pleural washout as a strategy to reduce pleural contamination.

Pre-transplant colonisation with multi-resistant or pan-resistant gram-negative bacilli, in isolation, is not an absolute contraindication to lung transplantation. Some transplant centres use multiple combination bactericidal testing (MCBT) synergy testing to identify an optimum peri-transplant bactericidal antibiotic combination.

The prevalence of methicillin-resistant staphylococcal strains (MRSA) has increased, reported in 20% of CF patients in the U.S., with attempted eradication recommended pre-transplant. Highly virulent strains, such as Panton-Valentine Leukocidin-positive (PVL+) MRSA have also emerged.

Burkholderia cepacia Complex (BCC)

BCC infection in CF is associated with a more rapid clinical decline, previously considered a contraindication for transplantation due to poor outcomes. Patients with non-cenocepacia BCC infection can be considered for listing, if other criteria are appropriate. Patients with *B. cenocepacia* (genomovar III) infection should only be considered by transplant centres applying novel research therapeutic strategies to eradicate infection post transplant. *B. gladioli* (which is not a member of the BCC) is increasing as a cause of chronic respiratory infection in CF, with significantly greater post-transplant mortality.

Fungal Disease

Aspergillus fumigatus, the most commonly cultured fungal species in the sputum of adult CF patients, is associated with increased early and late post-transplant invasive fungal infection and should be aggressively treated with anti-fungal therapy. The presence of large, multiple or peripheral mycetomas are a specific concern, and may preclude transplantation. *Scedosporium apiospermum* and *Pseudoallescheria boydii* are increasingly recognised as responsible for disseminated invasive pulmonary, skin, or central nervous system infections, with an associated poor prognosis. Early post-transplant prophylaxis with oral voriconazole, posaconazole, or caspofungin has been implemented with efficacy. Side effects have been noted with azoles, including frequent hepato-toxicity and photo-sensitivity. Inter-individual variability in voriconazole pharmacokinetics has lead to recommendations for interval azole blood level monitoring to ensure appropriate therapeutic levels are achieved. Careful monitoring for invasive fungal infection is required, as invasive fungal infection has been reported in the presence of, or following, cessation of voriconazole prophylaxis. Careful monitoring of calcineurin inhibitor levels is also required with introduction or cessation of azoles due to the recognised pharmacokinetic interaction.

Non-tuberculous Mycobacteria

An increased incidence of non-tuberculous mycobacteria (NTM)-positive sputum isolates has been noted in patients with CF, reported in 19% of patients referred for transplantation, emphasising regular surveillance. *M. avium* complex (MAC) and the *M. abscessus* complex are the most commonly isolated species. If a clinical decline unresponsive to standard treatment is noted with suggestive HRCT features, specific anti-mycobacterial therapy should be considered prior to transplant referral. Combination NTM regimens often include amikacin, cefoxitin, a macrolide, moxifloxacin, ethambutol or tigecycline, and adjunctive treatment with interferon gamma therapy can be considered. Progressive pulmonary or non-pulmonary NTM infection despite treatment, in particular with *M. abscessus*, or an inability to tolerate an NTM-specific therapeutic regimen, is a contraindication to transplantation.

Clostridium Difficile

CF patients have a high carriage of *C. difficile*, with the presence of pathogenic toxin-producing *C. difficile* strains present in 20–46.6% of stool samples from asymptomatic carriers. Severe *C. difficile*-associated disease has been reported in CF patients, particularly post-transplant, with high morbidity, where fulminant or pseudomembranous colitis can develop with a variable clinical presentation and a high requirement for urgent pan-colectomy and an associated 50% mortality rate reported [6].

Cystic Fibrosis: When to Refer for Transplantation

Lung transplant referral should be considered for patients with cystic fibrosis if:

- FEV1 <30% predicted, or
- Patients with advanced disease, and rapid decline in FEV1 despite optimum therapy (often females).
- Infection with non-tuberculous mycobacterial disease (NTM), or non-cenocepacia *B. cepacia* complex with/without diabetes mellitus.
- Six-minute walk distance <400 m.
- Evidence of pulmonary hypertension on echo (pulmonary artery systolic pressure >35 mmHg), or right heart catheter confirmed mean pulmonary artery pressure (mPAP) >25 mmHg.
- Increased frequency of exacerbations, particularly if associated with acute respiratory failure episode requiring non-invasive ventilation; increasing antibiotic resistance and failure to recover between exacerbations; declining nutritional state despite supplementation; pneumothorax; large volume haemoptysis despite bronchial embolization.

Cystic Fibrosis: When to List for Transplantation

- Established chronic respiratory failure:
  - Type 1: Hypoxia alone (PaO_2 < 8 kPa, 60 mmHg)
  - Type 2: Hypercapnia ($PaCO_2$ > 6.6 kPa, 50 mmHg)
- Established on non-invasive ventilation
- Pulmonary hypertension
- Frequent hospitalisation or home intravenous antibiotics
- Rapid lung function decline
- World Health Organisation functional class (WHO FC) IV
- Predicted 2 year survival <2 years.

Chronic Obstructive Pulmonary Disease (COPD)

Forty percent of lung transplants are performed worldwide for COPD and α1-anti-trypsin deficiency-related emphysema. Clinical disease progression is generally protracted, but often associated with significant limitation and impaired quality of life. The BODE score has been identified as a predictor of survival utilising a composite score that included body mass index (B), percentage predicted FEV1 as a measure of airflow obstruction (O), dyspnoea index (D), and functional exercise capacity (E). A BODE score of 7–10 is associated with an 80% risk of death at 4 years, and a score of 5–6 a mortality risk of 60% at 4 years.

A number of parameters were identified as predictors of survival in the National Emphysema Treatment Trial (NETT study). Surgical lung volume reduction (LVRS) and, more recently, bronchoscopic lung volume reduction (BLVR) has been shown to improve functional outcome for selected COPD patients. LVRS was considered as an initial therapeutic option prior to considering transplantation for COPD patients with a predicted FEV1 < 25% but >20%, DLCO >20%, and a heterogeneous distribution of emphysema on thoracic high-resolution CT scanning (HRCT). Previous surgery or endobronchial valve therapy does not preclude transplantation. Bilateral lung transplantation is the preferred procedure of choice for patients with COPD due to improved long-term outcomes.

COPD: When to Refer for Transplant

- Evidence of disease progression, despite maximum medical and interventional treatment including medication, oxygen, pulmonary rehabilitation, and lung volume reduction measures, if applicable.
- Candidates not suitable for surgical or endoscopic lung volume reduction intervention. Bilateral lung transplantation is the recommended operation for COPD patients.
- BODE index of 5–6.
- $PaCO_2$ > 6.6 kPa (>50 mmHg) and/or PaO_2 < 8 kPa (<60 mmHg)
- FEV1 < 25% predicted.

COPD: When to Consider Listing for Transplant

- BODE index $\geq$ 7.
- FEV1 < 15–20% predicted.
- Frequent severe exacerbations requiring hospitalisation.
- Severe exacerbation with hypercapnic respiratory failure requiring NIV.
- Moderate to severe pulmonary hypertension.

Pulmonary Arterial Hypertension (PAH)

An understanding of the natural history of pulmonary hypertension is important to guide optimal timing of listing for lung transplantation [7]. The increasing array of treatment options for PAH has markedly affected timing of referral of patients for transplantation. Connective tissue disease such as scleroderma-related PAH is associated with a poor response to targeted therapy. Lung transplant should be considered on an individual basis, with a careful assessment of co-morbid systemic disease entities.

A particular concern is the late referral of specific PAH patients for transplantation with prognostic markers of advanced disease, including evidence of hemodynamic instability, inotrope dependence, established severe right ventricle (RV) dysfunction, and renal or liver dysfunction. The presence of advanced PAH is likely to impact adversely on the patient's ability to survive on the waiting list to achieve transplantation and maintain physical conditioning sufficient for early postoperative rehabilitation. A number of markers identifying a poor prognosis for iPAH patients have been incorporated into the ISHLT referral guidelines for transplantation. Novel surgical strategies can be considered as a bridge to transplant for patients with rapid clinical decline despite maximal medical therapy, including balloon atrial septostomy, veno-arterial ECMO, or the pumpless Novalung® lung assist device with shunting conduits from the pulmonary artery to the left atrium which allows decompression and reverse remodelling of the failing right heart and improvement of right ventricular function prior to transplantation. Bilateral lung transplantation is the recommended operation for PAH, whereas heart-lung transplantation is reserved for selected patients with complex congenital heart disease.

PAH: When to Refer for Transplant Assessment

- Persisting NYHA FC III or IV symptoms.
- Optimal combination PH therapy including systemic prostanoid therapy.
- Rapidly progressive disease despite therapy.
- Suspected diagnosis of pulmonary veno-occlusive disease (VOD) or pulmonary capillary haemangiomatosis (PCH).

PAH: When to List for Lung Transplantation

- Persisting NYHA FC III or class IV symptoms despite optimal PH combination therapy including a systemic prostanoid.

- Six-minute walk distance <350 m.
- Cardiac index <2 L/min/m^2.
- Mean right atrial pressure (RAP) > 15 mmHg.
- Persisting adverse clinical features of right heart failure, including pericardial effusion, rising bilirubin, renal insufficiency, ascites.
- Significant haemoptysis.

Heart-Lung Transplantation

Combined heart-lung transplantation (HLT) is specifically considered for patients with an intrinsic severe pulmonary abnormality and irreversible myocardial dysfunction, with defects of cardiac valves or chambers not amenable to repair. HLT is performed most frequently for complex congenital heart disease. Timing of listing for HLT can be challenging for congenital heart disease, reflecting parameters of right heart failure including persistent NYHA FC IV in conjunction with poor haemodynamic parameters. Cardio-pulmonary sarcoidosis of a severe combined nature is ideally managed by HLT.

Lung Re-transplantation

Re-transplantation is associated with reduced long-term outcomes compared to primary lung transplant procedures, accounting for a small proportion of total lung transplant procedures performed [2]. Re-transplantation is performed most frequently for patients with advanced Bronchiolitis Obliterans Syndrome (BOS) phenotype of chronic lung allograft dysfunction (CLAD) demonstrating significantly better outcomes compared to patients with Primary Graft Dysfunction (PGD), early airway complications, or restrictive allograft syndrome (RAS). Candidates are selected on the basis of single-organ pulmonary failure, and an absence of other co-morbid risk factors. Single-lung transplant is often considered, but bilateral lung transplantation is often preferred, to remove any adverse potential for immunological stimulation or infection risk from the remaining failed allograft lung.

Donor Organ Optimisation Strategies

There remains a significant shortage of available donor organs, limiting the number of transplant procedures performed, which can lead to prolonged waiting list times for candidates, and affect the ability of rapidly declining candidates to survive to achieve transplantation. Ideal donor lung criteria include age less than 55 years old, less than 20-pack-a-year smoking history, absent chest trauma, clear chest radiograph, PaO_2/FiO_2 >300, and absence of purulent secretions or organisms on gram stain of respiratory samples.

A number of strategies have been developed to increase organ numbers for transplantation including: optimisation of national organ donation policies and legislation changes in certain countries (for example, opt out versus opt in for organ donation); the use of organs donated after cardiac death (DCD) in addition to organ donation after brain-stem death; use of extended criteria donor organs; the development of improved organ preservation solutions and techniques; and the use of *ex vivo* lung perfusion (EVLP) technology to optimise the function of donor organs with initial borderline function to a condition appropriate for later successful lung transplantation [8]. At the time of lung transplant assessment, candidates are counselled and consented regarding the precise extended donor organ criteria they would accept for transplantation. Personal preferences can be later revised as required, based on clinical status.

Donor Lung Allocation Policies

Lung allocation policies have been developed in the United Kingdom, Euro-transplant, and U.S.-based Organ Procurement and Transplantation Network (OPTN) to ensure equitable access to transplantation. Composite lung allocation scores (LAS) are implemented to improve the overall utilisation of donor lungs, facilitate urgent listing and early transplantation for patients at high risk of death on the waiting list, and identify those likely to benefit most from transplantation.

Clinical Decline on the Transplant Waiting List

The mortality on the transplant waiting list remains unacceptably high, currently approximately 20%. Intubation and prolonged mechanical ventilation should be avoided in the setting of clinical decline, as outcomes post-transplant for ventilated candidates are poor, resulting from the associated physical deconditioning and infection risk. Palliative care and symptom-control measures should be implemented in parallel for candidates with severe disease, where the later development of candidate frailty or co-morbid factors may preclude further consideration for transplantation due to futility.

Advanced Bridge to Transplant Strategies in Rapidly Declining Candidates

Carefully selected candidates can be considered for intensive care-based bridge to transplantation strategies. Ideally, patients should be psycho-socially and physically robust, free from adverse co-morbid factors, sepsis, or multi-organ dysfunction, and have been assessed, counselled, and accepted for lung transplant listing. Patients can be considered for support technology which may include Novalung® lung-assist device (LAD) or extra-corporeal membrane oxygenation (ECMO) [9]. The evolution of Novalung® and extra-corporeal membrane oxygenator (ECMO) membrane technology and vascular access cannulation devices has reduced ECMO-related complications, allowing prolonged patient support for weeks to months while awaiting lung transplantation, ideally in an awake, non-ventilated setting facilitating a degree of ongoing physiotherapy [10, 11]. The presence of high-circulating levels of pre-formed HLA antibodies may exclude transplantation. An urgent national lung allocation policy is important for early access to suitable donor organs to minimise the risk of intensive care complications affecting listing status.

The Novalung® lung-assist device has been applied as a bridge to transplantation for patients with hypercapnic respiratory failure, providing modest oxygenation but highly efficient CO2 removal, with cannulation involving the femoral artery and femoral vein [11]. It can be used in conjunction with non-invasive ventilation, avoiding intubation. Novalung® cannulation from pulmonary artery to left atrium has also been applied as a low-pressure oxygenating shunt device to bridge pulmonary arterial hypertension patients to lung transplantation, facilitating right ventricular reverse remodelling [7, 11].

Awake extra-corporeal membrane oxygenation (ECMO) is the preferred mode of bridging to transplant support for patients with severe hypoxia, preferably with the use of a single veno-venous Avalon® internal jugular central catheter device. If patients have hemodynamic instability then veno-arterial cannulation is required, with associated increased risk of ECMO-related complications including bleeding, thrombosis, infection, or cannulation-related problems including limb ischaemia with femoral cannulation. Development of multi-organ failure should be managed by palliative care.

Surgical Techniques

In general a bilateral thoracotomy, thoraco-sternotomy, or midline sternotomy approach is applied for lung transplantation, depending on surgeon preference and recipient-specific factors [12]. Cardio-pulmonary bypass or intra-operative ECMO is frequently required for transplantation due to intra-operative haemodynamic instability. Bilateral lung transplantation (BLT) is the procedure of choice for patients with cystic fibrosis and bronchiectasis, due to pulmonary sepsis, and increasingly for COPD/emphysema and interstitial lung disease, due to improved longer term outcomes. BLT is required for ILD patients with pulmonary hypertension, due to a higher risk of severe PGD.

Other procedures can be performed in specific circumstances for smaller recipients, specifically utilising lung volume-reduction measures for size matching: for example lobectomy or wedge resection; living-related lobar transplantation (less frequently performed now); or cadaveric bilateral lobar transplantation. These strategies have improved the options of achieving lung transplantation for smaller or paediatric lung transplant recipients where limited donor availability may lead to prolonged wait list times and associated clinical decline [12, 13].

Heart-lung transplantation is reserved for patients with complex congenital heart disease with Eisenmenger's physiology and defects not amenable to surgical repair (e.g. large atrial septal defect or ventricular septal defect), or candidates with co-morbid severe cardiac dysfunction.

Early Post-transplant Complications

Primary Graft Dysfunction

Primary Graft Dysfunction (PGD) is a severe form of ischaemia-re-perfusion lung injury process characterised clinically by pulmonary infiltrates, reduced PaO_2/FiO_2 ratio, and reduced lung compliance in the first 72 h post-transplant [14]. PGD affects between 10% and 25% of lung transplant recipients early post-transplant, with a 30-day mortality of 50% in severe grades of PGD. A higher incidence is noted in recipients with ILD and PAH, but also affected by donor characteristics and operative factors (use of cardio-pulmonary bypass or blood product transfusion). Treatment strategies are generally supportive, including the use of early inhaled NO, lung-protective ventilatory strategies, and avoiding fluid overload in the setting of capillary leakage. Early ECMO has been implemented with benefit in severe PGD associated with severe hypoxia and haemodynamic instability. An impact on long-term allo-immunity and reduced long-term BOS-free survival has been reported in severe cases independent of acute rejection episodes, lymphocytic bronchiolitis, or community respiratory virus infections.

Airway Complications

A main-stem bronchial anastomosis is performed for lung transplantation, with a tracheal anastomosis utilised for combined heart-lung procedures [12]. Airway anastomotic dehiscence is a rare but serious complication post-transplant, particularly if complicated by broncho-pleural fistula formation, and requires early surgical repair or stenting. Later airway complications include bronchial stenosis formation, either at anastomosis or bronchus intermedius, and are generally managed by serial bronchoscopic dilatation or airway stent placement.

Pulmonary Vascular Complications

Pulmonary artery or venous anastomotic complications are rare, but may be catastrophic. Early identification is important, requiring early surgical revision to avoid irreversible ischaemia of the transplanted lung in severe cases.

Infections

Infections are a frequent cause of morbidity and mortality post-transplantation (Fig. 20.1). Early extubation is preferred post-transplant, aggressive airway clearance physiotherapy and early mobilisation recommended, and intercostal drain removal reduces analgesia requirements. Tailored anti-microbial cover is applied depending on pre-transplant isolates and sensitivities, supported by multi-combination antibiotic synergy test results in specific centres.

Surgical wound infections with pre-transplant colonising organisms are a particular cause for morbidity in the early post-transplant period, specifically with bacterial or fungal organisms [4, 5, 15]. Invasive tracheo-bronchial, bronchial anastomotic, mediastinal, or pleural infections can result both early and late from Aspergillus, Candida, Fusarium or Scedosporium species, with risk of haematogenous dissemination. Specific tailored prophylactic anti-microbial regimens including fluconazole, posaconazole, voriconazole, caspofungin, taurolidine, or inhaled amphotericin B are employed in the early post-operative period to reduce the risk of infection [4, 12, 15]. Early identification by bronchoscopy with galactomannan testing and fungal culture, imaging with CT thorax, and prompt anti-microbial or required surgical intervention is important in the heavily immunosuppressed lung transplant recipient [16].

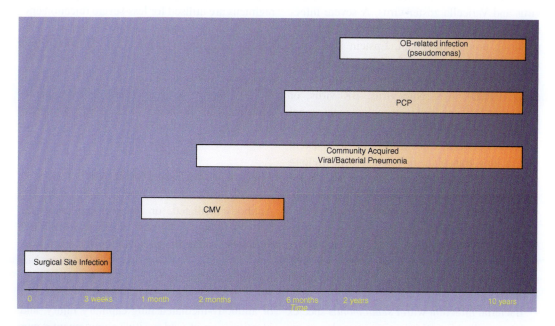

Fig. 20.1 Infectious complications frequently encountered in lung transplant recipients in the first year post-transplant

Cytomegalovirus (CMV) and Human Herpes Viruses

CMV is a common infection in lung transplant recipients with significant adverse and immunological effects on lung allograft function, clinically manifesting as viraemic symptoms of malaise, low-grade fever, myelosuppression, lung function decline, pneumonitis-related infiltrates, or gastro-intestinal upset. It most frequently develops from 1 to 4 months post-transplant, the timing affected by the precise valganciclovir prophylaxis regimen implemented, with specific risk dependent on the recipient (R) and donor (D) CMV antibody status at the time of transplantation. High-risk CMV recipient-negative and donor-positive transplant recipients are treated with prophylactic valganciclovir for 3–6 months post-transplant to reduce the risk of early CMV infection. Early post-transplant monitoring protocols are implemented with weekly quantitative blood CMV PCR blood levels to identify asymptomatic CMV viraemia, prompting early preemptive valganciclovir therapy administered to reduce CMV infectious consequences, while seroconversion and immunity develops [15].

Early prophylaxis with acyclovir is recommended to prevent infection with human herpes virus and Varicella zoster virus. A severe infection may develop in immunosuppressed patients, requiring prompt treatment. Epstein Barr virus infection can be associated with early development of post-transplant lymphoproliferative disorder (PTLD). West Nile virus, BK virus, or parvovirus B19 can lead to encephalopathy, renal infection, or red cell aplasia.

Pneumocystis jirovecii infection is a persistent risk in lung transplant recipients, with lifelong prophylaxis recommended. The recommended agents include cotrimoxazole, trimethoprim/dapsone, or less frequently, nebulised pentamidine.

Mycobacterium tuberculosis infection may occur due to re-activation or primary infection, requiring combination anti-mycobacterial regimen treatments that may interact with immunosuppressive therapy.

Bacterial infection with *Pseudomonas* species and Aspergillus fungal infection may also occur in the setting of chronic lung allograft dysfunction, with associated significant morbidity and accelerated lung function decline.

Acute Cellular Rejection

Acute rejection occurs in up to 36% of lung transplant recipients in the first year [17]. Patients may be asymptomatic, or the clinical presentation may be non-specific and include low-grade pyrexia, cough, dyspnoea, leukocytosis, pleural effusions or pulmonary infiltrates on chest radiograph, and/or a decline in oxygenation. Investigation with fibreoptic bronchoscopy is performed in the event of clinical decline, specifically with broncho-alveolar lavage to identify any bacterial, fungal or atypical infection, and transbronchial lung biopsy to confirm any suspected mild to severe acute vascular rejection which is graded A2–A4, by histological confirmation of peri-vascular lymphocytic infiltrates. Acute rejection in the first 3 months post-transplant, or severe episodes, are treated with augmented corticosteroids (10 mg/kg IV methylprednisolone for 3 days followed by gradual steroid taper from 1 mg/kg/day prednisolone, reducing by 0.2 mg/kg/week to maintenance levels). Oral tapering corticosteroid augmentation regimens are utilised for less-severe rejection episodes, with initial prednisolone dosing of 1 mg/kg/day. Occasionally, steroid-resistant, persistent, or recurrent cellular rejection may be noted, prompting the use of anti-thymocyte globulin (ATG), alternative T-cell depleting agents, or adjustment of the maintenance immunosuppression regimen.

Antibody-Mediated Rejection

Antibody-mediated, or humoral, rejection has been identified as a cause of allograft dysfunction, which may be suspected by the identification of *de novo* or rising titres of HLA class I or II donor-specific antibodies, the presence of lung allograft dysfunction, histological confirmation of antibody-mediated lung capillary injury, and identification of C4d positive complement deposition in lung parenchymal tissue. Humoral rejection may occur in parallel with a severe acute cellular acute rejection episode, and treatment of any associated cellular rejection with corticosteroids is recommended. Specific strategies for treatment of antibody-mediated rejection include antibody removal by sequential plasmapheresis or immune-adsorption followed by intravenous immunoglobulin therapy, and the subsequent use of rituximab (anti-CD20 monoclonal antibody) to deplete B cells and suppress antibody production. Bortezomib, a proteasome inhibitor which acts on plasma cells and eculizumab, a humanized anti-complement C5 antibody have been applied in highly selected resistant cases.

Immunosuppression and Associated Adverse Effects

Triple therapy immunosuppression is introduced early post-transplant in most transplant centres (Fig. 20.2) [16]. Protocol induction therapy is utilised by the majority of centres, but may be avoided in the presence of high-risk microbiology.

Induction therapy consists of a brief regimen of T cell-depleting therapy with the use of polyclonal anti-T cell preparations (anti-thymocyte globulin) or monoclonal antibodies aimed at lymphocyte surface molecules including CD3 (OKT3), IL-2R/CD25 (basiliximab, daclizumab), or CD52 (alemtuzumab). In brief, OKT3 prevents T-cell activation, daclizumab and basiliximab inhibit T-cell proliferation and differentiation, and alemtuzumab causes leukocyte depletion. A centre-specific triple combination immune suppression is commenced including a calcineurin inhibitor (CNI) (ciclosporin A or tacrolimus), a cell cycle inhibitor (azathioprine or mycophenolate mofetil), and prednisolone in slowly tapering doses.

The introduction of the mammalian target of rapamycin (mTOR) inhibitors (sirolimus and everolimus) has widened the range of combinations, but generally avoided early post-transplant due to impairment of wound healing. Randomized controlled studies have failed to indicate clear superiority of any of the above-named triple therapy regimens with respect to the development of chronic lung allograft dysfunction (CLAD), manifesting as bronchiolitis obliterans syndrome (BOS) or restrictive allograft syndrome (RAS), as discussed later. Immunosuppression is continued life-long, with frequent monitoring of levels, and regimens adjusted accordingly if adverse effects occur.

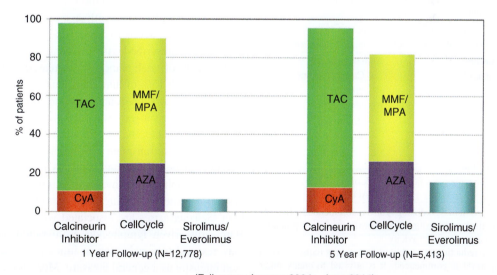

Fig. 20.2 Maintenance immunosuppression at time of follow-up for adult lung transplant patients under follow up by ISHLT Registry. Adapted from Ref [4] with permission

Calcineurin Inhibitors

Calcineurin inhibitors (CNIs) include ciclosporin and tacrolimus. Ciclosporin prevents IL-2-mediated CD4+ T cell activation and proliferation by binding to cyclophilin, preventing calcineurin de-phosphorylation of nuclear factor of activated T-cells (NFAT) and blocking nuclear translocation and transcriptional activity in the production of inflammatory proteins. Tacrolimus binds to immunophilin, an FK-binding protein, inhibiting calcineurin and preventing activation and translocation of NFAT with reduced IL-2 mediated proliferation of T-cells. CNIs are commenced early post-transplant, requiring frequent monitoring of CNI blood levels and awareness of drug metabolic interactions via the hepatic cytochrome P450 pathway for optimum dosing, and regular FBC, U&Es, and LFT checks required to identify side effects (Table 20.2).

CNIs are frequently associated with progressive nephrotoxicity that may range from mild renal dysfunction to end-stage renal disease (estimated GFR <50% in 37% of cases), requiring

Table 20.2 Immunosuppression medication interactions encountered in lung transplant recipients treated with a calcineurin inhibitor, such as ciclosporin or tacrolimus, requiring dose adjustment and more frequent trough level measurement

Drugs that increase calcineurin inhibitor[a] levels	Drugs that decrease calcineurin inhibitor[a] levels
Diltiazem	Anticonvulsants
Verapamil	– Carbamazepine
Antifungal azoles	– Phenytoin
– eg Voriconazole	Antibiotics
Macrolides	– Rifampicin
– Erythromycin	– Rifabutin
– Clarithromycin	
Cimetidine	
Risk of acute renal failure	Risk of acute rejection/CLAD[b]

A reduction in CNI dosing is also recommended when co-prescribed with sirolimus or everolimus due to potential for increased nephrotoxicity

A 75% reduction in azathioprine dosing is required when allopurinol is commenced. It is advised to check other new medications for potential interactions before co-prescribing

[a]Includes ciclosporin and tacrolimus

[b]Chronic lung allograft dysfunction (CLAD)

hemodialysis in 3.2% cases and renal transplantation reported in 0.7% at 5 years' post-transplant. Neurotoxicity is a common side effect of CNIs, manifesting more commonly as tremor, headaches, or peripheral neuropathy. Less common but more serious neurological manifestations include seizures and posterior reversible leuco-encephalopathy syndrome (PRES) which may require a switch to an alternative CNI, dose reduction strategies, or a switch to an alternative agent such as sirolimus or everolimus. Levetiracetam is a suitable medication in transplant recipients for seizure management, due to limited interactions with transplant immunosuppression. Other side effects of ciclosporin include electrolyte disturbances, hirsutism, gingival hyperplasia, and rarely, haemolytic uremic syndrome. However, tacrolimus is not associated with hirsutism, but increases the risk of post-transplant diabetes mellitus. At 5 years' post-transplant, recipients have developed complications (Table 20.3) including systemic hypertension (82%), dyslipidaemia (58%), and diabetes (41%).

Hypertension is preferably treated with the calcium channel blockers including nifedipine or amlodipine. Diltiazem and verapamil are avoided due to potentiating effects on circulating CNI blood levels. Angiotensin-converting enzyme inhibitors, losartan, or doxazosin are alternatives.

Hyperlipidaemia is a common side effect, routinely treated with statins, with atorvastatin as the preferred treatment due to a safer side effect profile when co-prescribed with CNIs.

The risk of malignancy is increased post-transplant with 15% of lung transplant recipients affected at 5 years, predominantly including skin malignancies in sun-exposed areas, emphasising avoidance measures and surveillance (Table 20.4). However, post-transplant lymphoproliferative disease can develop, manifesting as pulmonary nodules, lymphadenopathy, or affect other extra-pulmonary sites including the gastro-intestinal tract. Selected cases are associated with Epstein Barr virus-driven lymphocyte proliferation and may respond to a reduction in immunosuppression intensity as a general measure. More aggressive forms may require formal chemotherapy with interval rituximab or CHOP regimens, with significant associated infection risk and morbidity.

Table 20.3 Frequency of cumulative morbidity in lung transplant survivors within 1, 5, and 10 years post transplant. Follow-up from April 1994 to June 2014

Outcome	1 year	5 years	10 years
Hypertension	51.7%	80.7%	–
Renal dysfunction	22.5%	53.3%	71.9%
Abnormal Creatinine ≤2.5 mg/dl (220 μmol/L)	15.7%	35.3%	–
Creatinine >2.5 mg/dl (220 μmol/L)	5.0%	14.3%	18.7%
Chronic Dialysis	1.7%	3.0%	7.3%
Renal transplant	0.1%	0.8%	4.6%
Hyperlipidemia	26.2%	57.9%	–
Diabetes	23.0%	39.5%	–
Bronchiolitis Obliterans syndrome	9.3%	41.1%	64.6%

Adapted from Yusen RD, Edwards LB, Kucherayavaya AY, Benden C, Dipchand AI, Goldfarb SB, et al. The Registry of the International Society for Heart and Lung Transplantation: Thirty-second Official Adult Lung and Heart-Lung Transplantation Report – 2015; Focus Theme: Early Graft Failure. J Heart Lung Transplant. 2015;34(10):1264–77. With permission from Elsevier

Table 20.4 Cumulative post transplant malignancy percentage rates in adult lung transplant recipient survivors under follow-up from April 1994 to June 2014

Malignancy/type		1-year survivors	5-year survivors	10-year survivors
No malignancy		96.3%	83.4%	70.9%
Malignancy (combined)		3.7%	16.6%	29.1%
Sub-type	Skin %	36%	71%	72%
	Lymphoma %	35%	9%	9%
	Other[a] %	26%	24%	28%
	Type not reported %	3%	1%	0

[a]Other malignancies reported within each time period included adenocarcinoma (2; 2; 1), bladder (2; 1; 0), lung (2; 4; 0), breast (1; 5; 2); prostate (0; 5; 1), cervical (1; 1; 0); liver (1; 1; 1); and colon (1; 1; 0). Adapted from Yusen RD, Edwards LB, Kucherayavaya AY, Benden C, Dipchand AI, Goldfarb SB, et al. The Registry of the International Society for Heart and Lung Transplantation: Thirty-second Official Adult Lung and Heart-Lung Transplantation Report – 2015; Focus Theme: Early Graft Failure. J Heart Lung Transplant. 2015;34(10):1264–77. With permission from Elsevier

Cell Cycle Inhibitors

Azathioprine is an orally available antimetabolite, converted into 6-mercaptopurine via hepatic enzymes. It is recommended to test for thiopurine methyltransferase (TPMT) activity prior to use, as very low TPMT activity leads to accumulation of azathioprine and profound myelosuppression and toxicity (low TPMT levels found in 11% of population, with very low levels noted in 1 in 300 people). Azathioprine is administered pre-operatively (2 mg/kg, dose adjusted if reduced TPMT activity), and halts DNA replication and induces CD28 cell apoptosis, causing dose-dependent T-cell destruction. Myelosuppression may result in thrombocytopenia, leukopenia, and macrocytic anaemia. Hepatotoxicity and increased risk of malignancy are reported. Azathioprine has multiple drug interactions, most notable is allopurinol, an inhibitor of xanthine oxidase. Azathioprine dose reduction (by 75%), or cessation, is required if treatment of gout or hyperuricemia with allopurinol is commenced, as inhibition of xanthine oxidase leads to decreased metabolism of 6-mercaptopurine, with subsequent elevated circulating levels causing bone marrow toxicity.

Mycophenolate Mofetil

Mycophenolate mofetil (MMF) is an alternative agent with beneficial immunosuppressive effects, including the inhibition of *de novo* purine synthesis therefore blocking proliferation of T and B lymphocytes, and also induction of apoptosis of activated T-cells. MMF can be administered orally or intravenously. CellCept® (MMF) is an immediate-release product, whereas the related preparation, Myfortic® is enteric coated, helping to reduce the dose-limiting side effects of gastrointestinal upset and diarrhoea that are frequently observed. Other side effects include leukopenia and bone marrow suppression.

Mammalian Target of Rapamycin (mTOR) Inhibitors

mTOR inhibitors, including sirolimus and everolimus, are being increasingly used in CNI-sparing regimens in the setting of CNI-intolerance or side effects supporting dose reduction, such as nephrotoxicity, haemolytic uraemic syndrome, or neurotoxicity (e.g. reversible posterior leuco-encephalopathy). Sirolimus is taken once daily, and is less nephrotoxic than CNI therapy. When given in combination, ciclosporin dosing is reduced considerably as sirolimus can increase circulating levels of ciclosporin, potentiating nephropathy. Other side effects of sirolimus include dyslipidemia, hypertension, myelosuppression, skin fragility syndrome, and thrombotic microangiopathy. Specific pulmonary side effects have also been reported with sirolimus, including interstitial pneumonitis, organizing pneumonia, and alveolar haemorrhage.

Corticosteroids

Glucocorticoids are an essential requirement for the prevention and treatment of acute rejection due to their anti-inflammatory and immunosuppressive activity, albeit with a significant side effect profile. 500 mg iv Methylprednisolone is administered intra-operatively, and in the first 24 h post-transplant (125 mg eight hourly for three doses). Prednisolone (1 mg/kg/day) is subsequently administered in a gradually tapering fashion to a maintenance dose of 5–10 mg daily over the ensuing month.

Chronic Lung Allograft Dysfunction

Despite appropriate immunosuppression, approximately 50% of lung allograft recipients develop chronic lung allograft dysfunction (CLAD) at 5 years' post-transplant (Table 20.5) [18, 19]. Identified risk factors include early PGD, recurrent acute rejection episodes, cytomegalovirus (CMV) infections, the presence of donor-specific antibodies, and community respiratory virus infections. Most commonly, this manifests

Table 20.5 Phenotypes of chronic lung allograft dysfunction (CLAD) [18, 19]

Bronchiolitis obliterans syndrome	Restrictive allograft dysfunction
Obstructive (FEV1 ≤ 80% of stable)	Restrictive (TLC ≤ 90%), FEV1/VC ratio normal or increased
HRCT: Inspiratory and expiratory imaging Air trapping ± bronchiectasis; tree in bud opacities; minimal infiltrates	HRCT: Inspiratory and expiratory imaging Interstitial upper lobe infiltrates, ground glass, honeycombing ± bronchiectasis; air trapping
Histology: Obliterative bronchiolitis; difficult to diagnose by TBBx as patchy process BAL neutrophilia >15%	Histology: Parenchymal and pleural fibrosis ± obliterative bronchiolitis
Clinical course: Progressive but may stabilise	Clinical course: Frequently relentlessly progressive; may start or coincide with BOS
Potential co-existent chronic bacterial or fungal infection	Correlates with the presence of early diffuse alveolar damage post-transplant
May evolve to RAS	
Treatment: 40% azithromycin-responsive	Treatment: Poor response to azithromycin
Re-transplantation: Potential benefit	Re-transplantation: Poor outcomes

clinically as bronchiolitis obliterans syndrome (BOS) with symptomatic breathlessness, variable hypoxia, lung function decline with progressive small airflow obstruction, possible airway neutrophilia, and expiratory HRCT imaging confirming features of small airflow obstruction-related mosaicism and bronchial wall dilatation and thickening (Fig. 20.3). A proposed classification of CLAD post-transplant (Fig. 20.4) includes bronchiolitis obliterans syndrome (BOS), azithromycin-responsive allograft dysfunction (ARAD) with neutrophilia, [18, 20] and the more recently described restrictive allograft syndrome (RAS) (Fig. 20.5a, b and Table 20.5) which frequently progresses relentlessly despite treatment [18, 19].

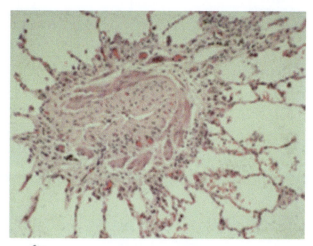

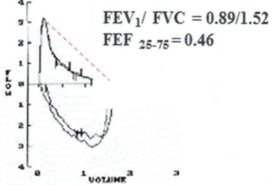

$FEV_1/\ FVC = 0.89/1.52$

$FEF\ _{25\text{-}75} = 0.46$

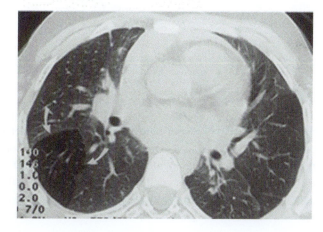

Fig. 20.3 Bronchiolitis obliterans syndrome phenotype of CLAD manifesting with patchy obliterative bronchiolitis histological lesions, airflow obstruction on flow volume loop, and small airway mosaicism on expiratory high-resolution CT thorax imaging

Fig. 20.4 Proposed phenotypic classification of chronic lung allograft dysfunction. From Suwara M, Vanaudenaerde BM, Verleden SE, Vos R, Green NJ, Ward C. Mechanistic differences between phenotypes of chronic lung allograft dysfunction after lung transplantation. Transpl Int. 2014;27(8):857–67. With permission from John Wiley and Sons

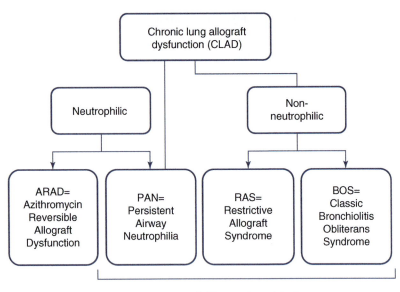

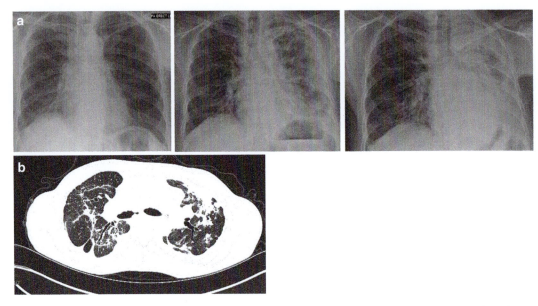

Fig. 20.5 Restrictive allograft syndrome (RAS) phenotype of CLAD manifesting as (**a**) progressive peripheral and upper zone radiographic infiltrates; (**b**) high-resolution CT thorax images of progressive pleuro-parenchymal upper zone infiltrates

BOS is defined as a persistent obstructive decline in FEV1 (≥20%) in two measurements taken at least 3 weeks apart. BOS is the clinical manifestation of an inflammatory bronchiolitis associated with fibrotic remodelling of the small and medium-sized airways, and is characterized by variable loss of allograft function with development of airflow obstruction and increased risk of bacterial and fungal infections. The importance of recognizing the specific phenotype of CLAD is suggested by the significantly worse survival of patients with RAS compared to recipients with BOS. Specific therapies of benefit for CLAD, therefore, include the use of low-dose

Fig. 20.6 Adult lung transplant survival demonstrating long-term outcomes post-transplant for different transplant indications [2]

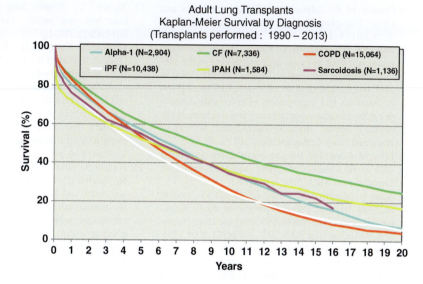

Adult Lung Transplants
Kaplan-Meier Survival by Diagnosis
(Transplants performed : 1990 – 2013)

alternate-day azithromycin, anti-reflux therapy, and total lymphoid irradiation (TLI).

Gastroesophageal reflux is common post-lung transplant, with recent studies suggesting that aspiration, characterised by the presence of pepsin and bile acids in bronchoalveolar lavage, may be present as early as 1 month post-transplant, supporting the need for early assessment of reflux and consideration of oesophageal fundoplication [21]. Early management with surgical fundoplication has been associated with greater freedom from BOS and improved survival.

The use of potent anti-inflammatory therapy with high-dose prednisolone or cytolytic therapy has not been shown to be of benefit and is generally avoided. Prompt treatment of *Pseudomonas* or fungal infection is important, as previous studies have shown that de novo colonization of the lung allograft by *Pseudomonas* is strongly associated with the subsequent development of BOS [22]. Methotrexate has been used to stabilise lung function in selected cases. Both total lymphoid irradiation (TLI) and extracorporeal photophoresis has been implemented to reduce the rate of decline in graft function associated with BOS, but less benefit was noted for RAS. TLI is administered in a total of 8 Gy over 10 sessions, being generally well tolerated apart from some transient myelosuppression, but few serious infec-

tious complications. Lung re-transplantation continues to be controversial, but may be considered in the setting of progressive CLAD.

Conclusion

The outcomes for lung transplant recipients have improved, with improved overall survival figures (Fig. 20.6). Future improvements in organ preservation technology, stem cell technology, and immunosuppression regimes will help to increase both long-term survival and quality of life for patients with advanced lung disease requiring transplantation.

References

1. Rutherford RM, Lordan JL, Fisher AJ, Corris PA. Historical overview of lung and heart-lung transplantation. In: Lynch JP, editor. Lung biology in health and disease; 2006. p. 1–16.
2. Yusen RD, Edwards LB, Kucherayavaya AY, Benden C, Dipchand AI, Goldfarb SB, et al. The registry of the International Society for Heart and Lung Transplantation: thirty-second official adult lung and heart-lung transplantation report--2015; focus theme: early graft failure. J Heart Lung Transplant. 2015;34(10):1264–77.
3. Weill D, Benden C, Corris PA, Dark JH, Davis RD, Keshavjee S, et al. A consensus document for the selection of lung transplant candidates: 2014 – an update from the Pulmonary Transplantation

Council of the International Society for Heart and Lung Transplantation. J Heart Lung Transplant. 2015;34:1):1–15.

4. Judge EP, Foweraker JE, Lordan JL. Infectious disease issues pertinent to cystic fibrosis patients in the pre-lung transplantation period. In: Mooney ML, Hannan MM, Husain S, Kirklin JK, editors. ISHLT monograph 5: diagnosis and management of infectious diseases in cardio-thoracic transplantation and mechanical circulatory support. Addison: International Society of Heart and Lung Transplantation; 2011.

5. Lobo LJ, Noone PG. Respiratory infections in patients with cystic fibrosis undergoing lung transplantation. Lancet Respir Med. 2014;2(1):73–82.

6. Yates B, Murphy DM, Fisher AJ, Gould FK, Lordan JL, Dark JH, et al. Pseudomembranous colitis in four patients with cystic fibrosis following lung transplantation. BMJ Case Rep. 2009;2009. pii: bcr11.2008.1218. https://doi.org/10.1136/bcr.11.2008.1218.

7. Lordan JL, Corris PA. Pulmonary arterial hypertension and lung transplantation. Expert Rev Respir Med. 2011;5(3):441–54.

8. Cypel M, Yeung JC, Liu M, Anraku CF, Karolak W, et al. Normothermic ex vivo lung perfusion in clinical lung transplantation. N Engl J Med. 2011;364(15):1431–40.

9. de Perrot M, Granton JT, McRae K, Cypel M, Pierre A, Waddell TK, et al. Impact of extracorporeal life support on outcome in patients with idiopathic pulmonary arterial hypertension awaiting lung transplantation. J Heart Lung Transplant. 2011;30(9):997–1002.

10. Fuehner T, Kuehn C, Hadem J, Wiesner O, Gottlieb J, Tudorache I, et al. Extracorporeal membrane oxygenation in awake patients as bridge to lung transplantation. Am J Respir Crit Care Med. 2012;185(7):763–8.

11. Fischer S, Simon AR, Welte T, Hoeper MM, Tessman R, Meyer A, et al. Bridge to lung transplantation with the novel pumpless interventional lung assist device NovaLung. J Thorac Cardiovasc Surg. 2006;131(3):719–23.

12. Hartert M, Senbaklavacin O, Gohrbandt B, Fischer BM, Buhl R, Vahld CF. Lung transplantation: a treatment option in end-stage lung disease. Dtsch Arztebl Int. 2014;111(7):107–16.

13. Aigner C. Lobar lung transplantation: more than bits and pieces. Eur J Cardiothorac Surg. 2014;45(2):370–1.

14. Christie JD, Carby M, Bag R, Corris P, Hertz M, Weill D, et al. Report of the ISHLT Working Group on primary lung graft dysfunction part II: definition. A consensus statement of the International Society for Heart and Lung Transplantation. J Heart Lung Transplant. 2005;24(10):1454–9.

15. Remund KF, Best M, Egan JJ. Infections relevant to lung transplantation. Proc Am Thorac Soc. 2009;6(1):94–100.

16. Husain S, Sole A, Alexander BD, Aslam S, Avery R, Benden C, et al. The 2015 International Society for Heart and Lung Transplantation Guidelines for the management of fungal infections in mechanical circulatory support and cardiothoracic organ transplant recipients: executive summary. J Heart Lung Transplant. 2016;35(3):261–82.

17. McDonnell M, Lordan J. Review of immunosuppressive treatment in lung transplantation. Turk Thorac J. 2014;15:94–101.

18. Vanaudenaerde BM, Meyts I, Vos R, Geudens N, De Wever W, Verbeken EK, et al. A dichotomy in bronchiolitis obliterans syndrome after lung transplantation revealed by azithromycin therapy. Eur Respir J. 2008;32(4):832–43.

19. Suwara M, Vanaudenaerde BM, Verleden SE, Vos R, Green NJ, Ward C. Mechanistic differences between phenotypes of chronic lung allograft dysfunction after lung transplantation. Transpl Int. 2014;27(8):857–67.

20. Corris PA, Ryan VA, Small T, Lordan J, Fisher AJ, Meachery G, et al. A randomised controlled trial of azithromycin therapy in bronchiolitis obliterans syndrome (BOS) post lung transplantation. Thorax. 2015;70(5):442–50.

21. Robertson AG, Ward C, Pearson JP, Smart T, Lordan J, Fisher AJ, et al. Longitudinal changes in gastro-oesophageal reflux from 3 months to 6 months after lung transplantation. Thorax. 2009;64(11):1005–7.

22. Botha P, Archer L, Anderson RL, Lordan J, Dark JH, Corris PA, et al. Pseudomonas aeruginosa colonization of the allograft after lung transplantation and the risk of bronchiolitis obliterans syndrome. Transplantation. 2008;85(5):771–4.

Index

© Springer International Publishing AG, part of Springer Nature 2018
S. Hart, M. Greenstone (eds.), *Foundations of Respiratory Medicine*,
https://doi.org/10.1007/978-3-319-94127-1

CPI Antony Rowe
Eastbourne, UK
December 21, 2018

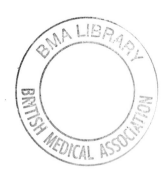